Grand Solar Minimum

D.L.Bjorngjeld

Published by D. L. Bjorngjeld
Forest Lake, Minnesota

ISBN #978-0-9981110-5-6

Layout & Design by Todd Anderson

Printed in United States of America

What is a Solar Cycle?

The sun is a huge ball of hot, fluid, electrically charged plasma. It is the most important source of energy for all life on Earth. It is continually moving, turning, and generating a powerful magnetic field. This magnetic field goes through cycles, called solar cycles, every 11 years.

During the 11 year cycle, the sun's magnetic field flips and makes its North Pole and South Pole switch. These cycles affect activity on the surface of the sun, such as sunspots, which are caused by the sun's magnetic field.

Solar cycles can be tracked as the number of sunspots increase. At the beginning of a solar cycle, the sun has the least activity and is called the solar minimum.

Over the next few years, solar activity and sunspots increase. The peak at the middle of the solar cycle is called the solar maximum, the time period when the sun has the most activity and sunspots.

As the cycle comes to an end, it fades back to the solar minimum again, then a new cycle will begin. We are currently coming to the end of Solar Cycle 24 (SC 24), which has been a cycle of very low sunspot activity. SC 25 is predicted to have even less solar activity and will be the 4th consecutive cycle of diminishing activity.

The possibility of a Grand Solar Minimum is gaining evermore support. Even Nassau appears to be on board with their recent SC 25 headline prediction:

June 18, 2019 NASA

NASA Predicts Next Solar Cycle, SC 25, Will Be Lowest in 200 Years (Dalton Minimum Levels Could Be Reached).

What is a Grand Solar Minimum?

The next three or four solar cycles are projected to be lower solar activity than the current one that's ending. This indicates SC 25, 26 and 27 will be cycles with very little or no sunspot activity. Extended periods of inactivity like this, is the definition of a Grand Solar Minimum. This minimum will likely cause Global Cooling and, perhaps, a mini ice age.

Russian Scientists originally thought the minimum would happen slowly, but according to researchers at the Lebedev Physics Institute in Moscow, it's already happening. Sunspots and associated solar storms are already diminishing.

"Based on the picture that we are seeing currently, the Sun is moving quickly toward low activity cycles that will likely be reached by the winter of 2019-2020," the Solar Scientists said in a recent statement.

According to researchers in Moscow, the regions of high activity will disappear, solar radiation will drop to near zero, and sunspots will nearly disappear in the very near future.

"Finally, at the minimum point, the solar magnetic energy almost completely vanishes. The sun will continue on in this condition for several months, and up to a year. Then new fluxes of the magnetic field begin to float from the depth of the Sun to the surface, the first spots appear, and the solar cycle starts a new 11 year curve."

The Little Ice Age (LIA) was dominated by four consecutive solar minimums: The Wolf, Sporer, Maunder, and Dalton solar minima. All of which lengthened the cooling of the LIA to 450 years.

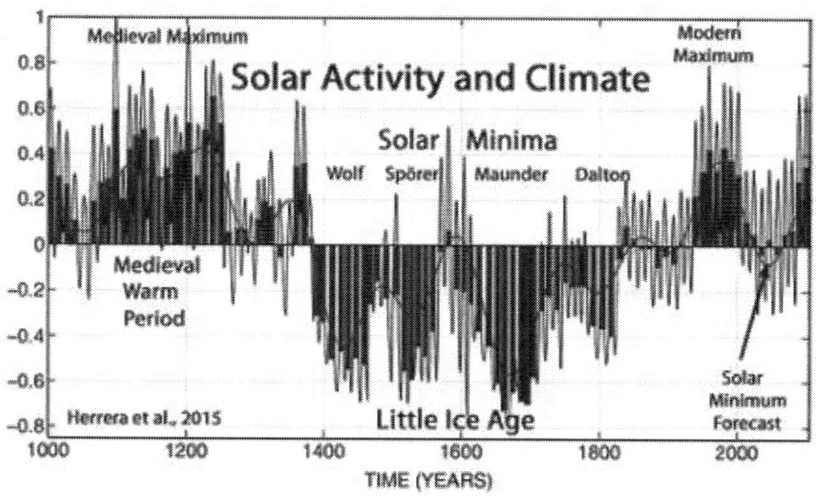

The **Wolf Minimum** was a period of low sunspot numbers in the 1300s.

The **Spörer Minimum** was a 90-year span of low solar activity, from about 1460 until 1550. It was named for the German astronomer Gustav Spörer.

The **Maunder Minimum** was from 1645 to 1715, during which sunspots became exceedingly rare. It was named for Astronomer E.W. Maunder.

The **Dalton Minimum** was a period of low solar activity, named after the English meteorologist John Dalton and lasted from about 1790 to 1830.

The Little Ice Age brought colder winters to Europe and North America. In the 17th-18th centuries, farms and villages in the Swiss Alps and in Norway were destroyed by encroaching glaciers. Canals and rivers in Great Britain and the Netherlands were froze, and many early settlers in North America reported exceptionally severe winters.

An Ice Age is triggered when summer temperatures in the northern hemisphere continually fail to rise above freezing for years. This means that winter snowfall doesn't melt, but instead builds up, compresses and, over time, starts to compact or glaciate into ice sheets.

Sunspots are somewhat cooler than the rest of the Sun, but when there are lots of sunspots, the Sun releases much more radiation. This greatly adds warming to Earth's climate. With fewer sunspots, the Earth's climate grows cooler over time.

High sunspot activity will make it warmer here on Earth. Low or no sunspot activity will cause cooling.

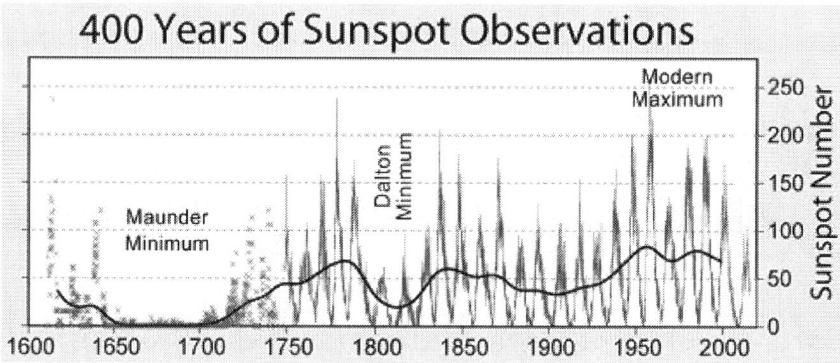

NASA is forecasting a possible return to the Dalton Minimum (1790-1830), *but gives no mention of the brutal cold, crop loss, famine, and death associated with it.*

Like the deeper Maunder and Spörer Minimums preceding it, the Dalton brought on a period of lower-than-average global temperatures. The Oberlach Weather Station in Germany, for example, experienced a 2°C decline in just 20 years, which devastated the country's food production. World-wide the climate became colder.

The "***Year Without a Summer***" also occurred during the Dalton Minimum in 1816. It was caused by a combination of already low temperatures plus the after-effects of the second largest volcanic eruption in 2,000 years. We are still currently in one of Earth's coldest periods and could face devastating cold if we enter a Grand Solar Minimum.

A Grand Solar Minimum is likely coming, and with it comes Global Cooling and maybe another mini Ice Age.

"Climate change continues (as it always has) however, there is verified scientific evidence that is pointing to a totally different result than the IPCC and Believers have been proclaiming."

Earth's Climate is a huge, immensely complex system. So far, however, there are strong indications *that we've ignored* a far greater factor in our climate than previously acknowledge. The factor that's been ignored is the influence that sunspots and solar activities have on our climate. We might well be ignoring this to our peril.

The frequency and intensity of sunspot activity has been shown to have a profound influence on Earth's weather systems, atmospheric temperature, ocean temperature, Gulf Stream flows and more. *It is also notable that the IPCC simply dismisses such influences as insignificant... A huge mistake.*

While governments and the United Nations have funneled Billions of dollars to the computer *modelers* to input various levels of CO2 in their models, *far too little attention has been given to the effect of the sun on earth's climate. At a minimum, in the interest of science if not our very survival, we need to remedy this.*

According to Prof. Masayuki Hyodo of the Research Centre for Inland Seas, Kobe University: *The United Nations' IPCC has discussed the impact that cloud cover and sunspots have on climate during their evaluations, but these phenomena have never been considered in their climate modeling or their predictions... All due to their insufficient understanding and inability to model them with accuracy.*

A Grand Solar Minimum and the Likely Effects on Climate.

If the predictions of the Russian Solar Physicists are accurate (and we will know in the next year or two, as opposed to the more than three decades of waiting for anything catastrophic to happen with the Warming Alarmism) we are in for a colder climate and unpleasant changes globally over the coming decades – perhaps until the 2050s – due to the onset of a new *Grand Solar Minimum.*

It is the conjunction of an 11 year cycle of declining sunspot numbers, with longer wave 100 year solar cycles. If this is so, the extreme weather conditions, severe cold waves, and more earthquakes, all could be predictors of what we'll be living with for the next 30–40 years, or longer. With that will likely come <u>shortened growing seasons around the world, harvest failures, and famine in poor areas of the world.</u>

A highly respected Solar Physicist studying solar cycles is Professor Valentina Zharkova, who teaches mathematics at Northumbria University in England. At a conference of the Global Warming Policy Foundation in October 2018, Zharkova presented findings that suggest, "***In 2020 a Grand Solar Minimum period could begin.***" (In the past, predictions from her models have demonstrated **95%** accuracy.)

Evidence, from independent scientists, suggest that we need to develop a better understanding of the sun and its effects on climate, if we are going to prepare for major climate catastrophes in coming years. ***(But the IPCC and Believers continue to assure us, "It's the CO2, Stupid.")***

Grand Solar Minimum: What If?

Climate events have been overly-dramatized by advocacy groups (particularly the political left and the United Nation's IPCC) contending that man-made global warming by the emission of CO2 is the cause. We've been inundated with proposals for new taxes in the Hundreds of Billions of dollars, taxes that we're told are needed to solve this problem." ***What if we are focused on the wrong problem?***

Recent research suggests that we have been too limited in our outlook and *are virtually ignoring some much greater influences in global weather than any man-made emissions.*

What is relevant to this discussion is the fact that *no climate model* used by the IPCC, or any of the hundreds of climate think tanks around the world, *are able to 'accurately model'* what is ***by far the greatest factor affecting our weather... The Sun.***

Currently, since 2018, we are experiencing a period of significant decline in solar activity. There is convincing evidence that this will bring us to what is called a Grand Solar Minimum, far more devastating than anything in our recent history.

According to Dr. Roy Spencer, "Clouds are the Earth's sun-shade, and if cloud cover changes for any reason, you will have global warming or global cooling." A Grand Solar Minimum will allow more Cosmic Rays to enter our atmosphere, having a direct effect on cloud cover.

The US Government's National Oceanic and Atmospheric Administration (NOAA) now tell us, "All weather on Earth, from the surface of the planet out into space, begins with the Sun." *(This is not what we've heard for the past three decades, when they were marching in stride with the "CO2 emissions are what is driving global warming" proclaimed by the IPCC and Believers.)*

What are the effects of less solar activity?

We will experience less solar energy or radiance reaching Earth. In addition to affecting cloud coverage globally, vital jet streams will be weakened and volcanic activity will be increased. We'll likely experience many more earthquakes and erratic unpredictable weather. The Jet Stream will shift south as it did in January, 2019 in North America, causing the record cold and snows across the region.

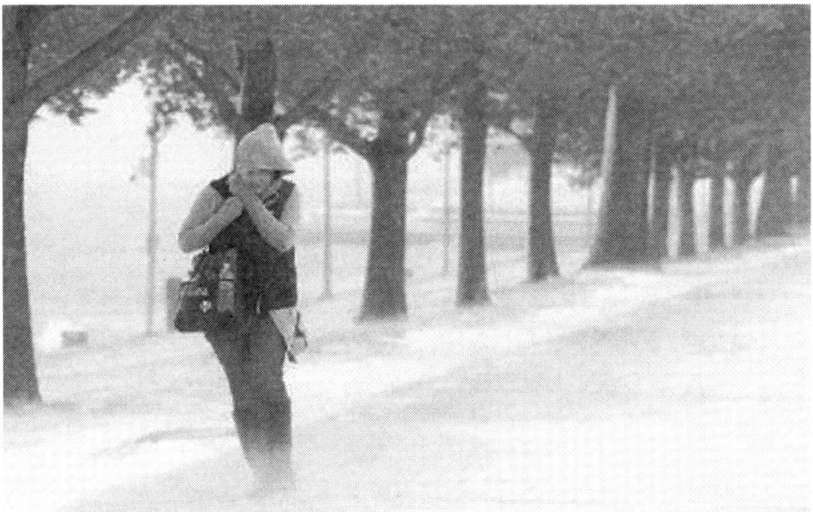

The Arctic blast that descended on a swath of the country stretching from the Rocky Mountains to New England continues, bringing record-breaking low temperatures, heavy snowfall in some Northeast areas, and school closings in the Mid-South. December, 2019.

The current solar cycle, designated by NASA as number SC 24 peaked in early 2014 before starting its measurable decline in annual sunspot activity. A Grand Minimum is predicted to take place in 2020 and could last for a few decades. Some predict it will cause a new "mini Ice Age."

The subject of sunspots is complex and vastly under-researched, as we have focused instead on man-made changes to our climate with simplistic computer models. *If the coming winter in the Northern Hemisphere is anything like the past one, it should prompt us to take this solar component of our climatic influences seriously.*

By refusing to promote vigorous new research, we run a real risk, in coming years, of being unprepared for dramatic cold resulting in harvest failures, and at a time when most governments have decided to eliminate emergency public grain reserves, and our food supply operates on a "just-in-time" system.

Science is about discovering the *truth*, wherever it leads and however controversial.

ANOTHER CLIMATE SCIENTIST WITH IMPECCABLE CREDENTIALS BREAKS RANKS WITH THE IPCC, SAYING: "OUR MODELS ARE SIMPLY MOCKERIES OF THE REAL WORLD"

Dr. Mototaka Nakamura received his Doctorate of Science from the Massachusetts Institute of Technology (MIT), and for nearly 25 years specialized in abnormal weather and climate change at prestigious institutions that included MIT, Georgia Institute of Technology, NASA's Jet Propulsion Laboratory, California Institute of Technology, and Duke University.

In his book titled, "The Global Warming Hypothesis is an Unproven Hypothesis," Dr. Nakamura explains why the data underpinning the Global Warmist science is doctored, untrustworthy, and cannot be verified or relied on.

From 1990 to 2014, Nakamura worked on cloud dynamics and forces mixing atmospheric and ocean flows on planetary scales. His home-bases were MIT (for a Doctor of Science in Meteorology), Georgia Institute of Technology, Goddard Space Flight Center, and the Japan Agency for Marine-Earth Science and Technology.

"Today's 'global warming science' is akin to an upside down pyramid which is built on the work of a few climate modelers. These 'few' claim to have demonstrated that human-derived CO2 emissions are the cause of recently rising temperatures and have then simply projected that forward. Every climate researcher thereafter has taken the results of these original models as a given. ***Merely testing their validity is regarded as heresy.***

With Nakamura, we have a highly qualified and experienced climate modeler with impeccable credentials ***rejecting the unscientific basis of the climate crisis claims***. But he's up against a big army. The activists seem to be winning at the moment, and they're now being fronted by scared, crying children; an unstoppable combination. One that's tricky to discredit without looking like a heartless bastard.

NAKAMURA ON DATA FALSIFICATION

When arguing against global warming, the hardest thing is *convincing people of data falsification, namely temperature doctoring*. If you don't pick your words carefully, or get your tone right, then it's very easy to sound like a conspiracy crank.

Now we have Nakamura, one of their own. He has accused the "climate scientists" of data falsification in the form adjusting historical temperature to *inflate today's subtle warming trend.*

Additionally, the climate models grossly simplify the way climate works. As well as ignoring the sun's effect, they drastically simplify ***large and small-scale*** **ocean dynamics**, ignore **changes that generate** ***clouds*** (cloud cover is one of the key factors determining whether we have global warming or cooling), and ***water vapor***.

NAKAMURA ON CO2

"Earth's climate system is far more complex than an absurdly simple system simulated by the 'models' that have been used for climate projections.

"The dynamics of the atmosphere and oceans are absolutely critical facets of the climate system if one hopes to ever make any meaningful prediction of climate variations.

"Solar input is modeled as a 'never changing quantity,' which is absurd.

NAKAMURA ON SOLAR FORCING (SOLAR INFLUENCE ON EARTH'S CLIMATE)

Solar output is not constant, which is what the IPCC insists. During solar minima, like the one we're entering now, the sun's magnetic field weakens and the outward pressure of the solar wind decreases.

This allows more Cosmic Rays from deep space to penetrate our planet's atmosphere. These CRs have been found to affect clouds, and clouds are a crucial player earth's climate. As Roy Spencer, PhD, writes: *"Clouds serve as Earth's sunshade. If cloud cover changes for any reason you will have global warming or global cooling."*

Cold times appear to be returning, as a result of ***historically low solar activity.*** NASA has warned that this next solar cycle (Cycle 25) will be "the weakest of the past 200 years":

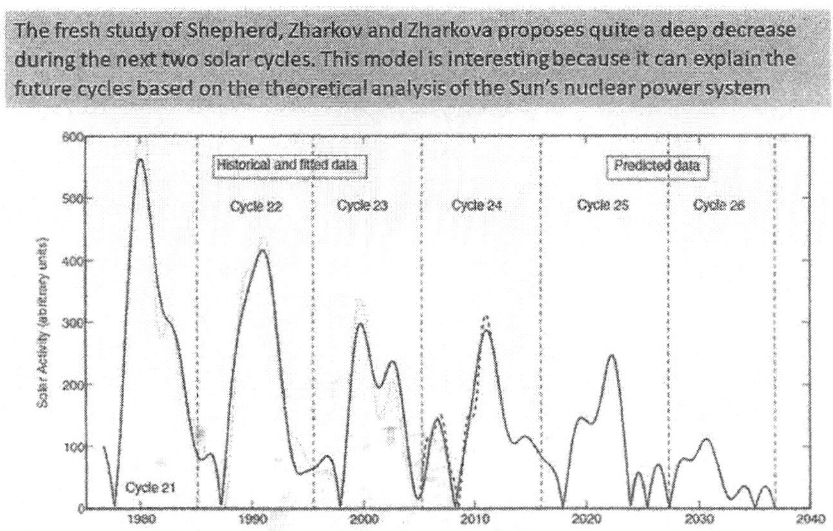

The Maunder minimum, AD 1645–1715, is the most recent Grand Solar Minimum, and the only one covered by telescopic sunspot observations.

The current cycle, SC 24, is the lowest sunspot cycle in 100 years and the third in a trend of diminishing sunspot cycles. Solar physicists expect cycle 25 to be even less active and expect the sun to move into a new solar minimum, one comparable with the Dalton Minimum. Studying such a minimum with available modern instruments could potentially answer a lot of the serious questions surrounding the influence of the sun on our climate.

Previously, researchers used the number of sunspots to represent the activity of the solar magnetic field. New technology takes advantage of direct observations of magnetic fields emerging on the surface of the Sun – data which has only existed for the last four solar cycles.

SC 25 may likely be a mere stop-off on our descent into the next Grand Solar Minimum. The excellent observation and analysis of Dr. Valentia Zharkova suggests that all four of the Sun's magnetic fields will go out of phase in 2020, which strongly suggests that we're headed into a very cold climate.

Professor Zharkova gave a presentation of her Climate and the Solar Magnetic Field Hypothesis at the Global Warming Policy Foundation in October, 2018. The information she unveiled should wake up the Warmists.

Zharkova was one of two scientists to correctly predict solar cycle 24 would be weaker than cycle 23. In fact, only 2 out of 120+ climate models predicted this correctly.

The last time we had a GSM (the Maunder Minimum) only two magnetic fields of the sun went out of phase. This time, all four magnetic fields are going out of phase.

Professor Zharkova's model has shown 95% accuracy and now is suggesting that a Grand Solar Minimum and global cooling will be headed our way beginning in 2020.

How cold might it get? Based on the study of previous sunspot reductions proceeding a grand minimum period, we will see a 7% reduction in the Sun's heat and light. This will likely result in bitterly cold winters and shorter summers in North America and parts of Europe.

Meanwhile, the United Nation's International Panel on Climate Change (IPCC) has countered all of this new information from the last couple of years, which shows a strong potential of Climate Cooling; AND the IPCC's poor reputation in their ability to model Earth's climate; AND the evidence of doctoring historical records to prop up their claims; with them producing and ***proclaiming an ever more frantic barrage of new, more extreme, and more fraudulent alarmism.*** The following is a good example of their frenzied alarmism and, many times, outright lying:

"We could be losing the race against climate change, new UN report says."

Sea walls all across the globe are being rendered useless by increasingly volatile seas all due to sea level rises.

Scientists behind a study of the links between oceans, glaciers, ice caps and the climate delivered a stark warning to the world: ***slash emissions or watch cities vanish under rising seas.***

The U.N. backed panel of experts has found that radical action may yet avert outcomes of global warming. The study was clear that allowing CO2 emissions to continue on their upward path would upset the balance of the great geophysical systems governing oceans and the ice regions of the earth so profoundly that no one would be untouched.

Are the sea levels continuing to rise? Yes they are... At an average rate of 2 mm/year, as they have since we've been keeping records. (A rise of 2 mm/year over ***12 years*** equals one inch of sea level rise.)

Sea levels are not, "rising at 10 times the rate seen in the 20th century."

We are not, "releasing enormous quantities of CO2 which will *unleash feedback loops driving ever faster warming."*

We are not, "causing oceans to get hotter, bringing on what are known as Marine Heat Waves that will damage ecosystems."

We are not, "heating the oceans and starving the upper layers of oxygen, suffocating marine life, creating growing dead zones, and disrupting the circulation of ocean currents."

If emissions do continue rising – as they have for the past 70 years – ***it will not*** "accelerate impacts so rapidly that they will overwhelm society's ability to cope."

Choose a descriptive word for the proclamations of the IPCC, their Believers and fellow alarmists:

Absurdity	Fabricated
Poppycock	Distorted
Horse-Feathers	Preposterous
Balderdash	Ridiculous
Baloney	Hogwash
Twaddle	Prattle

I'm afraid that we might be wishing for a bit of warming, if Dr. Zharkova is correct in her prediction of a coming Grand Solar Minimum.

My thoughts...

I'll take a little warming, like that of +0.8°C during the 20th century.

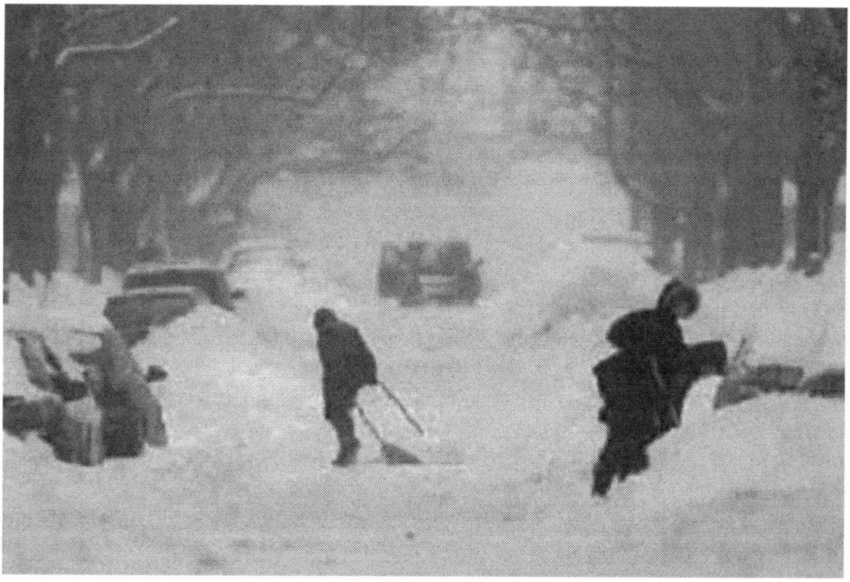

If a 'Grand Solar Minimum' happens and influences climate as it did in the 15th–19th centuries, we'll see lots of this. AND, what is the IPCC going to do about stopping it?

Made in the USA
Monee, IL
13 September 2026

62979534R00015

"Stella Gaon explores how the radicality of Derridean deconstruction lies in its unwavering fidelity to the very conditions of reason. This is what drives deconstruction to uncover the irreducible violence at the heart of every law, but also every moral claim, with far-reaching consequences for political and pedagogical theory and practice. For Gaon, deconstruction exemplifies critical thinking: the unflinching interrogation of the categories through which good and evil, fact and fiction, the righteous and the reprehensible are established. With admirable conceptual clarity Gaon's captivating book explores the pivotal ramifications of a deconstructive mode of analysis for pedagogy, politics and ethics."

—Elisabeth Weber, University of California, Santa Barbara

"Anyone still in doubt about the political and ethical relevance or force of deconstruction will have to read Stella Gaon's brilliant new work *The Lucid Vigil*. Gaon demonstrates with a stunning lucidity and attentiveness of her own that Derridean deconstruction was never a nihilistic attack on Enlightenment values but a relentless questioning of the foundations of ethical and political legitimacy in line with the most exacting demands of reason and self-critique. This work should set the record straight once and for all and should cause anyone interested in questions of ethics and politics to return to Derrida's work, both early and late, with renewed attention, passion, and urgency."

—Michael Naas, DePaul University, Chicago

The Lucid Vigil

Stella Gaon provides the first fully philosophical account of the critical nature of deconstruction, and she does so by turning in an original way to psychoanalysis. Drawing on close readings of Freud and Laplanche, Gaon argues that Derridean deconstruction is driven by a normative investment in reason's psychological force. Indeed, deconstruction is more faithful to the principle of reason than the various forms of critical theory prevalent today. For if one pursues the classical demand for rational grounds vigilantly, one finds that claims to ethical or political legitimacy cannot be rationally justified, because they are undone by logical undecidability. Gaon's argument is borne out in the cases of Kantian deontology, Deweyan pragmatism, progressive pedagogy, Habermasian moral theory, Levinasian ethics and others. What emerges is the groundbreaking demonstration that deconstruction is impelled by a quasi-ethical critical drive, and that to read deconstructively is to radicalize the emancipatory practice of reason as self-critique.

This important volume will be of great value to critical theorists as well as to Derrida scholars and researchers in social and political thought.

Stella Gaon is Professor of Political Science and Adjunct Professor of Women and Gender Studies at Saint Mary's University. She is the editor of *Democracy in Crisis: Violence, Alterity, Community.*

Psychoanalytic Political Theory

Edited by Matthew H. Bowker, Medaille College, and David W. McIvor, Colorado State University

Psychoanalytic Political Theory provides a publishing space for the highest quality scholarship at the intersection of psychoanalysis and normative political theory. It offers a forum for texts that deepen our understanding of the complex relationships between the world of politics and the world of the psyche.

1. The Lucid Vigil
Deconstruction, Desire and the Politics of Critique
Stella Gaon

For more information about this series, please visit: www.routledge.com/Psychoanalytic-Political-Theory/book-series/PPT

The Lucid Vigil

Deconstruction, Desire and the Politics of Critique

Stella Gaon

Routledge
Taylor & Francis Group
LONDON AND NEW YORK

First published 2019 by Routledge

2 Park Square, Milton Park, Abingdon, Oxfordshire OX14 4RN
52 Vanderbilt Avenue, New York, NY 10017

Routledge is an imprint of the Taylor & Francis Group, an informa business

First issued in paperback 2020

Library of Congress Cataloging-in-Publication Data
Names: Gaon, Stella, 1960- author.
Title: The lucid Virgil : deconstruction, desire and the politics of critique / Stella Gaon.
Description: New York, NY : Routledge, 2019. |
Series: Psychoanalytic political theory | Includes bibliographical references and index. |
Identifiers: LCCN 2018048147 (print) | LCCN 2018060850 (ebook) |
ISBN 9780429465574 (Master) | ISBN 9780429879043 (Adobe) |
ISBN 9780429879036 (ePub) | ISBN 9780429879029 (MobiPocket) |
ISBN 9781138610828 (hardback) | ISBN 9780429465574 (ebook)
Subjects: LCSH: Deconstruction. | Psychoanalysis and philosophy. |
Reason. | Political psychology.
Classification: LCC B809.6 (ebook) | LCC B809.6 .G36 2019 (print) |
DDC 149/.97--dc23
LC record available at https://lccn.loc.gov/2018048147

ISBN: 978-1-138-61082-8 (hbk)
ISBN: 978-0-367-66178-6 (pbk)

Typeset in Times New Roman
by Taylor & Francis Books

In memory of Harry Gaon

Contents

Acknowledgements

A section of Chapter Eight draws heavily on "Pluralizing Universal 'Man': The Legacy of Transcendentalism and Teleology in Habermas's Discourse Ethics," which was published in *The Review of Politics* Volume 60, 4 (Autumn 1998), 685–714, by Cambridge University Press. Chapter Ten includes a section of "Politicizing Deconstruction: On Not Treating *Specters of Marx*," which appeared in *Rethinking MARXISM* Volume 11, 2 (Summer 1999), 38–48. An earlier version of some parts of Chapter 11 originally appeared in *Mosaic, an interdisciplinary critical journal*, Volume 44, issue 4 (December 2011), 79–93. Permission to reprint revised versions of these materials is gratefully acknowledged.

I am thankful to the series editors, Matt Bowker and David McIvor, and to Natalja Mortensen, Senior Acquisitions Editor at Routledge, for their early and strong endorsement of this project. Three anonymous reviewers offered a thoughtful set of incisive comments. Their criticisms and suggestions provoked important clarifications and are much appreciated. Many colleagues and friends also spared time to read, discuss and comment upon various chapters, sometimes in multiple drafts. While I owe more appreciation than I will ever fully recall, I particularly want to acknowledge Dorota Glowacka, Geraldine Finn, Florian Bail, Silke Helmerdig, Anita Janzen, Teresa Heffernan, Bettina Bergo and Dominique Scarfone, who each read different parts of the book, highlighted unclear or misleading formulations and offered ongoing support and interest. I am indebted to Karyn Ball for pointing me to the work of Jean Laplanche. A special thanks to Catherine Kellogg, for all the conversations over all the years, and to my mother and brothers for always being there. Finally, Karen Asp provided not only meticulous work on the manuscript and the index, but ongoing critical and intellectual engagement with the arguments developed in the book. I am beyond lucky to have her unconditional encouragement and support. The responsibility for any errors or omissions is of course mine.

Introduction

This book concerns the relevance of Derridean deconstruction for critical political theory in general, and for the political idea of education as emancipation, in particular. It demonstrates that contrary to widespread misconceptions, the deconstruction of the philosophical discourse of modernity is not the effect of deliberate attacks on Enlightenment reason by Nietzschean sceptics, as Jürgen Habermas initially charged (1987). But nor is it the ethical embrace of difference, alterity or radically heterogeneous others, as Jacques Derrida's sympathizers tend to suggest (Critchley 1992; Butler 2004; Horowitz 2006). Rather, my thesis is that deconstruction marks the inevitable unfolding of the modern promise of reason. As such it embodies rather than refutes the Enlightenment's own substantive, ethical–political impulse. I argue on this basis that the epistemological crisis associated with deconstructive readings of Enlightenment philosophy issues from the critical, philosophical tenets of modernity themselves. The deconstructive approach to philosophy that appears to have caused this crisis, therefore, must be seen as the radicalization of reason as self-critique, and thus as in keeping with critical theory's most pointed emancipatory aims. It is in this respect that deconstruction qualifies as a certain form of "critique." Drawing on the psychoanalytic theory of Jean Laplanche, I show that it can be deemed "quasi-ethical" in a particular sense as well.

My central argument is that deconstructive strategies of reading fulfil, in a profound and utterly faithful way, the critical, emancipatory ethos of the European Enlightenment. They do so most especially when they reveal the groundlessness of philosophical claims to ethical–political legitimacy. For, as Derrida never ceased to underscore, what remains implacable in the ethos of Enlightenment is the necessity of a philosophically radical critique – an "unconditional theoreticism," as he calls it in "The University Without Condition" (2002b, 218) – a rational critique that takes *itself* to court, where it stands as both accuser and judged (Cachopo 2013, 66, 75, nt.12; Kant 1929, A xi–xii). This imperative, which Derrida refers to as the "enigmatic desire for vigilance, for the lucid vigil [*veille*], for elucidation, for critique and truth, but for a truth that at the same time keeps within itself some apocalyptic desire" (1983a, 22) regarding the metaphysics of all those norms we take for granted or seek to establish as foundational, was announced in Derrida's first speaking engagement in the United States. In the seminal essay he gave at the Johns Hopkins University in 1966, "Structure, Sign, and Play in the Discourse of the Human Sciences," Derrida writes,

> The substitute does not substitute itself for anything which has somehow existed before it. Henceforth, it was necessary to begin thinking that there was no centre, that the centre could not be thought in the form of a present-being … that it was not a fixed locus but a function, a sort of nonlocus in which an infinite number of sign-substitutions came into play. This was the moment when language invaded the universal problematic, the moment when, in the absence of a centre or origin, everything became discourse … that is to say, a system in which the central signified, the original or transcendental signified, is never absolutely present outside a system of differences. The absence of the transcendental signified extends the domain and the play of signification infinitely. (Qtd. in Kamuf 2002, 284, nt.5)

In other words, in one of his earliest formulations of what came to be called "deconstruction," Derrida had already underscored the impossibility of determining a foundational norm as a common standard of critique, or of legitimizing universal or unconditional validity, and this for logically ineluctable reasons that stem from the demand of philosophical criticism itself.

His attention to this impossibility is evident long before the so-called "ethical turn," which was by no means a departure from his initial work. Indeed, it was manifest at least as early as 1964, for example, in the groundbreaking essay "Violence and Metaphysics." There, Derrida argues that the 'unrelenting' interrogation of philosophy's own possibility is the only undertaking capable of founding a community "of those who are still called philosophers" (1978, 79) – even if that interrogation is exactly what can "make us tremble" (1978, 82). One finds his attentiveness to this issue in all the major texts of the 1970s and '80s – including *Margins of Philosophy* (1982 [1972]), *Limited Inc* (1988b [1972, 1977]), and "Of an Apocalyptic Tone" (1983a) – and one can thus track the normative impulse of deconstruction *into* the explicitly political writings of the 1990s and 2000s, such as "Force of Law" (1992a), *Specters of Marx* (1994), *Without Alibi* (2002c), *Paper Machine* (2005c) and *Rogues* (2005d). In fact, Derrida engaged tirelessly for over 40 years with the question of what it means when, "in the absence of a centre or origin, everything became discourse … a system in which the … original or transcendental signified is never absolutely present outside a system of differences" (ibid.). In each case he finds that it means *another* thinking is called for, one that arises from classical logic to reveal the limits of conceptual thought. As he put it in "Fichus," the address he gave upon receiving the Theodor W. Adorno prize in 2001, a "different thinking" is required in the face of our political responsibilities, one that "involves a deconstructive critique that is sober, wide awake, vigilant, and attentive to everything that solders the political to the metaphysical, to capitalist speculating, to the perversions of religious or nationalist feeling, or to the fantasy of sovereignty" (2005b, 179).

This is exactly why, in his response in *Limited Inc* to John Searle – who had accused Derrida of imposing an 'all or nothing' "choice between pure realization or self-presence and complete free play and undecidability" – Derrida begins by pointing out there can be no "completeness" where undecidability is concerned: both "pure realization" and "complete free play" issue from a fantasy of metaphysical absolutism. At the same time, however, "the alternative of 'all or nothing'" remains logically inescapable, because it is implied by "any concept that lays claim to any rigor whatsoever" (1988b, 116). He continues,

> In fact, not only do I find this logic [of all or nothing] strong, and, in conceptual language and analysis, *an absolute must* [*il la faut*], it must (this "it must" translates the faithfulness of my love for philosophy) be sustained against all empirical confusion, to the point where the same demand of rigor requires the structure of that logic to be transformed or complicated. (1988b, 122–3)

Indeed, he says,

> Whenever one feels obliged to stop doing this (as happens to me when I speak of *différance*, of mark, of supplement, of iterability and of all they entail), it is *better* to make explicit in the most conceptual, rigorous, formalizing, and pedagogical manner possible the reasons one has for doing so, for thus changing the rules and the context of discourse. (1988b, 117; emphasis his)

Derrida reiterates this point regarding his fidelity to the principle of reason and to the protocols of critical philosophy that it informs in an essay he wrote ten years later, in 1998. There, he says that his use of the "*quasi* or the 'ultra-transcendental'" was always "a way of saving, even while betraying it, the philosophical inheritance, namely, the demand for the condition of possibility (the a priori, the originary, or ground, all different forms of the same radical demand and of any philosophical 'question')" (2005a, 83–4). Saving it by virtue of an adherence to the demand for rigorous logic and vigilance; betraying it by virtue of exactly the same thing.

What was saved was philosophy's *critical* quality, in other words, at the cost of political certainty. For if what will always be "imperative" is, as Derrida says, "the question of the principle, the question of the principle*s*, and the question of *the* principle – of the principial [*sic*], of the sovereign prince, and of princedom" (2002a, 257; emphases his), and if one heeds this imperative stringently, one will be forced to concede that no concept is ever nameable "with a single name or a single word" (2005a, 83). Rather, "[t]he concept always demands sentences, discourses, work, and process: in a word, text" (ibid.). And, if every concept always demands 'text' – which is to say, *context* (1988b, 136) – then there is no way of knowing with certainty what one must responsibly or rightfully *do*.

That difficulty is thus not a consequence of deconstruction; it is inherent to critical thinking itself. That is why the attempt to establish legitimate political norms must be clearly distinguished from the rigorous interrogation of their solidity. Indeed, this book sustains the argument that the very demands for universality, for a common standard or for unconditional foundations may well end up, as João Pedro Cachopo has discerned, "obliterating what could be deemed … the core of a philosophically radical critique: the possibility of questioning its own conditions of possibility" (2013, 66). In other words, as Cachopo says,

> *Critical thinking*, for the sake of its political consequences (paradoxical as it might sound), is definitely not to be equated with the attempt to find an agreement on *what might be done*, or more generally put, to bring together the theoretical conditions that allow for normatively justified action. (2013, 73, emphases his; cf. Colebrook 2011, 63)

Rather, critical thinking ought instead to be recognized – "*for the sake of its political consequences*" – as what undoes the very righteousness of what is said to be normatively justified. What remains most faithful to the tradition of critical theory, in short, is not the determination of what is politically or ethically good. It is, rather, the interrogation of the categories of reality through which the righteous and the morally reprehensible, the good and the evil, the legitimate and the illegitimate, and the benign and the malevolent, are separated. For these distinctions have concrete political effects, and they are never neutral.

Ironically, it is precisely this, that which has been most radically and most pointedly political about deconstruction all along, that is most often misunderstood not only by detractors and critics, but by readers sympathetic to Derrida's work as well. This misunderstanding is rooted in early debates about which contemporary theorists are either unaware, or which they now see as over and done with. It is in order to correct this state of affairs that I have found it necessary to re-examine the most robust and explicit moments of the debate. In particular, it must be recalled, Jürgen Habermas notoriously dismissed "postmodernism" on the grounds that Derrida turned the difference between legitimate and illegitimate political–theoretical claims into an infinite 'free play' of textual semiosis, leaving the critical theorist with no way of determining legitimately what one ought to *do*. The question of the normative implications of deconstruction – which is vigorously debated in the field of Derrida studies today (Hägglund 2008; Anderson 2012; Haddad 2013; Gasché 2016) – was thus raised already then. It was taken up at the time by Simon Critchley (1992), who argued that *this* problem, this same problem of legitimation that Habermas erroneously diagnosed, could be solved by the addition of Levinasian ethics – that something like Emmanuel Levinas's turn to "alterity" could be brought on board to fill the gap that deconstruction supposedly produced, thereby providing an *alternative* normative basis for political action. Critchley's Levinasian solution appears to have been displaced since then, but his quintessentially 'modernist' question of how to provide *from* or *through* deconstruction the norms that political claims require remains very much alive in debates about deconstruction now.

This was always the wrong question, but in order to see why, it is necessary to return to the original controversy. For the Derridean insight regarding the instability of the legitimacy that underlines the Enlightenment conception of emancipation, and the significant problems that insight poses for emancipatory thought, only emerge clearly in the context of the so-called "modernism–postmodernism" debate. As we shall see, Derrida does show there is no way of determining legitimately what one ought to do. But this is not because he promotes rhetoric (or 'free play') to the privileged position within the dyad (Habermas's charge). It is because he *quasi-legitimately* reveals the impossibility of privileging *either* of its elements and, thus, of fully legitimizing anything. Derridean deconstruction, in other words, puts into question the modern philosophical assumption that a rational justification of political ends is possible in the first place. That this assumption tends to work behind the scenes more frequently than it works in front of them makes the issue all the more intransigent and necessary to root out.

Yet Derrida himself rarely engaged directly with these Habermasian charges, apart from some pointed remarks in *Limited Inc* (1988b); his comments appear in a footnote to the section entitled "Toward an Ethic of Discussion."[1] With somewhat uncharacteristic vehemence, Derrida there describes the shoddiness of Habermas's depiction of deconstruction in *The Philosophical Discourse of Modernity* (1987):

> Although I am not cited a single time, although not one of my texts is even indicated as a reference in a chapter of twenty-five pages that claims to be a long critique of my work, phrases such as the following can be found: "Derrida is particularly interested in standing the primacy of logic over rhetoric, canonized since Aristotle, on its head." (1988b, 156)

This claim, Derrida goes on to say, is unambiguously "false. I say *false*, as opposed to *true*" (157; his emphasis). He then adds,

> If I insist here on the example of Habermas, after that of Searle, it is not only because of the importance of the questions I have just evoked, in their very contents. It is to underscore a situation that is unfortunately typical – and politically very serious – at a juncture that I will not hesitate to qualify as worldwide and historic; which is as much to say that … it deserves serious analyses. Everywhere, in particular in the United States and in Europe, the self-declared philosophers, theoreticians, and ideologists of communication, dialogue, and consensus, of univocity and transparency, those who claim ceaselessly to reinstate the classical ethics of proof, discussion, and exchange, are most often those who excuse themselves from attentively reading and listening to the other, who demonstrate precipitation and dogmatism, and who no longer respect the elementary rules of philology and of interpretation, confounding science and chatter as though they had not the slightest taste for communication or rather as though they were afraid of it, at bottom. *Why? That is the real question. What is going on at this moment, above all around "deconstruction," to explain this fear and this dogmatism*? (157–8; emphasis added)

These comments confirmed my own sense that deconstruction is impelled by an "ethic," that is, by the adherence to a deep understanding of scholarly and, more specifically, of philosophical responsibility. Derrida's constant insistence on the need to confront dogmatism, and his unceasing appeal to the classical philosophical norms of "proof, discussion, and exchange" for this purpose, thus underlie the entire trajectory of my argument.

Generally, however, Derrida did not tend to engage with uninformed or unscholarly attacks on his work or his character. Instead, he undertook a series of philosophical analyses that have significant ethical–political stakes. As I explain in what follows, he says that his objective was not to choose between logic and rhetoric or concept and metaphor, but simply to recognize what he calls "the old solidarity" between these "antagonists" (1983a, 16). My own objective, in distinction, is to explicate the normative quality and the political significance of that recognition. So, the central issues at hand concern the nature of the form of deconstruction that Derrida practised, and the question of whether a normative case can be made to describe it.

With a view to defending the argument that deconstruction constitutes a certain form of normative critique, I begin by explaining the fear and the dogmatism that gave rise to charges against it – charges concerning the relationship between 'logic and rhetoric,' let us say – which were freely dispensed not only by Habermas, but also by various Marxists, feminists, and defenders of early Frankfurt School critical theory. Indeed, Habermas was far from alone in dismissing deconstruction as a nihilistic, negative, aesthetic or relativist approach to politics at the time, even if other critics did not share his particular understanding of critique. Peter Dews and Gillian Rose, for example, both posited an "incompatibility" between Derrida's deconstruction and the critical theory of Max Horkheimer and Theodor Adorno. While Dews and Rose both sought to rescue first-generation critical theory from its second-generation inheritors – specifically as represented by Habermas, ironically enough – their shared understanding of deconstruction is virtually identical with his. Like Habermas, Dews and Rose present deconstruction as the aestheticization of politics or as negative theology (Dews 2004, 142), and as issuing in nihilism (Rose 2008, 202). Indeed, Dews specifically associates *différance* with Foucaultian "unreason" and "negativity" (2004, 138), whereas Rose associates it with "lack" (2008, 205). One need only recall that Rose's important book on the topic was entitled *Dialectic of Nihilism* (1984), and that Dews's was the *Logics of Distintegration* (1987), to expose the association with Habermas's characterization of "postmodernism." In other words, Rose and Dews both rejected deconstruction and argued for its differences from critical theory on the same grounds as Habermas; what differs is merely the version of critical theory they defend in its stead.

Among all the various responses to so-called "postmodernism" in general, therefore, I focus most directly on Habermas's views because he provides the most fully developed and trenchant version of this critique. Habermas's interpretation of deconstruction was so influential, in fact, that deconstruction is now almost entirely off the radar in North America as far as normative political theory is concerned. Few political theorists appear to have read Derrida's work for themselves – beyond an acquaintance with such explicitly political texts as "Force of Law" (1992a) or *Specters of Marx* (1994) – or to have any deep sense of its critical implications for politics. I believe this is because the interpretation of deconstruction that Habermas first espoused is so often simply taken as read – it is deployed, as it were, rather than challenged. In this sense, the Habermasian characterization of deconstruction has largely become the mute common sense through which Derridean thought is understood by critical political theorists today.

That characterization, I argue here, is blind to deconstruction's normative quality and its real political consequences. What is political about deconstruction, most importantly, is its "negative" work, namely, the way in which it reveals how "writing" – which is to say, text, textuality and thus context – destabilizes even while it makes possible the determination of every conceptual claim. As Geoffrey Bennington explains, "Derrida's simple insight, with its almost unimaginably, fractally complex implications" (2016, para. 6) is that,

> Identities in general (of whatever kind, at whatever level) arise out of difference, but difference is not itself any identity or indeed any thing at all. It is not that there are first things, and then differences and

> relations between them: the "things" emerge only from the differences and relations, which have an absolute priority, and that emergence is never complete. It's that insight that led to the neologism *différance*. In the beginning is *différance*, which means that there is no simple beginning or origin. And the *différance* never ends, which means that there is no simple end. Derrida's simple claim, then, is that nowhere ever is there anything simple. (2016, para. 3)

My view corresponds with Bennington's. I maintain that deconstructive readings push reason to the edges of its own limits, thus rendering impossible the Enlightenment dream of a rationality that can establish legitimately (and universally) what we ought to do, because they put into question the very boundaries of truth's distinction from ideology, from rhetoric or from dogma. Deconstructive readings show that the "simple," the origin or the root can never be obtained, because it never obtained to begin with. This aporia is what I call the "impossible-necessity" of critique.

If one could simply eschew metaphysical foundations and move on, of course, none of this would matter. But the point I elaborate at length in the first part of this study is that one cannot simply move on. In his most recent book, Rodolphe Gasché underscores the same point. What Derrida shows, Gasché writes, is that,

> The belief that one can cut all ties with the system of metaphysics, especially from a position outside the system, *is an illusion fostered by metaphysics itself* (to reabsorb the critic better, as it were). The intra-metaphysical distinction between an inside and an outside is the conceptual and formal template of such an illusion. (2016, 19; emphasis added)

Gasché continues, "The force of deconstruction does not consist in overthrowing metaphysics, through which metaphysics would be replaced by something else, its other, non-Western thought. The force of deconstruction delimits the system of metaphysics from within" (2016, 20). This is as clear a statement as there could be of why the lesson of deconstruction is not that epistemological foundations are impossible. It is that *notwithstanding* their impossibility, *an evocation of foundations is necessary for critical theories aimed at emancipatory political ends nonetheless.* This radical challenge to the modernist belief in legitimacy is the real lesson of "postmodernism." The political–theoretical question is not, therefore, 'what *other* normative term, if any, can deconstruction be said to privilege (if not logic *or* rhetoric)?' – which is what so many Derrida scholars tend to ask now. Rather, it is, 'what are the *political implications* of the thesis "that no responsibility could ever be taken without equivocation and without contradiction? Or that the self-justification of a decision is impossible, and could not, a priori and for structural reasons, be absolutely answerable for itself?"' (Derrida 1992b, 9–10).

This question concerning the equivocality of ethical–political responsibility implicates two conjoined dimensions of the *political* idea of Enlightenment reason. On one hand, what is at stake is the tradition of ideology critique – from Marx, through Horkheimer and Adorno, up to Habermas and beyond – insofar as ideology critique entails unmasking the interestedness of thought that purports to be *disinterestedly* neutral. If the evocation of foundations is unjustifiable but nonetheless irreducible, and if, therefore, interestedness goes all the way down, then where does this leave critical theory? On the other hand, the idea of Enlightenment also informs the emancipatory educative project, which involves the inculcation of critical reason as a political, democratizing force. Specifically, I argue in Chapter One that the move whereby Immanuel Kant establishes a moral principle on epistemological grounds is absolutely vital because, with it, Kant substantiates a notion of (practical) reason as critical – which is to say, as normative, and not merely as axiomatic or deductive – in nature. By virtue of Kant's intervention, Enlightenment comes to mean both education *and* emancipation: education, because it is a question of *learning* to use one's reason, and emancipation because it is a matter of learning to use it to overcome biases, partialities and dogmas (of a local or given point of view) that are imposed, thereby limiting the *freedom* of our decisions, our values, and our acts. As I explain below, this opposition between justice and ideology underlines characterizations of the school as one of the founding sites of liberal and/or radical democracy. If "the self-justification of a decision is impossible," as Derrida says (cited above), then the "postmodern" critique of modern epistemology will undermine the emancipatory *educational* ideal as well.

This is why the purported eschewal of logic and its replacement with rhetoric was, and is still, deemed so 'dangerous' for political and educational theory alike. My analysis of that danger constitutes the basis for my argument in Chapter Two, which is that Habermas's charges are indeed "false" – a point that comes across clearly in Derrida's reading of Kant's essay on the 'apocalyptic tone of philosophy.' The purpose of this demonstration is to open up the questions of exactly how, and at what *political* cost, that "solidarity," that 'mutual contamination' of the categories, is denied. These questions are explored in Chapters Three and Four, where I provide a thoroughgoing analysis of Jean-François Lyotard's diagnosis of the "postmodern condition," and I develop the implications of this analysis for the Kantian conception of "critique." My conclusion in Part One is not that the Enlightenment protocols of truth and reason no longer hold, but – on the contrary – that their groundlessness emerges only when we hold to them most tightly. Rational determinations are always contestable by virtue of reason's own demand for grounds – for non-contradiction and for completeness, in Leibniz's terms – and they only come under scrutiny on that basis at all. This is because a modality of reason that purports to be critical entails the radical "demand for the condition of possibility;" it honours the philosophical inheritance of critique by seeking the origin, root or ground of epistemological and ethical judgements. It is the philosophical discourse of modernity itself, therefore, with its ethos of criticality, which issues in its own postmodernization.

This argument raises an immediate and obvious question: why would this Kantian problematic implicate emancipatory theories that purport to have left the Enlightenment metanarrative behind? The problematic I am referring to encompasses the issues that attend Kant's explication of "critique" as a philosophical procedure, and the use of that procedure to ground ethical judgements ("practical reason") on the logical principle of freedom. Certainly, there are many contemporary theorists who are aware of this problematic, and who make no apparent appeal to Kant's ethics or his metaphysics. Critical political theorists often draw instead, for example, on such diverse philosophical resources as Deweyan pragmatism, Freirean liberation theology, Habermasian communicative ethics, or Marxist, feminist or anti-racist critical theories of society. Such approaches would thus appear to be free of metaphysical foundations, since they explicitly reject any direct reliance upon them.

The argument I provide in the chapters that comprise Part Two, however, is that the explicit rejection of transcendental reason and universal subjectivity (two of the basic pillars of Enlightenment metaphysics) is belied by a much more basic Kantian assumption that implicitly remains in play. It is that a legitimate standard of critique can be determined without recourse to ideology, mere opinion or culturally-contingent mores. What rests at the core of the Kantian idea of Enlightenment in its emancipatory sense, in other words, is the assumption that a legitimate standard of ethical–political judgement is something we can teach because it is something we can know. This deep link between the emancipation aims of Enlightenment reason and the specific question of education is why critical educational and pedagogical theory is such a propitious site for the elaboration of the political idea of Enlightenment as emancipation. For, regardless of one's specific position on Kant, one must presuppose the possibility of moral legitimacy in general – that is, the possibility of knowing in a valid way how the line between justice and injustice can be drawn – if the educative dimension of Enlightenment is to be advanced, because a non-ideological conception of the good is what the concept of emancipation through education needs.

Part Two therefore comprises my treatment of a series of critical educational theories that aim to bypass Kant's foundationalism and his transcendentalism without sacrificing the political goal of emancipation. As will become clear, this treatment applies to political theory in general, notwithstanding the focus on educational theory in particular, because what is at issue in both cases is the emancipatory ideal of Enlightenment. To this end, I analyze the approaches of those who feel no need to appeal to Enlightenment reason, on the grounds that Kantian metaphysics have already been (or can in principle be) surpassed. I refute these strategic approaches by demonstrating both what is at stake in the separation between logic and rhetoric for the field of critical educational theory, and at what political cost the inseparability of these categories is (in each case) obscured. My discussion encompasses both modern (typically, philosophy of education) and so-called "postmodern" (typically, critical pedagogy) approaches to progressive educational thought, because my aim is to bring out the political significance of the philosophical deconstruction of "critical reason" for the emancipatory project of the Enlightenment. In each of the cases I analyze, the logic of deconstruction reveals ideological dimensions of emancipatory thought that other critical methods overlook, and it does so in a way that no other form of critical analysis can.

Specifically, I demonstrate, where norms and beliefs are explicitly held as provisional and revisable (as in pragmatism and fallibilism, for example), they fail as critical standards of critique; for, if they cannot be epistemologically legitimated, they cannot be generalized or taught. I also show, on the other hand, that where norms and beliefs are not held as provisional and revisable, or where they are only ambivalently so held, they necessarily embody the very foundationalism they purport to disavow. This means that critical pedagogical and critical political theorists who advocate any particular standard of judgement – whether in the name of feminism, anti-racism, multiculturalism, the rights of the poor or just simply "difference" – are caught on the horns of a dilemma. If they assume that moral legitimacy *is* possible and then seek alternative epistemological grounds on which to establish it, they will have repeated the Kantian move they explicitly repudiated and will have purchased a critical standard at the cost of covering up its own impossible conditions. Conversely, if – purporting to break from Kant – they reject the possibility of moral legitimacy, they must also give way to the charges of partiality, particularism or belief that could rightfully be brought against them. These claims are supported through a treatment of each theoretical case in turn. The conclusion of Part Two is that emancipatory thought aimed at addressing political oppression will remain in a bind until it becomes more deeply attuned to the challenge that deconstruction actually poses to the modernist assumptions underlying critical theory, and to the resources it can actually provide.

These resources involve a new way to understand the aim and the nature of political–theoretical "critique." To be sure, it is widely assumed that if critical theory cannot appeal to an unconditioned ground, the critical–theoretical enterprise has nowhere left to go. And indeed, I show, the demand for the origins, grounds or roots of the critical endeavour can never be satisfied, because no grounds or simple origins are there to be found. But critical political theory cannot just eschew the demand for the legitimation of its moral determinations either, because reason as self-critique demands a lucid vigilance with regard to the possibility of its own conditions. This is the very meaning of intellectual or scholarly responsibility, and its obligation is ineluctable; the alternative is an unwitting lapse into relativism or dogma, where no theorist will willingly go. The revelation of this "impossible-necessity" at the root of critical thought, therefore, cannot be reduced to "critique" in either a "traditional" or "critical" sense (Horkheimer 2002), since what is revealed is neither a set of determinable, logical principles in the abstract, nor a set of determinable, social and political conditions in the concrete. And yet, paradoxically, the interrogative character of deconstructive readings does answer to the demand *for* legitimacy, the demand *for* "a centre or origin" that has characterized critical thought all along. What thus becomes clear is that the deconstruction of what Derrida calls the "critical idea" itself (2005d, 142) – namely, the philosophical idea that legitimate judgements are possible in the spheres of epistemology and ethics, most notably, and that these judgements can be applied to politics – is neither strictly critical nor strictly uncritical, neither clearly inside nor clearly outside the spheres of legitimacy that it contests. It is in this particular sense, I contend, that a deconstructive inquiry constitutes a *certain* form of critique.

Importantly, then, the critical–political status of deconstruction does not concern the link between the demonstration of undecidability and the putative impossibility of political decision. In this regard, Critchley misrepresented the issue significantly when he posited an impasse between the ethics of a deconstructive *reading* and the activity of political judgement as a desirable *end* (1992, 190). To say this is to forget that what is radical about deconstruction is its fidelity to the conditions of reason – to the question of the principle*s* and the question of *the* principle (Derrida 2002a, 257, cited above) – and that it is only because of one's fidelity to the injunction to seek the 'root' that one discovers that the centre is spectral and that, consequently, no good conscience, no unassailable critical position, can be had. This political revelation *is* the core, and the inescapable consequence, of a philosophically radical critique.

To undertake a deconstructive reading is thus to inherit and put to work the *critical* potential of reason in its most classical sense, reason as non-contradiction and completeness, with respect to every last judgement and every ethical–political end. At the same time, however, this undertaking has no authority of its own, because the practice of deconstruction cannot account for itself – not if what are in question are precisely "the traditional categories of responsibility," and even "the form of the question" (Derrida, Gadamer, Lacoue-Labarthe 2016, 23). The implication of Derrida's paradoxical formulation concerning the duty to deconstruct, in other words, is this: if what imposes itself enigmatically "in the name of the Enlightenment to come" (2005d, 142) and appears as "an absolute must" (1988b, 122) is the *desire* for an unrelenting, lucid vigilance with regard to the (impossible) conditions of critical reason itself, then such an obligation cannot be rationally authorized, because it will have preceded the very reason *at* which its interrogations are aimed. The responsibility that Derrida upholds is thus still a responsibility to reason, but it is a logically impossible one. In what, then, can *its* forceful impulse be said to consist? The normative status of deconstruction thus emerges *as* a question (the question of its own status as "critique") when the "modernist" belief in the possibility of rational legitimation is challenged in the way that deconstruction, understood as "postmodernism" in this very restricted sense, actually challenges it. This brings us back to Derrida's own question: 'what could be the responsibility, the quality or the virtue of responsibility' *of* "a consistent discourse" (i.e., deconstruction) that *reveals* the necessary equivocality and the contradictory nature of all claims to responsibility (1992b, 9)? *What is the status of that undertaking itself*?

My answer is provided in the third and final part of the book. It is that the obligation (*il faut*) that permeates Derrida's oeuvre is neither a call to celebrate difference nor, relatedly, a duty to welcome the other with unconditional hospitality. It is instead only what Derrida calls the "law and the destiny" not to "forgo the *Aufklärung*" (1983a, 22). And, once it is recognized that deconstruction is impelled by a desire for Enlightenment that exceeds reason's own bounds, it becomes necessary to move beyond the Derridean text. I turn to the discourse of Freudian psychoanalysis at this juncture, because I hold that what is "enigmatic" about the desire for reason is that its motivation does not and cannot appear *as such* to conscious, rational thought. Specifically, my hypothesis is that what drives deconstruction is in fact a *drive* (*Trieb*, in the psychoanalytic sense), and not a rational principle at all. This is how one should understand the "apocalyptic tone" that Derrida describes (1983a) – the tone that opens philosophy with a groundless and soundless affirmation in the form of the gesture, "come" (1983a, 24), or the "yes, yes" that precedes any question (2005a, 74) – that derives from an unknown and indeterminable source.

Indeed, Derrida himself opens the door to a psychoanalytic reading of the 'ethics' of deconstruction insofar as he refers to the way in which "a certain madness must watch over thinking" (1995a), to the Kierkegaardian idea that "the instant of decision is madness" (qtd. in Derrida 1978, 31), to the way in which "deconstruction is mad for justice" (1992a), and so on. These regular references to "madness" pertain, on my view, to the possibility that deconstructive readings are driven by an unconscious (ultimately non-rational) *attachment* to rationality – that is, by a psychological investment in the principle of reason that remains opaque to consciousness. It is this attachment, I aver, that impels the deconstructive exposure of the logical structure and irreducible effects of *différance*.

Interestingly, Gasché propels Derrida scholars in a psychoanalytic direction as well. Gasché writes that because "the violence of arche-writing, originary violence, the writing that has always already occurred, cannot possibly be avoided," because "[w]ithout it, there would be nothing rather than something," and because it is for this reason "a fundamental, structurally necessary violence," it follows that a "second violence is inevitable, as well" (2016, 78). This "second violence," he goes on to say, "which both protects against and, in protecting, confirms the originary violence, *is inevitable insofar as the latter is experienced in consciousness*" (2016, 79; emphasis added). This "second violence" is

> a function of the way the originary violence is perceived and experienced; that is, it is linked to what Derrida calls in this context, but also throughout *Of Grammatology*, "consciousness." *This problematic of consciousness in the context of an analysis of violence and writing would require an independent treatment.* For the time being, let me offer only the following: the originary division of all proper names and, hence, of their proper referents is coextensive with the dream of self-proximity, self-presence, self-affection, and self-consciousness. (Gasché 2016, 78; emphasis added)

The psychoanalytic study I undertake in Part Three provides the very "treatment" that Gasché, with his reference to the "problematic of consciousness," invokes. I directly relate the covering over of *différance* – that is, both the psychological (egoic) denial of the originary, *différantial* structure of subjectivity and the political–theoretical denial of the originary *différance* of linguistic meaning – to the "dream of self-proximity, self-presence, self-affection and self-consciousness" – that is, to the need in both spheres for the appearance of completeness and non-contradiction. My turn to psychoanalysis dovetails with the first-generation Frankfurt School's interest in Freud. More specifically, I take my cue from a note by Adorno in *Negative Dialectics*: "in idealism," he submits, "identity designates the point of indifference of the psychological and logical moments. Logical universality, as the universality of thought, is tied to individual identity, without which it would not come into being" (1973, 142nt.).

Just as the idealist dream of self-identity violently overwrites the originary violence of arche-writing, so deconstruction's own "force" can be understood through a psychoanalytic lens as well. For it constitutes a "third violence," as Gasché calls it, one which essentially consists in the *disclosure* of the originary violence, that is, in the "tearing apart the veil that social consciousness has [violently] drawn [over it] in the shape of a moral law" (2016, 80). As Gasché writes,

> deconstruction violently transgresses the law [understood as] as a violent concealment of the originary violence involved in naming … in order to acknowledge the originary dividedness and differentiation of all self-sameness, and to bring to light the secondariness of anything pretending to be proper. (2016, 86)

As a tertiary violence directed at the second violence, in other words, deconstruction uncovers the violence that instantiates "self-presence, self-affection and self-consciousness," a violence which, in "target[ing] difference ... is capable of producing such evils as xenophobia, racism, sexism, chauvinism, and so on" (2016, 79). The vigilance of deconstruction is characterized by its unrelenting attention to those forms of political violence and yet, paradoxically, what motivates it is the same *différantial* structure of subjectivity that gives rise to them in the first place.

The need to explain deconstruction's motivation emerges most clearly in Chapters Nine and Ten. There, I challenge the Levinasian interpretation of the ethics of deconstruction, particularly as it was applied by Drucilla Cornell to the field of critical legal studies. As I show, there is an internal limit to the extent to which the impulse to deconstruct can be explained in normative terms, and Derrida's own responses to this question fall short. In *Specters of Marx* (1994) for example, he relates the Marxist spirit of radical critique to a "*critical wanting-itself*" (to be open to its own transformation), but Derrida does not explain what this is or where it comes from, save to say that this desire is "not yet critical," but nor is it "pre-critical" (1994, 88). One can certainly understand this desire as "originary" in a Derridean sense (that is, as a 'non-originary origin,' or an origin 'under erasure'), but this still does not tell us very much about the nature of the force that opens critique to its own possibility. For the purpose of addressing this specific lacuna in Derrida's oeuvre, a psychoanalytic account is indispensable.

The argument developed in Chapters 11 and 12 thus begins from the psychoanalytic insight that, as with critique, so with the psychological subject: "identities in general (of whatever kind, at whatever level), arise out of difference," and "nowhere ever is there anything simple" (Bennington 2016, para. 3, cited above). In other words, the deconstructive explanation of how self-identical meaning appears in language, even though it cannot obtain, applies equally to the way in which self-identity appears in individuals: there is nothing simple *there.* This claim is supported through a careful reading of Freud, which on the one hand instructively brings the aporetic structure of the subject to light. Indeed, I show in Chapter 11, many of Freud's most essential categories and distinctions are vulnerable to a deconstructive analysis, just as Derrida has frequently proposed (1978, 196–231; 1987; 1998). My intent in undertaking this demonstration, however, is not to dismiss the Freudian account of subjectivity; rather, it is to complicate that account from a deconstructive point of view. The complication that ensues, specifically, is the paradoxical character of egoic coherence that Freud attempted to describe.

This demonstration paves the way for a discussion of Jean Laplanche's radical reconstruction of Freudian thought, which I develop in Chapter 12 and which I mobilize to make sense of the paradox without reducing it. As the chapter makes clear, Laplanche's account is surprisingly congruent with deconstruction, mobilizing as it does the temporal logic of the "always already" (*après coup*) that characterizes the Derridean notion of *différance*. Specifically, Laplanche shows that the threat of fragmentation or incoherence will mean to the ego (as-subject) its death. Thus, while there can be no "completeness" where subjectivity is concerned either (as was the case with undecidability in language), the logic of "all or nothing" imposes itself again. Specifically, my thesis is that modern individuals are impelled by a psychological drive to preserve themselves – that is, by a compulsive desire to cohere (more or less) as unified and complete egos or "selves" – and that the protocols of reason are essential to the process through which this impulse is met. If there is indeed an "apocalyptic desire" *for* reason, foundations and truth that characterizes critique, in short, it is rooted in the psychological constitution of the subject, and it stems from an unconscious drive to cohere.

The consequence of this analysis for critical political and educational thought is that advocates of the principle of reason (including Derrida *and* Habermas) can be shown to be mobilizing more than an idiosyncratic notion of moral obligation when they demand or appeal to the unconditional. For critical theory takes its normative bearing from those subjects who, as products of Western modernity, are (unconsciously) desirous of subjective coherence and, concomitantly, of logical coherence as well. Such a theory will therefore be committed to reason and its logical demand for grounds, or else it *will* be irresponsible. The argument thus supports the claim that deconstruction mobilizes more than a relative notion of the good, without implicating anything transcendental. It does not suggest, however, that deconstruction simply replaces the universal subject of the Enlightenment with the "decentred" subject of postmodernity. For when the ethical dimension of political theory (its quasi-responsibility) is taken in the sense that I propose, it necessarily sacrifices the possibility of universal or unconditional grounds. As a psychological imperative, the responsibility to reason that critical theory enacts is historically, socially and politically produced, and must be limited to this more modest sense.

Neither the logic of modern epistemology nor that of "postmodern" deconstruction, I therefore conclude, ultimately can justify the critical–theoretical ideal of the "true" good or the "real" nature of injustice, and so neither can reaffirm that opposition between justice and ideology that modernists and certain putative postmodernists hold so dear. Rather, what remains of the emancipatory discourse of Enlightenment in the wake of its "postmodernization" is an ineluctable imperative to question our ethical and political norms, and to do so in the most vigilant, rigorous and unrelenting way possible. In other words, I maintain that responsibility – the ability and the impulse to respond by giving a moral account – extends in the final analysis to a (quasi-ethical) imperative to question, rather than to determine, our moral ends. From this it follows that critical theory is 'good' neither when it promises the logical mastery of rhetorical undecidability, nor when it suggests that rhetoric can master logic. Instead, theory is 'good' (quasi-responsible) only insofar as it takes responsibility for its 'apocalyptic' opening by remaining lucidly vigilant about its own ideological closures, and this means both taking a risk and offering an emancipatory chance. The nature of ethical–political critique ultimately requires no less.

Note

1 The book *Philosophy in a Time of Terror: Dialogues with Jürgen Habermas and Jacques Derrida* (Borradori 2003) does not contain a direct exchange between the two philosophers.

Part I

Naming the Stakes

1 The Danger of Rhetoric

> That deconstruction could contribute something to the question of justice, possible or impossible, is taken as either self-evident or met with outrage these days (and hence in both cases remains unthought) … Deconstruction's ethico-political pertinence is either (1) taken for granted (often but by no means always presumed to be "progressive") with an appeal to its thematic or referential considerations of issues (democracy, torture, "race," feminism, the university and teaching, apartheid) or to its formal homologies with political interventions (the deconstruction of authority as emancipatory or as ideology-critique), or (2) condemned (as nefariously antipolitical or paralyzing) because it appears to ruin the categories on which political discourse has tried to found itself for as long as anyone can remember: subjectivity and agency, and the reliable knowledge (meaning, whether positively, theologically, or hermeneutically determined) that "allows" it to act.
>
> (Keenan 1995, 263)

Education has long been considered to be one of the most fundamental cornerstones of liberal, democratic society. Indeed, modern Western European ideals of education are imbued with the Enlightenment belief that human reason is the ultimate faculty through which human beings (qua "Man") can achieve not only epistemological truth, but moral goodness and social reform. For, as I will show, when Immanuel Kant first formulated the "categorical imperative" – when, that is to say, he made the strong argument that moral values can be logically determined in rational, universal terms on the basis of the pure use of (practical) reason – he clearly linked ethics to that same logic, or "true" knowledge, on which modern epistemology depends. For theorists and philosophers of education this link has been decisive: both the traditional (modernist) project of education *of* the people and, alternatively, various critical and progressive projects of education *for* the people, have founded emancipation from "natural want and social injustice" (Misgeld 1992, 125) upon the acquisition of knowledge and the enhancement of critical reason.[1] Within this tradition, moreover, criticism, knowledge and justice ("the good") are sharply opposed to ideology, opinion and injustice (the unethical). This opposition between justice and ideology continues to underline characterizations of the school as one of the founding sites of liberal and/or radical democracy.

Not surprisingly, therefore, the epistemological "crisis" of postmodernity – the so-called "postmetaphysical" or post-enlightenment position that there is no universal subject whose "truth" can be determined absolutely – has thrown the educational ideal into radical question. In other words, the argument that representations of almost any kind of "truth" are contingent in a variety of ways (historically, culturally, racially, in respect of gender or class, etc.) – and, hence, are to some extent implicated in ideology, opinion and injustice – has led some intellectuals to the conclusion that if rational truth is contestable, then the moral values which have been founded upon it are only relative.

This apprehension – and it is one shared not only by many theorists of education, but also by critical theorists more generally – stems, I shall argue, from a mistaken, though unfortunately common, belief about the normative implications of so-called "postmodernism."[2] It is the belief that theorists who have "decentred" the modern (universal) subject and thereby relativized the truth, such as Jacques Derrida, Michel Foucault, Jacques Lacan or Jean-François Lyotard, have effectively annihilated the very basis of a modernist ethico-political sensibility. Such theorists are charged, in effect, with endangering the social reform (the democracy) promised by traditional and progressive educational or political projects alike. It is this charge – or, more accurately, the ethico-political assumptions that underline it – that the present inquiry is intended to address.

Political philosopher Jürgen Habermas, for example, mobilized just these assumptions when he first accused Jacques Derrida of "levelling the genre distinction between philosophy and literature" and with thereby 'robbing' "philosophical thinking" of its "seriousness" and its "substance" (Habermas 1987, 185, 210). Indeed, the specific accusation that Derrida and other poststructuralists have made philosophy into, merely, a kind of literary or aesthetic object that is infinitely open to interpretation has become such a standard rebuttal to Derrida and other contemporary French philosophers that its mere citation is often accepted as an adequate conclusion to any substantive discussion.

Consider, for instance, Axel Honneth's claim that the "theoretical framework of interpretation" of the "postmodern conception" may be "a Nietzschean tinged concept of aesthetic freedom" (Honneth 1992, 164), or Christopher Norris's belief that it is the "desire to make reality over into an aesthetic phenomenon – to collapse the whole range of *ontological* distinctions between life and art, fact and fiction, history and poetry, truth and appearance – which typifies the current postmodernist drive against the Enlightenment and all its works" (Norris 1993, 63, 253; my emphasis). By the same token, Seyla Benhabib has asserted that "contextualism and post-modernism ... reject that criticism of validity and legitimacy can be formulated, and transform philosophy into literary criticism, aphorism, or poetry" (Benhabib 1986, 15). Amy Gutmann, similarly, has characterized what she calls "deconstructionism" as a "dangerous," "anti-intellectual, politicizing threat" to academies of higher learning – those bastions of "knowledge, understanding, intellectual dialogue and the pursuit of reasoned argument" (Gutmann, ed., 1994, 19, 20).

These examples illustrate the wide agreement that "postmodernism" in general and deconstruction in particular "relativize" or "aestheticize" those truths on which democratic political projects must be based. Gutmann is particularly clear on this; she finds deconstruction single-handedly responsible for turning all claims to political validity into unmitigated bullying or posturing. In fact, Gutmann argues, the deconstructionist view even "deconstructs" itself, for "the less powerful cannot possibly hope to have their standards win out, especially if their academic spokespersons publicize the view that intellectual standards are nothing more than assertions or reflections of the will to power" (1994, 19). Thus, Gutmann provides a more precise specification of Habermas's concern; the advent of "deconstructionism" in the university threatens the loss of the training in reasoned argument that schools provide and, concomitantly, the evisceration of the promise of a justice that transcends politics. "Deconstructionism," in short, threatens the very lifeblood of a democratic society (Gutmann 1994, 23–4).

One response to such dire predictions, to be sure, would be to take issue with each one of these charges on a case-by-case basis. For just as Benhabib's and Habermas's assertions that Derrida is engaged in a purely literary levelling of philosophical reflection can be countered on the basis of a careful reading of Derrida's work, so Honneth would be hard-pressed to demonstrate, rather than merely to assert, that all critics of the Enlightenment necessarily follow Nietzsche. Similarly, it could well be argued that Gutmann's characterization of all critics of the liberal arts canon as "deconstructionists" will not hold up to scrutiny, while Christopher Norris, for his part, might find it as difficult to defend the absolute purity and autonomous status of his classical, "ontological distinctions," as he would to substantiate his generalization that there is currently a "postmodernist drive" to "collapse" them.

While the formulation and substantiation of specific counterarguments is undoubtedly important, however, I do not propose to treat each of these debates in all their particulars here. For what I want to underline is that, taken together, such ethico-political fears about deconstruction and/or "postmodernism" evidence a profound misunderstanding of what relevance specific critiques of reason – and especially those undertaken by Derrida – might have for critical political theory in general, and for critical theories of education in particular. This misunderstanding is most clearly articulated by Christopher Norris, who writes,

> postmodernism can do nothing to challenge … forms of injustice and oppression since it offers no arguments, no critical resources or

> validating grounds for perceiving them *as* inherently unjust and oppressive. In the end, all this rhetoric of "plurality" and "difference" comes down to just another, more radical-sounding version of Rorty's neopragmatist message, that is to say, his advice that we should cultivate the private virtues … and cease the vain effort to square those virtues with a sense of our larger (public, social, ethical or political) responsibilities. Postmodernism cannot do other than promote this view insofar as it rejects the principle advanced by critical-enlightenment thinkers from Kant to Habermas. (Norris 1993, 287)

If this misunderstanding of Derrida's work[3] still persists so many decades after the publication of *Of Grammatology* (Derrida 1976 [1967]), this may be because references to the "aestheticizing" and hence "apolitical" nature of deconstructive writing are often accepted as an adequate end to the dispute. This itself should stand out as a point of interest. For the most remarkable thing about these accusations is not that one group of scholars disagrees vehemently with another, but rather that the charge is taken to speak for itself.

Among the critics cited here, for example, Honneth relies on only a few scant references to Jean-François Lyotard's *The Postmodern Condition* and Jean Baudrillard's, *Die Agonie des Realen* to support the claim that a Nietzschean, "aesthetic model of human freedom is what underlies, in one way or another, *all* versions of a theory of the 'postmodern'" (1992, 167; emphasis mine), Gutmann (1994) neglects to cite a single theorist in support of her claims, and Habermas's treatment of Derrida is largely given over to a discussion of literary critics Jonathan Culler, Hillis Miller and Geoffrey Hartman – on the basis, he says, that Derrida "does not belong to those philosophers who like to argue" and that the discussion between Derrida and John Searle is "somewhat impenetrable" (Habermas 1987, 193, 194).[4]

If Christopher Norris (who has investigated Derrida's thought comprehensively) is a notable exception among this group, it is not because he treats the relationship between the discourses of the European Enlightenment and the discourses of the (so-called) "postmodern" in a more nuanced way. Rather, it is because, in contrast to his colleagues, Norris places Derrida squarely on the side of modernity. Norris takes issue, for instance, with the Habermasian charge that Derrida eschews argumentation in favour of literary 'tricks,' arguing that such a criticism "involves the kind of typecast binary thinking that refuses to see how a 'literary' text – or one which exploits a wide range of stylistic resources – might yet possess sufficient *argumentative* force to unsettle such deep-laid assumptions" (Norris 1992, 190, emphasis his; and 1993, 89).[5] To the extent that Derrida's strategies of reading reflect, on Norris's view, "a distinctly Kantian form of argument," Norris declares that "Derrida has distanced his own thinking from a generalized 'post-modern' or post-structuralist discourse"

(1992, 167) and that "deconstruction, properly understood, belongs within that same 'philosophical discourse of modernity' that Habermas sets out to defend against its present-day detractors" (1992, 170). For Norris no less than the others, therefore, it can be taken as read that the line between the modern and the "postmodern" can be clearly delineated; if Derrida *were* to be guilty of that "aestheticizing" tendency characteristic of the "postmodern" in general (Norris 2004, 353), the French philosopher might be as easily dismissed. Indeed, Norris says, one can add "post-structuralism, postmodernism, Foucaldian 'genealogy' (or discourse-theory), and at least one variety of deconstruction as practised by (mainly American) literary critics," to a "catalogue" of thinkers for whom,

> it is a high point of doctrine that "truth" is nothing more than what counts as such according to the codes, cultural conventions, power/knowledge interests, "intertextual" relationships and so forth which make up the conditions of intelligibility within this or that field of "signifying practice." (1993, 102–3)

How is it that one need only cite one of a series of charges (of formulas, in effect) which distinguish 'good' from 'bad' philosophy? How is it that such widespread dismissiveness can overcome scholarly debate? The answer, one can only surmise, is that there is at work a powerful and deeply-held set of assumptions behind these claims. The question at hand, therefore, is what kind of assumption or, rather, what set of assumptions, might serve to render the scholarly requirements of textual substantiation, argumentative rigour and careful attention to content and form moot in these responses to a particular body of scholarship?

One such assumption, to be sure, is the Enlightenment belief that ethical and political 'goods' can be established in rational and hence universal terms. The "postmodern" postulation that what counts as "truth" may be determined on the grounds of racial, gender-related, class-based, historical, cultural, religious or otherwise contingent interests profoundly challenges this belief, and this challenge has in turn resulted in widespread fears concerning the political perils of "postmodern" theorizing. Yet this assumption should and can be made more precise in light of a significant clue provided in Habermas's reading of Derrida. For Habermas specifies that what is more narrowly at issue in deconstruction – and, presumably, in any form of "postmodern" theorizing that shares its ostensible "aestheticizing" tendency – is that "Derrida is particularly interested in standing the primacy of logic over rhetoric, canonized since Aristotle, on its head" (Habermas 1987, 187). Thus, the Kantian link between ethics and epistemology (via logic) that is taken for granted in the dominant response to "postmodernism" is anteceded by a prior philosophical conviction; *viz*, that logic has a traditional and justifiable standing over rhetoric, and that this status has been (illegitimately) overturned. As Johann Michel asserts, for example, "Derrida's philosophy ... should be understood as traditionally metaphysical, since it seeks only to *substitute* 'difference, separation and alterity, for a thought of presence, unity, and identity'" (Michel, qtd. in Purcell 2015, para. 8; emphasis added).

It is the illegitimate nature of the deconstructive reversal, then, or more accurately, the bald assumption that Derrida and other French philosophers have undertaken it, that apparently authorizes critics to engage in what appears as a decidedly dismissive approach. For, as I now want to show, the "primacy of the logical over the rhetorical" predates and grounds that very link which "postmodernism" is taken to threaten: the link between a critical epistemological ideal of reason freed from ideology and injustice, on the one hand, and a modern political ideal of progressive, social reform – which is to say, an ethico-political ideal of the 'good' – on the other. Precisely because it is so well established in the history of Western philosophy, in other words, the priority of logic over rhetoric pre-empts, and is regularly taken to have the authority to pre-empt, the modernism–postmodernism debate. The question that must be addressed first, therefore, is how the priority of the logical over the rhetorical – or, in Habermas's formulation, the primacy of the "problem-solving" capacity of *philosophy* over the "world-disclosing" capacity of fiction or the *literary* – ensures the a priori legitimacy of the modernist position and, relatedly, whether that primacy is in fact as secure as is supposed.

It is particularly significant, therefore, that in an essay that predates Habermas's "Excursus" on deconstruction by some five years, Paul de Man goes a substantial way towards answering these questions. He writes,

> The most misleading representation of literariness, and also the most recurrent objection to contemporary literary theory, considers it as pure verbalism, as a denial of the reality principle in the name of absolute fictions, and for reasons that are said to be ethically and politically shameful. (de Man 1982, 11)

Here, de Man is especially concerned with the question of what it is "about literary theory that is so threatening that it provokes such strong resistances and attacks" (1982, 11). This resistance to the 'literary,' he asserts, "is a resistance to the use of language about language. It is therefore a resistance to language itself" – which is to say, "to the possibility that language contains factors or functions that cannot be reduced to intuition" (1982, 13). For de Man, in fact, "literariness" is just this possibility; it refers to "the use of language that foregrounds the rhetorical over the grammatical and the logical function" (1982, 14).

Yet the excess of language beyond determinate meaning will always persist. As de Man remarks, the form taken by these difficulties in the present scene, and the contemporary resistance to them, "is only one more particular version of a question that cannot be reduced to a specific historical situation and called modern, post-modern, post-classical or romantic" (de Man 1982, 12). Thus, the term "language" itself – the very term we use to denote the possibility of denotation – brings us to the heart of the difficulty in Habermas's assumption that philosophy's logical mode of discourse must, for ethical and political reasons, be privileged over the rhetorical or the 'literary.' For, even if we begin with "the most familiar and general" of all models of language, the classical Greek *trivium*, we will soon encounter difficulties which no logical analysis can resolve (1982, 13). The *trivium*, it will be recalled, is the tripartite division of the sciences of language into grammar, rhetoric and logic. First formulated by Boethius in sixth century Greece, these "sciences of language," together with the sciences of number, or the *quadrivium* (arithmetic, geometry, astronomy and music), comprised the seven liberal arts, or *artes liberales* (Carr 1997, 317).

As de Man's analysis makes clear, the importance of the *trivium* as a linguistic model goes far beyond the fact that it is the classical (if skeletal) basis of the contemporary university curriculum (Carr 1997, 318). For the hierarchical arrangement of the three "sciences" of language – and particularly the standing of logic over rhetoric – establishes the original possibility of "scientific and humanistic knowledge" (de Man 1982, 15) – the very possibility, that is to say, that "postmodernism" in general, and deconstruction in particular, appears to threaten. Specifically, de Man argues that the condition of moving freely between the sciences of language and the sciences of nature or the phenomenal world (1982, 14) is the subjugation of rhetoric to logic within the *trivium*. And this is because it is first and foremost *logic* which links together the domains of the *trivium* and the *quadrivium*.

> In the history of philosophy, this link is traditionally, as well as substantially, accomplished by way of logic, the area where the rigor of the linguistic discourse about itself matches up with the rigor of the mathematical discourse about the world. Seventeenth-century epistemology, for instance, at the moment when the relationship between philosophy and mathematics is particularly close, holds up the language of what it calls geometry (*mos geometricus*), and which in fact includes the homogeneous concatenation between space, time and number, as the sole model of coherence and economy … This is a clear instance of the interconnection between a science of the phenomenal world and a science of language conceived as definitional logic, the pre-condition for a correct axiomatic-deductive, synthetic reasoning … [T]his articulation of the sciences of language with the mathematical sciences represents a particularly compelling version of a continuity between a theory of language, as logic, and the knowledge of the phenomenal world to which mathematics gives access. (1982, 13–14)

Yet, de Man continues, even if we grant the arguable claim that a theory of language as logic can guarantee the link to the phenomenal world of the natural sciences, the relationship between grammar, logic and rhetoric "within the confines of the *trivium* itself" is by no means securely established (1982, 14).

One can, de Man agrees, maintain a relatively close and relatively comfortable connection between grammar and logic, since grammar, like logic, must be virtually universal in its application, or else it does not satisfy the essential demand that it account for a potentially all-inclusive number of texts. Therefore, for an entire tradition of linguistic theorists, "the grammatical and the logical function of language are co-extensive. Grammar is an isotope of logic" (de Man 1982, 14). With regard to the relation between grammar and rhetoric, however, the case is not so clear. On the contrary, the instability of this relationship is apparent "in the uncertain status of figures of speech or tropes, a component of language that straddles the borderlines between the two areas" (1982, 15). If semiologists have attempted to master and to clarify meaning by extending grammar to include the "para-figural dimensions" of a text, for example – if they have thereby aimed to replace rhetorical with grammatical terminology – this strategy will nonetheless leave "a residue of indetermination that has to be, but cannot be, resolved by grammatical means, however extensively conceived" (1982, 15, 16).

As an example of just such undecidability, de Man considers the figure, or "trope," that forms the title of Keats's epic poem, "The Fall of Hyperion." This trope, it emerges, can be read in any one of a number of ways, none of which can be conclusively shown to be correct on the basis of a grammatical or a logical analysis. For instance, we can read "The Fall of Hyperion" as variously referring to "Hyperion's fall" – the defeat of Hyperion by Apollo – or as "Hyperion falling," which is to say as the "more disquieting evocation of an actual process of falling, regardless of its beginning, its end or the identity to whom it befalls to be falling." de Man asks,

> Does the title tell us that Hyperion is fallen and that Apollo stands, or does it tell us that Hyperion and Apollo (and Keats, whom it is hard to distinguish, at times, from Apollo) are interchangeable in that all of them are necessarily and constantly falling? Both readings are grammatically correct, but it is impossible to decide from the context (the ensuing narrative) which version is the right one. (1982, 16)

Moreover, de Man continues, we might also offer an 'intertextual' reading of the figure, whereby we refer this poem to an earlier one by Keats, also unfinished, called "Hyperion." In this case, one can read the title differently again, this time as,

> telling the story [either] of the failure of the first text [or] as the success of the second, the Fall of *Hyperion* as the Triumph of *The Fall of Hyperion* … The undecidability involves the figural or literal status of the proper name Hyperion as well as the verb falling, and is thus a matter of figuration and not of grammar. (1982, 16)

"Faced with the ineluctable necessity to come to a decision," he concludes, no grammatical or logical analysis can help us out (1982, 16).

de Man's point is that the tropological dimension of language, the effect of "rhetoric" on grammar and logic that is clearly in evidence here, "*can be revealed in any verbal event when it is read textually*" (1982, 17; emphasis mine). Thus, far from being contained or being (in principle) containable within the dictates of grammar and logic, rhetoric undoes the possibility of theory – which is to say, it undoes the possibility of *logic* as a "universal system of philosophy" (1982, 8). The resistance to "theory," therefore, is a resistance to that reading which focuses on the 'literary,' because the 'literary,' rhetorical or tropological dimension of language "undoes the claims of the *trivium*" and thus "disturbs the stable cognitive field that extends from grammar to logic to a general science of man and of the phenomenal world" (1982, 17). The problem with the "literariness" of literature, in short – and indeed of any "verbal event" – is that literariness undermines the a priori claim that language functions according to the same (logical) principles as phenomena. "It is therefore not *a priori* certain," de Man continues, "that literature is a reliable source of information about anything but its own language" (1982, 11).

In terms of the present argument, the most interesting aspect of de Man's analysis is that it reveals two irreconcilably different, and yet inextricably bound, notions of the term "theory." Rhetoric *as* literary theory, he says, undoes the possibility *of* theory. On one hand, then, there is the classical understanding of theory as a universal knowledge system (theory_1), based on the *trivium*. Theory_1 presumes the immediate, referential function of language – the unproblematic correspondence between the name and the thing – which is in turn based upon intuition, and which "implies perception, consciousness, and all its correlatives" (1982, 8, 10). The most important of these correlatives, of course, is the possibility of a logical relation between language and the phenomenal world, for this relationship is understood as the very basis of scientific and humanistic knowledge, expressed as a universal system of philosophy.

Significantly, rhetorical readings are themselves theory_1 in this sense, de Man asserts, insofar as they can be *taught* – which is to say, insofar as they are "generalizable and highly responsive to systematization" (1982, 20). But they are and are not theory at the same time. For, as the systematic disruption of systematicity, "literary" readings (theory_2) also undo just this possibility of universalizable or systematizable knowledge. A theory_2 of rhetorical reading, in other words, is always to some degree both teachable and unteachable, for it is the "methodical undoing of the grammatical construct and, in its *systematic* disarticulation of the *trivium*, will be *theoretically*[$_1$] sound as well as effective" (1982, 20; my emphasis). Just as theory$_1$ will therefore necessarily "resist" the advent of literary theory$_2$, therefore, it follows that theories$_2$ of reading rhetorically which are *teachable* (and hence, share the qualities of theory$_1$) will also resist the very reading they advocate. Theory$_1$, de Man concludes, is thus none other than this resistance (1982, 20), because it embodies the methodological assumption of the possibility of a stable and universal field of knowledge "that extends," as we have seen, "from grammar to logic to a general science of man" (1982, 12, 17). Theory$_2$, on the other hand, is the inevitable disruption – what I will hereafter call the "deconstruction" – that destabilizes this knowledge due to the uncontainable nature of language's tropological effects.

I have elaborated this discussion at some length, because it is necessary to clarify the tension within the concept of "theory" that de Man elucidates in order to treat the objections to the purported "aestheticizing" tendency of deconstruction with which I began. Specifically, de Man's mobilization of a distinction between what I am calling theory$_1$ and theory$_2$ points towards a parallel tension within the concept of the aesthetic. It is this *tension* within the aesthetic, not the aesthetic *per se*, which deconstructive practices of reading threaten to reveal. The equivocality of the concept of the aesthetic, in other words, is what common objections to deconstruction aim to conceal.

The aesthetic, as de Man has noted, has occupied a "prominent though never dominant place" (1982, 8) within theory$_1$, because the aesthetic concerns precisely the phenomenology of meaning (the meaning of the "beautiful" for us, based on its effects upon the senses, or intuition) in terms of the understanding. In other words, aesthetics – at least since Kant – is a part of, rather than extraneous to, a universal system of philosophy, because it assumes the same relation between theory and phenomenality that is expressed by the system as a whole. Thus, de Man writes, "in such a system the place of aesthetics is preordained, and by no means alien, provided the priority of logic, in the model of the *trivium*, is not being questioned" (1982, 14).

Yet a questioning or destabilization of the primacy of logic within the *trivium* is precisely what theory$_2$ does. When effective, therefore, rhetorical readings "void" rather than affirm the categories of the aesthetic, because they disarticulate that system in which such categories form a well-established part. This is perhaps what de Man has in mind when he suggests that "the assumption that there can be a science of language [i.e., semiology, or structural linguistics] which is not necessarily a logic leads to the development of a terminology which is not necessarily aesthetic" (1982, 8). Indeed, in the classical model of language, rhetoric itself was presumed to serve a merely "aesthetic" or "ornamental" role within the *trivium* – precisely, that is, insofar as it was possible to "ignore its epistemological thrust" and to keep it subjugated as a lesser value within the semantic function (1982, 15). The "literariness" which rhetorical (or deconstructive) readings uncover are thus properly speaking neither aesthetic nor mimetic, from de Man's point of view, but strictly linguistic.

Once it is acknowledged that the aesthetic is part and parcel of a system of philosophy premised upon the primacy of logic within the *trivium*, it is no longer plausible to claim that the problem with deconstructive or rhetorical readings of textual undecidability is that they express an "anti-intellectualism" (Gutmann), or that they *simply* "aestheticize" political philosophy (Honneth, Norris). For the concept of the "aesthetic" itself already presupposes that same priority of logic required to link the sciences of language to the sciences of number, and thus in no way threatens classical epistemology. On the contrary, the aesthetic so understood is already contained within the very philosophical system that Habermas, Honneth, Norris, Benhabib and Gutmann have tried to defend.

If it is not the rhetorical *qua aesthetic* that deconstruction threatens to elevate illegitimately, therefore, it is all the more interesting that this is precisely the heading under which deconstruction is so regularly dismissed. In revealing exactly that aspect of writing that *cannot* be expressed with traditional aesthetic terminology, its "literariness" or its 'rhetoricity,' deconstruction is hung on the charge of "aestheticizing." It is in this sense that de Man's distinction between theory as universal knowledge (theory$_1$) on the one hand, and a literary theory of rhetorical reading which undoes it from within, on the other (theory$_2$) – points to a tension, or rather a split, within the category of the aesthetic as well. The split becomes evident once it is noticed that deconstruction both does and does not "aestheticize," because rhetoric properly understood both is and is not an aesthetic effect. Deconstruction *does* aestheticize philosophy, that is to say, insofar as the primacy of logic within the *trivium* is given, for on this view deconstruction is seen to elevate illegitimately the rhetorical function – traditionally understood as mere "ornament" – above the functions of grammar and logic. Yet it is equally possible to argue that deconstruction does *not* aestheticize philosophy, insofar as the inclusion of aesthetics within the philosophical system depends upon the subordination of rhetoric within the *trivium*, and this subordination, in turn, is unstable. The rhetorical aspect of writing, when revealed, thus reflects that "aesthetic" 'something' that remains "aesthetic" only insofar as its effects are properly subdued; once brought to light, rhetoric threatens to upset the system as a whole.

In responding to this analysis, Norris avers that the threat posed by rhetoric to the *trivium* – and by extension to the place of the aesthetic within a stable and universal system of knowledge – is falsely premised upon an erroneous and vastly overstated reading of the Kantian sublime. Specifically, Norris argues that postmodernists in general, Paul de Man and Hillis Miller in particular, can only 'blithely decouple' the terms of logic, grammar and rhetoric "to the point where 'textuality' (or 'unlimited semiosis') takes over from the old repressive regime of reality, truth and reference," if they assume that 'reality' is merely a "figment" – an imaginary, fictional or artistic construct – of a wholly arbitrary linguistic system (1993, 198, 227). According to Norris, however, this premise is falsely authorized by a wilful misreading of the Kantian text. Indeed, he asserts, antifoundationalist, postmodern philosophers,

> go far beyond anything warranted by the Kantian text when they relegate the beautiful (the realm of enlightened consensus-judgement) to a distinctly subordinate role, and promote the sublime – the figure of disjunction, radical alterity, "gulfs," "chasms" etc. – to an eminent position where it works to disarticulate the entire doctrine of the faculties. (Norris 1993, 253)

Sceptics – including "postmodernists, deconstructionists, [and] counter-enlightenment ideologues of various colours" – thus "[lean] over into a strain of downright contempt for the truth claims of enlightened ethical reason" (1993, 230, 203).

If this characterization is somewhat overdrawn, as I will show, Norris is not wrong to insist on the necessity of stabilizing the place of the sublime in Kant's third *Critique*. For the relationship between the beautiful and the sublime re-entrenches exactly that relationship between rhetoric and grammar expressed in the *trivium*. It does so precisely to contain the very danger that rhetoric first represented, namely, the epistemological challenge to logic that rhetoric, with its potential to disrupt a universal system of philosophy, is said to entail. For example, whether or not one wishes to make the kinds of radical claims that (for instance) Lyotard makes with regard to the sublime's disruptive potential within the *Critique of Judgment* (see Norris 1993, 15–18, passim, 219), it remains that the sublime clearly occupies a crucial and yet remarkably indeterminate place within Kant's treatment of reflective judgement. Specifically, the discussion of the sublime is bracketed as an "Appendix" within the first Division of the text (i.e., within the "Critique of Aesthetic Judgment"); within this Division, moreover, the Appendix is positioned between the "Analytic of the Beautiful" (which alone provides the principle of the "pure" aesthetic judgement), and the "Deduction of Pure Aesthetic Judgments." If the discussion of the sublime is thus not strictly included within the argument concerning pure judgements of taste, however, its positioning prior to the second division of the text (i.e., the "Critique of Teleological Judgment") indicates that it is not a teleological judgement either. Yet notwithstanding this equivocality, in fact, because of it, the analysis of the sublime plays an integral role within the argument of the third *Critique*.

In an important sense, 'bracketing' is exactly the treatment the sublime demands. For on one hand, it must be recalled, the effect of the sublime is not said to lead to a pure aesthetic judgement of taste, but rather to a judgement concerning the primacy of practical reason among the faculties of the noumenal subject. The sublime is thus not strictly a part of the critique of aesthetic judgement, since only the beautiful results in a 'purely' aesthetic, "*disinterested*," judgemental end. On the other hand, however, the sublime is an indispensable "supplement"[6] to the analytic of the beautiful, because it serves the crucial role of marking the limits of imaginative, aesthetic engagement. The judgement of the sublime, in effect, is the judgement that the imagination has failed, and this failure in turn allows us to know what beauty is *not*. Both as a condition of the meaning of the beautiful, therefore, and as a phenomenal effect, the judgement of sublimity can no more be divorced from the critique of pure aesthetic taste than it can be contained within it.

The unstable positioning of the sublime within the *Critique of Judgment* is evident not only in relation to the pure aesthetic judgement of taste, but in relation to the principle of teleological judgement as well. For, if we look to what the third *Critique* is intended to accomplish as a whole within the Kantian system rather than merely to the first division concerning the pure judgement of "beauty," it is clear that it is ultimately the judgement of the sublime, not the judgement of the beautiful, that furnishes the link between the first and the second division of the text (between aesthetic and teleological judgements) that is necessary to connect the "domains" of nature and freedom (i.e., the "domains" of theoretical and practical reason). This connection between nature and freedom is required in order to solve the problem that, while neither the principle of nature nor the principle of freedom can legislate in the other's domain, the purposes governed by the law of freedom *must* be realizable in nature. As Kant says, "the concept of freedom *is* to actualize in the world of sense the purpose enjoined by its laws" (Kant 1987, 15; emphasis his). And while the beautiful is said to "prefigure" this possibility, it does not fully establish it. Norris himself is careful to claim only this 'prefiguration' of freedom with regard to the systemic import of the judgement of the beautiful, even though he wants to argue that Kant's reflections on the beautiful bring to the fore "ideas of an enlightened community of judgment," in which "rational subjects are enabled to agree upon mutually-acceptable standards of taste" (1993, 246, 245). It is unfortunate, therefore, that Norris does not explore the consequence of "beauty's" limited capacity to relate pure to practical reason (what Norris calls "knowledge-constitutive interests" and those of "practical [ethico-political] reason"; 1993, 243); that is, the consequences of the problem that a judgement of pure taste merely 'prefigures' but does not actually confirm a link between beauty and morality. For this means that the "gulf" between the two cognitive domains (theoretical and practical reason), which Kant explicitly set out to bridge, still remains.

The discussion of the sublime intervenes at just this juncture; it is an important key to the Kantian system as a whole. Specifically, the experience of sublimity is said to provide the sensible moment of reason's supremacy over the imagination and the presentational powers in general (see esp. Kant 1987, 99, 129). The judgement of this sensation thus entails a transition between the two cognitive faculties by virtue of the fact that it is said to provide a *sensible* experience (i.e., it mobilizes the relation between imagination and the understanding that is in effect in theoretical modes of judgement) of 'our' *supersensible* (moral) vocation (which is to say, it also mobilizes the relation between the imagination and reason, which is in effect in practical modes of judgement). The feeling of sublimity can be contrasted with the feeling of the beautiful, therefore, which makes the link between nature (theory) and freedom (practice) only by analogy, and which requires a "predisposition" for the morally good in order to do so (Kant 1987, §§42 and 59).

The analysis of sublimity thus anticipates the critique of teleology and provides a crucial key to the way in which Kant's critique of teleological judgement articulates the critical system as a whole. Nonetheless, the experience of the sublime is no better described as a teleological judgement *per se* than as a pure, aesthetic judgement of taste. For Kant, the experience of the sublime is simply the experience of what the imagination *cannot* present. As that which is judged to be "contrapurposive" by the faculty of judgement, the sublime is that aesthetic (i.e., sensible, or available to intuition) 'something' that establishes in a negative way the limits of the merely cognitive, or theoretical, faculty of reason.

It is certainly arguable, therefore, that just as rhetoric cannot be contained within or finally subjugated to the ostensible primacy of logic or grammar within the *trivium*, and just as what de Man calls "literariness" can neither be circumvented by, nor assimilated to, a theory$_1$ of language, so the experience of the sublime can be neither included in nor excluded from the critique of aesthetic judgement. In other words, the judgement of the sublime is neither an aesthetic nor a teleological judgement *per se*. It is, rather, a structural requirement (a condition of possibility) for both of those particular, judgemental modes. What is required for judgement is an experience whereby the imagination fails, rather than succeeds, to determine (reflectively) any *thing*. In this sense, the sublime can be said to signal precisely that equivocality within the concept of the "aesthetic" that rhetoric, when understood as de Man suggests, provokes within the concept of "theory." If the sublime is thus said to undermine the supremacy of the beautiful within the aesthetic and thereby to threaten the disarticulation of the Kantian architectonic (Norris 1993, 253), however – just as rhetoric is said to undo the cognitive field promised by the traditional configuration of the *trivium* – this is not to say that the sublime can any more be elevated to a place of primacy within the Kantian text than can rhetoric within the *trivium*. This is where both proponents and critics of "postmodernism" (such as Lyotard *and* Norris and Habermas, respectively) go astray.

With regard to the ostensible primacy of the rhetorical brought about by deconstruction, for instance, both Norris and Habermas fail to notice that de Man's aim is not to *reverse* the relationship between rhetoric and logic, but rather to show that the priority of logic cannot be sustained. One need not jump from this to the conclusion that linguistic reference is therefore a fiction, or that theory *qua* knowledge is impossible, simply because its status is not absolute. In making this leap, critics such as Norris fail to remark that it is theory$_1$'s *resistance* to a literary theory$_2$ of the tropological dimensions of language – and not the impossibility *of* theory$_1$ altogether (the impossibility of systematic "truth") – that de Man set out to explore. In fact, as the closing paragraph of the essay clearly states, de Man does *not* conclude that knowledge or truth are themselves impossible, merely because their status has been destabilized. On the contrary, he claims, because theory$_2$ *is* the destabilization of knowledge, it cannot and will not ever come to take the place of theory$_1$. At the same time, if theory$_2$ is to be a *knowledge* of knowledge's impossible conditions, and if it is a *systematic* undertaking of this attempt, then theory$_2$ is, paradoxically, among theory$_1$'s own 'loftiest aims' (1982, 20). Moreover, "*nothing* can overcome the resistance to theory," because "theory *is* itself this resistance" (de Man 1982, 20; first emphasis mine). In other words, since it remains that any *theory* of reading rhetorically – any theory$_2$ which aims to understand *with* logic the rhetorical challenge *to* logic – will partake in that resistance as well (that is, will speak *as* that resistance), the possibility that rhetoric will take the place *of* philosophy is ruled out of court.[7]

A similar argument applies to the Kantian sublime. That is, insofar as the sublime – the experience of the "contrapurposivity of the presentational powers" – is required to mark the limits of the beautiful so that the latter may in turn be judged as "purposive" (for us), the sublime undoubtedly does destabilize the possibility of a *pure* universal judgement of taste. In this sense, moreover, to acknowledge the sublime is to disrupt from within that "community" postulated by Kant, that is, the community of those who share the universal "common sense" (*sensus communis*) that aesthetic "pleasure" ostensibly evokes. Nonetheless, one still cannot conclude that the sublime *qua* "ultimate heterogeneity" (Norris 1993, 21, citing Lyotard) *takes the place of* the beautiful as an alternate aesthetic – which is to say, as a variant phenomenal meaning. For the sublime could not be said to be a proper (anti-)aesthetic judgement without partaking in that very thing which necessarily keeps it at bay; namely, a system in which it is already preordained that the aesthetic *qua* meaningful phenomenon *requires* the bracketing of, or the resistance to, the unimaginable *qua* sublime. Theorists who attempt this kind of a straightforward reversal, consequently, are rightly charged with the accusation that they are involved in a kind of "performative contradiction" (Norris 1993, 70; Burbules 1996, 41).

This is why the crucial question is not whether the rhetorical or the sublime *displaces* the logical or the aesthetic, since this move is impossible in principle. The question, rather, is what is accomplished by the insistence on keeping these troublesome possibilities (i.e., rhetoric and the sublime) in their subordinate and customary place. What is accomplished, I submit, is the a priori legitimacy of the modernist assumption that a reason free of ideology is the *sine qua non* of any legitimate, ethico-political notion of the good. For what the critique of aesthetic judgement achieves – provided it can contain the tension between the beautiful and the sublime – is precisely that universal system of knowledge promised by the *trivium*. Unlike classical conceptions of knowledge, however, the Kantian system also includes moral reason within the concept of knowledge as a systematic science. That is to say, for Kant morally (as opposed to merely technically) "practical" reason differs from reason called "theoretical" when – and only when – it can be *logically* distinguished from the latter; when the logical principle that legislates over determinative moral judgements is the supersensible principle of freedom rather than the sensibly-conditioned principle of nature, which legislates over theoretical judgements of the understanding. For Kant, therefore, practical reason is based on a different logical principle than is theoretical reason, but it is by no means a different kind of judgement altogether (e.g., Kant 1987, 12).

Importantly, however, the priority of logic entailed by theoretical and practical judgement alike is maintained only insofar as the disruptive potential of rhetoric and (or as) the sublime – the internal deconstruction of the system – is contained. In other words, the positioning and containment of the sublime as the "interior–exterior" of the third *Critique*, and the primacy of the logical mode of judgement that is thereby confirmed, are necessary features of the Kantian analysis. For it is only by controlling a potentially destabilizing force within the concept of the aesthetic – for example, by bracketing the sublime between the "aesthetic" and the "teleological" divisions of the text – that Kant can posit the autonomy of the pure judgement of taste. This judgement must remain pure, for it alone can provide the logical principle of reflective judgement in general – the principle of "*subjective* purposiveness" (purposive for us) – which, in turn, is what is said to be mobilized when we make a reflective *teleological* judgement that nature is designed "as though" in accordance with a supersensible will "like" our own (i.e., as "*objectively* purposive"). The teleological, reflective judgement can thereby establish the link between the spheres of nature and freedom (theory and practice) that Kant had been aiming at all along, but it can do so only on the basis of a principle first discovered in the critique of pure, aesthetic judgements of taste.

Significantly, even if we ignore the role of the "Critique of Teleological Judgment" in the architectonic as a whole and focus exclusively on the first division of the *Critique*, the autonomy of pure judgements of taste can still be seen as a necessary condition for universal, ethico-political judgements that are rational in kind. For example, Hannah Arendt (1982), Ronald Beiner (in Arendt 1982) and Onara O'Neill (see Norris 1993, 182–256, 318 nt.2) have all capitalized on Kant's suggestion that the pure aesthetic judgement of taste, in particular, evokes a universal, communal sense (i.e., *sensus communis*). These theorists again suspend Kant's analysis of the sublime, in other words, in order to argue that aesthetic judgements evoke a common public sphere and thereby provide a principled basis for the universality on which legitimate ethico-political judgements depend. With or without accounting for the critique of teleological judgement, therefore, the priority of logic over rhetoric can be said to have been transferred from the classical *trivium* to the modern, Kantian architectonic with one decisive difference: what modern philosophy adds to the classical formulation is the *scientific* possibility that ethico-political values can be determined in rational, universal terms.[8]

This move, whereby ethics and not merely theoretical cognition is systematized as a logic, should be seen as nothing less than pivotal for critical theorists and philosophers of education, as I have claimed. For in linking the supersensible domain of practical (ethico-political) reason to the sensible domain of pure (theoretical) reason by way of the aesthetic, Kant substantiates a notion of reason as *critical* – which is to say, as normative, and not merely as axiomatic or deductive – in nature.[9] Indeed, as Dieter Misgeld has rightly noted, the Kantian "ideal of critical reason and the notion of critical inquiry," first formulated in "What is Enlightenment," "displays the interconnectedness of ideas of emancipation, reason, and education" (Misgeld 1985, 81). For this reason, he continues, the term *Enlightenment* can clearly be understood as referring to both

> the historical process of the generation of scientific rationality *and* [the] universal principles of practical judgment ... The Enlightenment's confidence in cognitive learning, in both the theoretical disciplines and practical-moral ones, is the normative basis of social and political emancipation. (Misgeld 1985, 81; emphasis added)

The significance of the Kantian connection between an ethical and a theoretical mode of judgement via the third *Critique* (and, more specifically, via the bracketing of the experience of the sublime), in short, is that it establishes the basis of modern emancipatory thought.

For critical and educational theorists alike, therefore, the primacy of logic first instantiated in the classical *trivium* and later re-entrenched in the Kantian architectonic serves to ground and thus to legitimize the modernist position within the modernism–postmodernism debate. This is why logic's priority over rhetoric is taken by Habermas to be both self-evident in and indispensable to the discourses of modernity. And it is why "postmodernism" is seen as dangerous across the fields of critical theory. In allegedly challenging the supremacy of logic over rhetoric, "postmodern" thinkers – if they are not ruled to have gone beyond the boundaries of reasonable discussion altogether – are deemed to spell the end of any kind of normative or critical political engagement.

This is the danger of rhetoric that is evoked implicitly in the "modernism–postmodernism" debate. As I have argued, however, the pre-emptive charge that deconstruction "aestheticizes" philosophy is premised on a profound misunderstanding of the nature of deconstruction, and therefore misconstrues its relevance for critical political thought. Yet, if this misconstrual has escaped the notice of deconstruction's critics, this is largely because it is not only the question of the primacy of logic that is begged. More importantly, the charge that deconstruction "aestheticizes" philosophy also begs the question of logic's autonomy or *purity* with regard to language's tropological effects. The accusation that the categories can simply be reversed, in short, already suggests they are distinct. It is therefore to this second (though logically prior) presupposition that I now want to turn.

Notes

1 For a classic formulation of the modernist project of education see R.S. Peters (1967). See also Hare and Portelli, eds. (1988). With regard to critical and progressive projects of education, McLaren (1989a), Shor (1992), Freire (1970 and 1973), Aronowitz and Giroux (1991), and Giroux (1991) may fairly be taken as representative.

2 Although the terms "postmodern" and "postmodernism" famously popularized by Jean-François Lyotard (1984) occur regularly in contemporary social, political and educational thought, my practice here is to specify the theorist under discussion whenever possible. To be sure, continental philosophers such as Michel Foucault, Jacques Lacan and Jacques Derrida can be characterized as intervening in, or even as radicalizing, a structuralist problematic and, to this extent, might fairly be grouped as "post-structuralists." For example, while Derrida claims that he has personally "never used this word," he does acknowledge that, "[deconstruction] is a questioning of a certain structuralism that presupposes a closed structural system, which brings about its effects without opening itself up" (in Rötzer, ed. 1995, 45; cf. Derrida 1988a, 2–3). In contrast to the structuralist–post-structuralist relationship, however, it is by no means clear how each of the theorists included in the common appellation post-*modernist* should actually be situated vis-à-vis the broader "discourses of modernity" (Habermas 1987). On the contrary, the issue of Derrida's own relation to Enlightenment discourses, and to the ethico-political ethos that informs them, is a central concern of the present study. It is fair to ask, therefore, to what end the characterization "postmodernism" is so regularly deployed. Judith Butler has persuasively suggested, for instance, that this "assemblage" variously called "postmodernism" and/or "poststructuralism" – the conflation of significantly different theoretical approaches, such as "French feminism, deconstruction, Lacanian psychoanalysis, Foucaultian analysis, Rorty's conversationalism and cultural studies" – may reflect an "effort to colonize and domesticate these theories under the sign of the same, to group them synthetically and masterfully under a single rubric"; it may, in fact, signal "a simple refusal to grant the specificity of these positions, an excuse not to read, and not to read closely" (Butler

1992, 5). In light of this tendency, as well as the plethora of views concerning what either of the terms "post" or "modern" properly signify, "postmodernism" is enclosed in quotation marks throughout.

3 While Norris does not include Derrida in this characterization, he does include deconstruction in general.

4 For the most complete text of this exchange in one volume (excluding Searle's rebuttal), see *Limited Inc* (Derrida 1988b). For a careful discussion of why Derrida's work should not be collapsed into that of the "Yale School" of deconstruction treated by Habermas, see S.P. Mohanty (1986). Habermas's chapter on Derrida ("Beyond a Temporalized Philosophy of Origins: Jacques Derrida's Critique of Phonocentrism"), to which his "Excursus on Levelling the Genre Distinction between Philosophy and Literature" is attached, does reference the Derridean corpus more directly, if only in the end to announce that "all denials notwithstanding, [Derrida] remains close to Jewish mysticism" (1987, 182, 184). Moreover, Habermas seems not ever to have wavered from this position. In the conclusion to a paper he presented in 2000, for example, Habermas writes, "This surprising end [to Derrida's book on Heidegger] seems to indicate that Derrida's own appropriation of Heidegger's later philosophy rests on a ground that is theological rather than Pre-Socratic, and Jewish rather than Greek" (Habermas 2007, 154). I address the charge of Derrida's 'Jewish mysticism' in Chapter Two.

5 Judith Butler has recently reiterated this claim in almost identical terms. She writes, "And so we find that one of the defining features of *Of Grammatology* is the coining of new phrases and terms, as if we cannot stay content with the ordinary language practices that we have. They are pervaded, or sedimented, with this [Western] framework, and only through a revolutionary practice of writing can that framework begin to become dislodged. *So this practice of coining new phrases unsettles those discourses pervaded by the metaphysics of presence*, the speculative attribution of a substance or a subject to every possible concept, but also enacts the claim that language is in a process of becoming" (2016, xvi; emphasis added).

6 On this term, see Derrida's analysis of Rousseau's treatment of the relationship between speech and writing. Derrida shows that for Rousseau writing has the character of a "supplement": i.e., it is a necessary and yet unassimilable 'something' without which a given system cannot function, but with which the system cannot be logically reconciled (1976, 141–64). As Robert Bernasconi explains, not only is "the supplement both addition and substitute," but "what is added to take the place of a lack or default is itself a lack" (1992, 145). Similarly, beauty lacks the capacity to demarcate the limits of the imagination. Insofar as the imagination is shown to be limited precisely to the extent that it fails to encompass the sublime, the sublime can be said to 'add' to (to supplement) our knowledge of the beautiful, but only negatively so, in terms of a lack.

7 See S.P. Mohanty, however, for an alternate reading of de Man's analysis. Mohanty argues that de Man bases his argument concerning 'literariness' on a "fallacy of simple referential determination," which allows de Man to hypostatize rhetoric and to define "all" language as accordingly "*primarily* figural" (Mohanty 1986, 164, 158 and 160; emphasis added). Mohanty therefore finds de Man guilty of the reversal (of logic and rhetoric) described above.

8 By "scientific" Kant specifies "systematic." Kant writes, "As *systematic unity is what first raises ordinary knowledge to the rank of science*, that is, makes a system out of a mere aggregate of knowledge, architectonic is the doctrine of the scientific in our knowledge, and therefore necessarily forms part of the doctrine of method" (Kant 1929, 653; my emphasis). His usage of the term thus corresponds with the notion of "theory$_1$" as a universal *system* of knowledge.

9 Omid Payrow Shabani makes a similar observation (2003, 17).

2 The Apocalyptic Tone of Philosophy

The assumption that deconstruction and other forms of post-structuralism represent a straightforwardly "anti-Enlightenment" discourse is based on the erroneous belief, whether explicit or not, that the aim of a deconstructive analysis is to *reverse* the classical subjugation of rhetoric – to elevate the "poetic function" *over* the "normal" function of language by engaging exclusively in a "critique of style" (Habermas 1987, 202–3, 189). Such a reversal is strictly speaking impossible, I have argued, since both knowledge (in the case of a theory of literature) and phenomenal meaning (in the case of the aesthetic) are always already constituted on the basis of the subjugation of the rhetorical and the sublime (respectively). Rhetoric and (or as) the sublime are not extrinsic to the logical and the aesthetic, in other words, but rather occur inevitably; they provoke the "resistance" that de Man calls "theory." If this provocative force was ever to take the place *of* knowledge or aesthetic meaning, it would cease being the force of theoretical 'undoing' that it is. Deconstruction therefore cannot be said to "aestheticize" philosophy – not even in the narrow sense of overvaluing the sublime – because such an undertaking is essentially incoherent.

Yet it is not only the primacy of logic over rhetoric, but the very autonomy of these categories to begin with, that is crucially at stake in the modernism–postmodernism debate. Moreover, once both the primacy and the autonomy of logic vis-à-vis rhetoric are challenged, the emancipatory conception of critique must be rethought as well. For the issue at stake in the modernism–postmodernism debate is not merely the premature rejection of an important body of work. It is that the dismissal of deconstruction – based on the assumption that "postmodernism" replaces enlightened judgement with imaginative 'free-play' – pre-empts the possibility that deconstructive readings may entail a substantive, ethico-political critique *of* reason, and so may point towards a form of critical theory that is genuinely responsive to developments in continental philosophy.[1]

It is exactly this possibility that the present study investigates. I argue that by virtue of its unwavering acknowledgement of, and its strict accounting for, the way in which rational modes of discourse *cannot* be divorced from the tropological or figural dimensions of language, Derrida's work embodies a version of reason as self-critique. In other words, in what I will provisionally characterize here a "radicalization" of critical reason, Derrida reveals the ethical and political interests served *by* Enlightenment formulations of reason as "pure." More specifically, he exposes the contingency of the particular cultural, historical, national, racial, sexual and class-related (*inter alia*) interests that are conveyed – carried, communicated and delivered – by the figures or tropes supporting a (universal) philosophical argument, but that are never acknowledged, as such, within it. The interests that those tropes convey are covered over by the insistence that the rhetorical elements of speech are "tamed" by the problem-solving, logical function of "illocutionary" speech acts (Habermas 1987, 209). Here, for example, Habermas is evoking a gender-loaded split between culture (as that which "tames") and nature (as that which is "tamed"). The metaphor is itself endemic to the discourse of modernity. For example, the project of Enlightenment has been characterized in terms of a narrative in which, "becoming human is a learning process whereby knowledge 'tames' natural instincts and replaces them with reason" (Usher and Edwards 1994, 125).[2]

In undertaking the "critical" work of exposing the interests embedded in tropes, Derrida's writings can be fairly characterized as "responsible"; moreover, it is a form of ethico-political "responsibility" that can be instructively contrasted with the understanding of those who dismiss "postmodernism." Specifically, the Enlightenment understanding of this term is one whereby,

> Grounding and subjectivity figure each other, thanks to the essential assumption of the subject's capacity to "master its discourse," to "author its acts or ideas" – in other words, its capacity to be an author by virtue of the articulation of ideas with acts, the coordination of cognition with performance in a subject. The signature (of an "author") marks the connection of knowing with doing, the mastery of the linguistic field (discourse) in which they can come together, and the ability to sign is what is called responsibility. (Keenan 1997, 135)

Paradoxically, I shall argue, the normative or ethico-political dimension of Derrida's work consists in its interrogation of this very ideal. However, this normative dimension cannot be recognized as such if we leave unchallenged the modernist presupposition regarding the autonomy of language's logical function. In other words, by contesting the belief that the responsible agent is the 'master of the linguistic field,' or that the rational mode of discourse is pure/free of language's tropological effects, it becomes possible to outline much more precisely what are and are not the normative consequences of "postmodernism" vis-à-vis the modernist discourse of critique.

It is necessary to demonstrate, therefore, why language in its logical mode (as philosophy or science, for example) cannot be understood as autonomous or separable from rhetoric. And for this purpose there is perhaps no better text than Derrida's "Of an Apocalyptic Tone Recently Adopted in Philosophy" (1983a), as Christopher Norris rightly observes (1992, 187). For, in contrast to de Man's essay, which was concerned with the specific field of literary theory, Derrida's essay concerns the field of philosophy at large.

It is interesting that Habermas himself does not discuss this text, given that it treats precisely that conflict within philosophy that seems to have defenders of modernity so vexed; namely, the conflict between an enlightened discourse of reasoned philosophical persuasion, on the one hand, and a mystical or rhetorical, and ultimately unintelligible discourse of apocalypse and catastrophe on the other. Habermas might otherwise have observed that Derrida had already composed a carefully stated response to the charge of turning philosophy into literature, only in this case as it was issued by Kant against those who adopt an "overlordly tone in philosophy" (Derrida 1983a, 6). Unlike those "postmodernists" characterized by Norris, however, Derrida's purpose is "not to take sides or come to a decision – I shall do no such thing – between metaphor and concept, literary mystagogy and true philosophy, but for a start to recognize the old solidarity of these antagonists or protagonists" (1983a, 16). In this sense, Derrida goes one better than both Kant and his 'mystagogical' interlocutors; he offers a reading which challenges the very ground of their dispute. In so doing, I will argue, he challenges the basis of Habermas's critique as well.

To be sure, the essay begins with an acknowledgement of where Kant and his interlocutors differ: on the distinction between the philosophical ideal of tonal neutrality, on the one hand, and the "overlordly" tone adopted by those "mystagogues" who deign to take on airs (who behave in an "overlordly" fashion) by presuming to announce the end of philosophy, on the other. As quickly becomes clear, however, it is not for Kant the mere fact that there is tonal marking at all that spells the "death of all philosophy" (1983a, 7). In the first place, Kant's own essay is marked by "polemical or satiric verve" and, in the second place, the "tonal loftiness" to which Kant objects is a "metaphoric loftiness," not a literal one. What Kant objects to, then, is not that there is some tone rather than none, but that those who would say *certain* things about philosophy – that it is in danger or that it is coming to an end – display a kind of inappropriate presumptuousness (1983a, 7). Those mystagogues who presume to announce the end of philosophy – and who do so, moreover, by mimicking the tone of the overlord (thereby "usurping signs of social membership" [1983a, 10]) – exalt themselves as among the privileged few who are "above their colleagues or fellows (*Zunftgenossen*)" (1983a, 10–11).[3]

This, then, is the "mystagogic," or "apocalyptic" tone that provides the focus for this essay. Yet, as readers familiar with Habermas's own indictment of deconstruction will observe, Kant's satirical polemic bears some remarkably contemporary resonances. For example, what is so unacceptable to Kant about those who pronounce the death of philosophy is that they presume to be in "immediate and intuitive relation with the mystery." As Derrida paraphrases,

> [T]hey wish to attract, seduce, lead toward the mystery and by the mystery. *Mystagogein* is indeed this: to lead, initiate into the mystery; that is the mystagogue's or the initiatory priest's function. This *agogic* function of the leader of men, of *duce*, of *Führer*, of *leader* places him above the crowd he manipulates through the intermediary of a small number of followers gathered into a sect with a crypted language, a band, a clique or a small party with its ritualized practices. The mystagogues claim to possess as if in private the privilege of a mysterious *secret* ... (1983a, 9).

In this context, it is interesting to return to the Habermasian charge that Derrida "remains close" to some form of (Jewish, Christian or Pagan) mysticism (1987, 182, 183, 184). As Habermas writes,

> Derrida's grammatologically circumscribed concept of an archewriting whose traces call forth all the more interpretations the more unfamiliar [i.e., "secret" – SG] they become, renews the mystical concept of a tradition as an ever *delayed* event of revelation. Religious authority only maintains its force as long as it conceals its true face and thereby incites the frenzy of deciphering interpreters. Earnestly pursued deconstruction is the paradoxical labour of continuing a tradition in which the saving energy is only renewed by expenditure: The labour of deconstruction lets the refuse heap of interpretations, which it wants to clear away in order to get at the buried foundations, mount ever higher. (1987, 183)

Similarly, as Derrida explains, for Kant the voice of reason "speaks to each without equivocation (*deutlich*)" and "gives access to scientific knowledge" whereas, in contrast,

> the voice of an oracle (*die Stimme eines Orakels) always lends itself to all kinds of interpretations* (*Auslegungen*). The priest-mystagogues are also interpreters; the element of their agogic power is the hermeneutic or hermetic seduction ... The overlordly tone dominates and is dominated by the oracular voice that covers over the voice of reason, rather parasitises it, causes it to derail or become delirious. (Derrida, 1983a, 12, 11; my emphasis)

As these citations begin to indicate, the "oracular" voice portrayed by Kant is a virtually precise match for the "labour of deconstruction" Habermas describes. Both deconstruction and the "mystagogical" voice in philosophy not only ostensibly presume an esoteric and privileged access to knowledge but both, putatively, eschew scholarly argumentation (Derrida 1983a, 9; Habermas 1987, 193, 194) for "cryptopoetics" (Derrida 1983a, 14), both replace "evidences and proofs with 'analogies' and 'versimilitudes'" (Kant, cited in Derrida 1983a, 15; Habermas 1987, 189),[4] and both thereby 'rob philosophical thinking of its seriousness and its substance' (Habermas 1987, 185, 210) threatening, in effect, to 'emasculate' it (Kant uses the word *Entmannung*; qtd. in Derrida 1983a, 16). As Norris remarks, "when Derrida offers his own free paraphrase of Kant's case against the mystagogues it could easily be taken for a passage from one of Habermas's chapters on Derrida in PDM [Habermas 1987]" (1992, 188).

Both the deconstructionists targeted by Habermas and the Romantics with whom Kant took issue, are seen as mystagogues because they displace the ideal of a universal truth based on reason, and available to all, with a privileged notion of truth based on revelation and available, consequently, only to a few. Importantly, however, the "apocalyptic" tone is not merely an errant and unfortunate possibility that philosophy has faced, according to Kant, ever since it lost its "primitive signification" as, "literally, a wisdom of life regulating itself according to knowledge or science (*wissenschaftlichen Lebensweisheit*)" (cited in Derrida 1983a, 8). Rather, Derrida shows, the tone described by Kant is actually intrinsic to the philosophical endeavour as such. Indeed, this is why Derrida himself speaks "of/in" (both "of" and "in") 'an apocalyptic tone in philosophy' (1983a, 3, 5).

Derrida's initial analysis of the term "apocalypse" already points towards the inscription of the apocalyptic within the philosophical. For, it must be recalled, Kant uses the term "apocalyptic" to designate a tone he calls "overlordly"; this is the tone that mimics loftiness, presuming as it does to speak of the "end" of philosophy. This tone which warns of imminent ends is, in Derrida's terminology, an "apocalyptic tone." Now, the "apocalyptic" first meant disclosure, not catastrophe, as it has come to connote; *apokalupsis* is an ancient translator's choice of a Greek equivalent to the Hebrew word "*gala*," or "unveiling." As a more recent translator of John's Apocalypse writes, "YHWH can be the agent of this disclosure." In this sense, "the Apocalypse is essentially a contemplation (*hazôn*) or an inspiration [*neboua*] at the sight, the uncovering or disclosure of YHWH and, here, of Yeshoua the Messiah." Thus, the term "apocalypse" occurs regularly in the Hebrew Bible to signify, specifically, the unveiling or disclosure of God the messiah (André Chouraqui, cited in Derrida 1983a, 4). The word "apocalyptic" itself, therefore, is an early signifier of philosophical contemplation (i.e., contemplation of the truth).

But here again, if Derrida proceeds to play on this word "gala," whereby "gala" becomes "galactic," "milky ways" and, later, "galatic ostentation" (1983a, 5, 30), he is not merely offering a "literary" and hence an "aesthetic" (or "rhetorical") reading of philosophy. On the contrary, in addressing the question of translation and the linguistic deviation it presupposes – the question, in effect, of the firmness (or, more precisely, the lack thereof) of the bond between the sign and the thing (the referent) – Derrida underlines the difficulty in finding the "true" meaning for (or of), in this case, the word for the revelation of God (*gala*). And this difficulty, in turn, leads to a 'revelation' (so to speak) of the *logical* difficulty inherent in distinguishing, finally and definitively, between the philosophical truth (of reason) and the mystical truth revealed by God.

In particular, it becomes clear that the opening of philosophy promised by the unequivocality of scientific discourse cannot be strictly opposed to those 'equivocal,' 'apocalyptic' discourses of the end. Consequently, it is impossible to maintain the Kantian dualism between scientific truth as the one voice (tonality) which speaks equally to all, and that mystical polyvocality which speaks variously, and only to the few. For Derrida's analysis shows that the equivocal and polyvocal voice of "mysticism" – of that "exalted vision" (Kant, qtd. in Derrida 1983a, 20) – is the condition of possibility for the philosophical 'opening.' A discourse of the "end," in effect, does not mark the "closure" of philosophy, but rather its inception (1983a, 20–21). Derrida writes,

> But if Kant denounces those who proclaim that philosophy has been at an end for two thousand years, he has himself, in marking a limit, indeed, the end of a certain type of metaphysics, freed another wave of eschatological discourses in philosophy. His progressivism, his belief in the future of a certain philosophy, of another metaphysics, is not contradictory to this proclamation of ends and of the end. (1983a, 20)

On the contrary, Derrida elaborates, Kant thereby inaugurated a "powerful program" and an "untransgressible contract among discourses of the end," of which "the themes of the end of history and the death of philosophy represent only the most comprehensive, massive, and gathered forms" (1983a, 20). Thus, even though there are obvious differences between the Hegelian, Marxist and Nietzschean eschatologies, Derrida claims, these can all be seen to "take the form of a going-one-better in eschatological eloquence, each newcomer, more lucid than the other, more vigilant, and more prodigal too" (1983a, 20).

On this basis, Derrida wonders "if eschatology is a tone, or even the voice itself." "Isn't the voice [of language] always that of the last man?" (1983a, 21).

> There is light, and there are lights, the lights of reason or the *logos*, that are not, for all that, some other thing. And it is in the name of an *Aufklärung* that Kant, for example, undertakes to demystify the overlordly tone. In the daylight of today we cannot not have become the heirs of these *Lumières*. We cannot and we must not – this is a law and a destiny – forgo the *Aufklärung*, in other words, what imposes itself

> as the enigmatic desire for vigilance, for the lucid vigil [*veille*], for elucidation, for critique and truth, but for a truth that at the same time keeps within itself some apocalyptic desire, this time as desire for clarity and revelation, in order to demystify or, if you prefer, to deconstruct apocalyptic discourse itself and with it everything that speculates on vision, the imminence of the end, theophany, parousia, the last judgment. (1983a, 22)

As I shall argue in the third part of this study, this desire for clarity and revelation – this desire which we "heirs" of the Enlightenment "cannot *not*" share – must be explained, not merely announced, if we are to appreciate fully the normative nature of Derrida's work. At this point, however, I want to emphasize that what Derrida is pointing towards here is the co-implication of philosophy *qua* scientific discourse and apocalyptic discourse *qua* (mysticism or) revelation.

It is especially important to underline this claim, for it seems to represent that aspect of Derrida's work that is most difficult to convey. For example, although he cites a section of the passage I have just quoted as well, it is not clear that Norris reaches the same conclusion I have just identified, or that he understands its deepest implications; namely, that there is something *in* or *of* the desire for Enlightenment – the desire *for* reason – that is in principle incapable of being 'lit' or illuminated *by* reason.

Certainly, it is clear that Norris has studied Derrida carefully, as his reading of Derrida's "Of an Apocalyptic Tone" indicates (Norris 1992). Yet Norris argues that, to the extent that Derrida's "essay itself is shot through with apocalyptic figures and devices, among them various mystical injunctions from Jewish and Christian source-texts," Derrida is asking us to see the limits of or, as it were, an exterior to the "ethos of Kantian civilized reason" (1992, 189–90). Moreover, it seems that Norris's belief that "deconstruction belongs with that 'philosophical discourse of modernity'" defended by Habermas is based on the assumption that Derrida's insistence on the intermingling of "'ordinary' language" and "various extra-ordinary styles, idioms, metaphorical usages, 'expert' registers and so forth," is intended to "*defamiliarize* our commonplace beliefs" (1992, 170, 190; my emphasis). It is impossible to know just what Norris has in mind, but these comments lead one to suspect that he views Derrida's unorthodox 'style' as an additional resource that is *philosophically* valid, just not fully appreciated by Habermas and that, consequently, deconstruction too can be seen to aim at *more* Enlightenment. Norris apparently misses or overlooks the point: deconstructive strategies of reading reveal (they illuminate or 'en-lighten') the way in which the progressive aim of more enlightenment is undercut by, although never replaced with, a regressive tendency that inheres in the Enlightenment project itself.

To substantiate this claim, it is necessary to look more directly at the tone of apocalyptic discourse. If we do so, Derrida argues, what we will notice is that this tone is, above all, that which is taken to announce the truth. The "overlordly" or "mystagogical" tone is always "the revelatory of some unveiling in process" (1983a, 24) – the tone, one might say, of "disclosure." Furthermore, the apocalyptic tone is (always) the tone that discloses something to the following (for example) effect:

> The end is soon, it is imminent … I see it, I know it, I tell you, now you know, come. We're all going to die, we're going to disappear … We're the only ones in the world. I'm the only one able to reveal to you the truth or the destination. I tell you it, I give it to you, come, let us be for a moment, we who don't know yet who we are, let us be for a moment, before the end the sole survivors, the only ones to stay awake, it'll be the stronger for it. We'll be a sect, we'll form a species, a sex or gender, a race (*Geschlecht*) all by ourselves, we'll give ourselves a name. (1983a, 24–5)

The regular characteristic of the apocalyptic tone is not simply that it announces (reveals) the truth which *is*; what is significant is not merely that "truth itself is the end, the destination, and [the fact] that truth unveils itself is [itself] the advent of the end" (1983a, 24). More importantly, the apocalyptic tone names *into* being, so to speak, the "we" (a "sect," a "sex," a "gender" or a "race"), the privileged few, who are witnesses *to* the truth as this end. This "we" survives the end because "we" is determined *by* the apocalyptic tone that announces the end; the "we" survives, that is to say, as an "as such" (as being 'this' or 'that,' here now, or, as we here name ourselves now *as* witnesses to this particular apocalypse). In this sense, the apocalyptic tone is the tone that says, "come." Come and be (present, here now, and as such) witness to the end that is coming. The apocalyptic tone, then, is the *gesture*, in speech, that conveys this "come."

Once understood in this way, it can be seen that an apocalyptic discourse (any apocalyptic discourse) – or more precisely, as Derrida says, the tone he has "translated into discourse" (1983a, 25) – "always cites or echoes in a certain way" the scene of John's Apocalypse:

> I know your works:
> you are renowned for living,
> but you are dead.
> …
> Stay awake! [*Esto vigilans* says the Latin translation][5]
> Strengthen what remains, so near dying.
> If you do not stay awake,
> I shall come like a thief:
> you will not know at what hour I shall come upon you.
> [3:1–3] (cited in Derrida 1983a, 25)

Yet if we try to determine who, exactly, says "come" in this originary scene – from whence issues this directive (to stay awake, to watch, to witness as an "us" the coming of the end) in the Johannine text itself – we see that this is exactly what cannot be decided. Thus, Derrida returns to the Apocalypse of John (to the text) in order to trace the original meaning (the truth) of the apocalyptic tone (the tone which comes to say the truth) discussed by Kant.

What Derrida finds is that John receives the revelatory dispatch from an unnamed and indeterminable, "narratorial" voice.[6] For even before the scene in which John is seen to be writing what Jesus dictates (i.e., the injunction to "Stay awake"), Derrida says, "there was a preamble without narrative, or in any case narratorial voice, a kind of title or name tag come from one knows not where ..." (1983a, 26). This preamble, which is "come from one knows not where," announces the announcement dictated by "Yéshoua" and written by John. Derrida cites,

> Disclosure of Yéshoua the messiah (*Apokalupsis Jesou Khristou*)
> Elohim gives of him
> to show his servants
> what will arrive quickly.
> He signifies it by sending it through his messenger
> (*esemanen aposteilas dia tou angelou autou,*
> *significavit, mitten per angelum suum*)
> to his servant Yohanân [1:1–2] (1983a, 26).

Based on this reading, Derrida concludes that the biblical discourse of the apocalypse reflects a certain "unmasterable polytonality" (1983a, 23); it cannot be determined, finally, who is saying/writing what, or consequently, where this apocalyptic tone, this gesture "come," comes *from*. It thus emerges that the 'truth' of the apocalypse can be traced to an originary division ("*pli*" or fold, as well as "envelope, letter, habit or message" [1983a, 28]) within the narrative message of the apocalyptic vision. A non-truth, then, at the source of truth. Or, as Derrida says, an apocalypse without vision, without apocalypse.

> One does not know (for it is no longer of the order of knowing), to whom the apocalyptic dispatch [*envoi*] returns; it leaps [*saute*] from one place of emission to the other (and a place is always determined *starting from* the presumed emission); it goes from one destination, one name, and one tone to the other; it always refers to [*renvoie à*] the name and to the tone of the other that is there but as having been there and before yet coming, no longer being or not yet there in the present of the *récit*. (1983a, 27)

Two consequences can be drawn from this discussion. The first is that if the "come" that this apocalyptic discourse signals is the gesture that names *into* being the presence of the truth (the truth as 'presence' or revelation of the "we," the being, that is its witness), then this would be a structural gesture of discourse as such, and not merely of apocalyptic discourse – which would only be "an example, an *exemplary* revelation of this transcendental structure" (1983a, 27). For the naming into being (the claim "it is") is what discourse does. The second consequence is that if the "come" itself is unrevealable in principle – because the "come" does not come from an identifiable subject, a narrator, a source that can be unveiled or disclosed or revealed as such (as *an* 'as such') – then as Derrida asserts, "there is no certainty that man is the exchange of these telephone lines or the terminal of this endless computer" (1983a, 27), because there is no sovereign voice which masters it.

> [A]s soon as one no longer knows who speaks or who writes, the text becomes apocalyptic. And if the dispatches [envois] always refer to other dispatches without decidable destination, the destination always remaining to come, then isn't this completely angelic structure, that of the Johannine apocalypse, isn't it also the structure of every scene of writing in general? (1983a, 27)

The structure, that is to say, and not the content.[7] For the discursive gesture "come" is the opening *of* discourse (of philosophy). It brings into being the witness, presently (here now), as the survivor of the end who can speak of it; the one(s), namely, who can tell us what *it is*. (It is always this apocalypse, here now – the end of man, of philosophy, of religion or of metaphysics, for example). The saying of "what *is*" (any saying of "what is") is thus conditioned by the "come." "Come" as apocalyptic gesture, therefore, can neither be attributed to an identifiable subject, nor determined within the "grammatical, linguistic, or semantic categories" (1983a, 34) it sets in motion.

This marks one of the limits to the demystification that "we *Aufklärer* of modern times" (1983a, 29) might attempt; the ultimate irrecuperability in discourse of the gesture "come" that opens discourse means that the task of 'denouncing false apocalypses' is interminable. The apocalypse is always already with us, in our speech. As Derrida says, "All language on apocalypse is also apocalyptic, and cannot be excluded from its object" (1983a, 30). On one hand, to be sure, apocalyptic language embodies a potentially radical, progressive "challenge to the established receivability [*recevabilité*] of messages and to the policing of destination" (1983a, 30), insofar as it is irreducible to the strictures of metaphysical presence. On the other hand, however, a second limit emerges here as well. For insofar as it is itself apocalyptic, an analysis of the apocalyptic tone will be received according to conventional codes of discourse. Here we find Derrida's most pointed rebuttal to Habermas:

> We could even say that every discord or every tonal disorder, everything that detones and becomes inadmissible [*irrecevable*] in general collocution, everything that is no longer identifiable starting from established codes, from both sides of a front, will necessarily pass for mystagogic, obscurantist, and apocalyptic. It will be made to pass for such. (1983a, 30)

The second limit of any attempt to demystify by undertaking a deconstruction, in other words, is that it will be received as the very 'mystagogy' it attempts to reveal. This is precisely why, I suggest, "postmodernism" in general and deconstruction as it is characterized by Habermas in particular are so often considered to present irrational, irresponsible or nihilistic approaches to politics.

In contrast to this, I contend that ethico-political "responsibility" of deconstruction consists in its unwavering insistence on recognizing and accounting for the rhetorical, the tropological or (in this case) the apocalyptic dimensions of discourse. At the same time, however, it remains that the demystifying endeavour undertaken by Derrida cannot be identified (*pace* Norris) with "a simple progressive demystification in the style of the Enlightenment" (Derrida 1983a, 30). Recall, first, that the apocalyptic tone is the tone which announces the imminence of the end. If "translated into discourse," moreover, it can be seen that the apocalyptic tone says "come," and in this way, names into being the "we" that witnesses the end. So understood, "come" is a *gesture* of speaking, not a content of speech; therefore, it cannot be recovered in discursive form. To this extent, it follows, there is a certain apocalyptic dimension (an apocalypse *without* end, without apocalypse) that is intrinsic to all discourse, including the philosophical. Moreover, this tone which says "come" (this apocalyptic tone *of* philosophy) is the very condition whereby philosophical discourse can offer an end to discourses deemed apocalyptic or mystagogical. And, if there is no possible self-presentation of the apocalyptic, discursive gesture ("come") itself, the analysis of mystagogy will be interminable rather than final.

This is one of the implications of Derrida's distinction between the "closure" and the "end" (1983a, 21). As I have shown, Kant's own discourse offers another beginning or opening to philosophy – not simply by refuting mystagogical pronouncements of philosophy's end but, on the contrary, by marking the 'end' of a certain mystagogical metaphysics and the beginning of an era of "enlightenment." The discourse of ends or of apocalypses, therefore, even the most careful, precise or rigorous of deconstructive discourses, do not close the debate, for they cannot exhaust the "overdeterminations and the indeterminations of apocalyptic strategems" (1983a, 29), among which deconstruction itself must be included.

Unlike the project of Enlightenment *simple*, then, deconstruction does not aim at a horizon of ultimate closure or an ideal of perfect translatability (*qua* scientific univocity). In fact, deconstruction does not "aim" at all, since it is always already the destination of philosophy (its ends, or its 'good' of a reason that is 'pure') that it questions. It does so by revealing the way in which the "apocalyptic" tone *is* the tone of philosophy – or, rather, is that which crosses *through* philosophy *as* its perpetual opening – not its determinate exterior.

What this analysis demonstrates, therefore – what it illuminates or enlightens – is that the logical function of language cannot be said to bear a strictly autonomous status with regard to its rhetorical or tropological dimensions. Significantly, this also means that deconstruction no more belongs *to* "that same 'philosophical discourse of modernity' that Habermas sets out to defend" (Norris 1992, 170), than it is a purely *anti*-Enlightenment discourse, as Habermas and others contend. Deconstruction does not impose the rhetorical in or on philosophy, but rather reveals (en-lightens) the rhetorical (the apocalyptic) as the necessary, unacknowledged (non)original condition *of* the modern philosophical enterprise *qua* Enlightenment. Thus, just as the rhetorical undoes, without replacing, the primacy of logic within the *trivium*, and just as the sublime destabilizes the category of the aesthetic within the Kantian system or architectonic, so the apocalyptic tone emerges as the very condition of that "knowledge or science" by virtue of which life "regulates itself" in the original signification of the term "philosophy" (Kant, in Derrida 1983a, 8; cited above).

Only when this is understood is it possible to outline what are and are not the normative consequences of so-called "postmodernism" for political–theoretical critique. In particular: if deconstructive strategies of reading do not *replace* logic with rhetoric, the aesthetic with the sublime, or philosophy with mysticism, and if they do not do so because they cannot – both because a purely rhetorical, sublime or mystical discourse is strictly unintelligible, and because (even before this) the categories are not strictly autonomous to begin with – then it cannot be the case that challenges to the philosophical premises of modernity will endanger the very possibility of progressive (or democratic) social and political reform. This cannot be the case because, if logic and rhetoric (or, for example, $theory_1$ and $theory_2$) are thoroughly co-implicated from the start, then any democratic project that was founded upon the strict configuration of the classical *trivium* was bound to be misguided, up to a point. That point is precisely the moment at which the unacknowledged interests that are buried within particular philosophical arguments (by virtue, for example, of their rhetoric) are actually the ones at stake.

While he is primarily concerned with the controversy over deconstruction within the field of literary theory, for example, de Man is by no means unaware of these broader, ethico-political, implications. On the contrary, he argues that "what we call ideology is precisely the confusion of linguistic with natural reality, of reference with phenomenalism" (1982, 11).

According to de Man, this distinction between reference and phenomenalism can be exemplified as follows:

> no one in his right mind will try to grow grapes by the luminosity of the word "day," but it is very difficult not to conceive the pattern of one's past and future existence as in accordance with temporal and spatial schemes that belong to fictional narratives and not to the world. (1982, 11)

From this point of view, it follows that

> the linguistics of literariness is a powerful and indispensable tool in the unmasking of ideological aberrations, as well as a determining factor in accounting for their occurrence. Those who reproach literary theory for being oblivious to social and historical (that is to say ideological) reality are merely stating their fear at having their own ideological mystifications exposed by the tool they are trying to discredit. They are, in short, very poor readers of Marx's *German Ideology*.[8] (1982, 11)

de Man's suggestion makes clear that the *critical* significance of deconstruction should not be understood in terms of an either/or choice: either we embrace what Jean-François Lyotard calls a "metadiscourse" or a "grand narrative" of modernity on the one hand (Lyotard 1984), or we postulate its reversal into negativity, and concomitantly, the absolute absence of any critical resources or grounds whatsoever with which to combat injustice (Norris 1993, 287), on the other.

Where the significance of deconstruction for a critical political theory *is* to be found, I propose, is rather in its provocation to rethink the very foundations of our beliefs about ethics and politics, and, more specifically still, in its provocation to reconsider the consequences of the fact that emancipatory political thought necessarily reflects those original, Enlightenment ideals. Specifically, the Kantian inauguration of a notion of reason as critical – as ethico-political, or as normative in nature – is the bedrock on which the project of Enlightenment as emancipation rests, and this ideal, in turn, is deeply indebted to a classical conception of logic's primacy within the sciences of language and the sciences of the natural world. Thus, the decentring of logic vis-à-vis rhetoric impels a fundamental reconfiguration of both the classical and the modern ideal. In the next two chapters, we will see precisely how Kant's own conception of critical reason works, despite itself, to cover over contingently-determined, historically-specific and politically-loaded interests and claims. Such an analysis cannot but have profoundly important implications for a political or educational theory that understands itself as a form of critique.

Notes

1 Rudi Visker (1995) has made a similar argument on behalf of Michel Foucault – arguing, in effect, that genealogy is a critique of that very "reason" which, traditionally, has authorized the critical enterprise.
2 Derrida analyzes the culture–nature dualism effectively in *Of Grammatology* (1976).
3 All italics, translations and textual insertions within quotations in what follows are Derrida's or his translator's, unless otherwise noted.
4 The citation to which I refer here is as follows: "Derrida does not proceed analytically, in the sense of identifying hidden presuppositions or implications," but instead, "proceeds by a critique of style, in that he finds something like indirect communications, by which the text itself denies its manifest content, in the rhetorical surplus of meaning inherent in the literary strata of texts that present themselves as nonliterary" (1987, 189).
5 In Latin, then, the phrase would seem to indicate the imperative to "remain vigilant," or to keep watch: do not cease bearing witness to.
6 Derrida specifies the "'narrative voice' in order to distinguish it from the narratorial voice, that of an identifiable subject, of the narrator or determinable sender in a narrative, a *récit*" (1983a, 25). Derrida's suggestion seems to be that the "narrative voice" refers to the whole narrative – to all its voices as an overall narrative effect – *within* which the "narratorial" voice is "that of an identifiable subject." The term "narratorial" is borrowed from Maurice Blanchot; see Pierre Joris's preface to *The Unavowable Community* (in Blanchot 1988, xii).
7 This distinction appears to parallel the Levinasian distinction between the "saying" and the "said" in terms of the difference between that whose source (or destination) is indeterminable, and that whose source is determined as ontologically present. Interdeterminable "saying" corresponds to ethics, for Levinas, which takes priority over the ontological, or the "said."
8 Charles Taylor's justification of the spatial metaphor in *Sources of the Self* exemplifies the ideological confusion between fictional narratives and the world (reference and phenomenon) that de Man has in mind. For Taylor, spatial orientation is an "analogue" (or, a trope) that *figures for* moral orientation. To understand ourselves in terms of this trope is thus to take our fictional or narrative "frameworks" *as* "ontologically basic"; that is, it is precisely to take our fictions as a fundamental feature of what "is," or of what is 'phenomenally *there*,' in the world. These phenomenal/fictional frameworks are thus the phenomenal/figurative "space" of the questions in which we literally and/or figuratively "stand" as human agents (see Taylor 1989, 29).

3 Redefining the "Postmodern"

> [N]either modernity nor so-called postmodernity can be identified and defined as clearly circumscribed historical entities, of which the latter would always come "after" the former. Rather, we have to say that the postmodern is always implied in the modern because of the fact that modernity, modern temporality, comprises in itself an impulsion to exceed itself into a state other than itself. And not only to exceed itself in that way, but to resolve itself into a sort of ultimate stability, such for example as is aimed at by the utopian project, but also by the straightforward political project implied in the grand narratives of emancipation. Modernity is constitutionally and ceaselessly pregnant with its postmodernity.
>
> (Lyotard 1991, 25)

Kant's incorporation of ethics into a logical system (or "science") of knowledge was decisive for the emancipatory conception of education, I have suggested, because it was through this move that reason took on its quintessentially modern sense of "critique": its sense as normative or, in Kant's terminology, as "practical" (as having a moral as well as a theoretical interest). Kant's explication of practical reason is centred on the tenet that legitimate moral judgements are universal determinations derived from an a priori, logical principle of freedom; these are explicitly contrasted with judgements that stem from contingent local beliefs based on tradition or authority. Importantly, then, Kantian practical reason entails that the legitimate moral judgement is rational in kind, that the capacity for rationality is the true, the essential and the highest feature of the human subject (i.e., "universal man") and, concomitantly, that an ideal realization of justice (a "kingdom of ends") entails universal moral agreement. From this it follows that the enhancement or 'education' of the capacity for independent, rational thought – the inculcation of the capacity to 'universalize' on one's own, as it were – is the normative thrust of the Enlightenment. The ability to undertake such moral "work" is precisely what an educational practice aimed at democracy was (and largely still is) intended to instil.

In Kant's well-known formulation, "enlightenment" already entailed this political dimension: "enlightenment" is, "man's release [or emancipation] from his self-incurred tutelage," wherein the term "tutelage," in turn, is defined as that "inability to make use of [one's own] understanding [or 'intelligence'] without direction from another" (Kant 1959, 85).[1] Consequently, as Dieter Misgeld remarks, "the Enlightenment concern with education must follow from its interest in emancipation" (Misgeld 1985, 81). Wilfred Carr has observed this correlation between the political good of social emancipation and the educative project of Enlightenment as well. He writes,

> Historically, the cultivation of this capacity for rational independent thought has been the aim of liberal education – a form of education that was first developed by the Greeks to meet the needs of the "free man" capable of making rational judgements as a member of an educated public. In eighteenth and nineteenth-century Britain, access to a liberal education was the exclusive preserve of an aristocratic élite. But as democracy replaced aristocracy, so the need to extend to all the kind of intellectual development that a liberal education is designed to promote has increasingly been seen as a political obligation of the democratic state. (1995, 75)

As Misgeld and Carr clarify, the idea of Enlightenment as emancipation – and, more specifically, as the political good of progressive social reform for all (rather than merely for a select elite) – was always intrinsically educative in nature. Paul Smeyers summarizes the point:

> For the Enlightenment, education was the road to becoming human; i.e., rational. Rationality, as the proper end of what being human is, does not necessitate means-end reasoning. In becoming free from one's own inclinations and passions, one realises one's true nature: one puts oneself under the guidance of reason, which is never alienating, given that to be rational is the same for everyone. (1995a, 111)

Taken together, these observations reflect a general recognition: in relating the question of knowledge to the possibility of a universal ethical and political 'good' in terms of a normative notion of "practical reason," Kant effectively mobilized the classical primacy of logic over rhetoric for the Enlightenment project in its paradigmatically *political* sense. It was at the onset of modernity, specifically, that education first came to be understood in a way that is still reflected in formulations of "critical" pedagogy today, namely,

> as the vehicle by which modernity's "grand narratives," the Enlightenment ideals of critical reason, individual freedom, progress and benevolent change, are substantiated and realized. The very rationale of the educative process and the role of the educator is founded on

> modernity's self-motivated, self-directing, rational subject, capable of exercising individual agency. (Usher and Edwards 1994, 2)

Significantly, this view of the political project of Enlightenment hinges directly on the relationship between logic and rhetoric that was analyzed above.

Since the work of Jacques Derrida, Michel Foucault and Jacques Lacan reflects the kind of "incredulity" towards this particular narrative that is said to characterize the "postmodern condition" in general (Lyotard 1984, xxiv), critical educational theorists are right to take it quite seriously. For these philosophers have undertaken a series of complex, careful and often pointed critiques of the transcendental, rational subject whose critical agency the modern epic of emancipation depicts. For example, by providing an analysis of an inescapable structure of undecidability that is logically prior to determinate, theoretical (or practical) judgements (Derrida), of the imbrication of knowledge with power (Foucault), or of the unavoidable ways in which unconscious desire both conditions and undermines subjective mastery over discourse (Lacan), Derrida, Foucault and Lacan have problematized the universality promised by a unified theory of knowledge. And, in suggesting that the 'good' of universality itself can give rise to ideological distortions, they therefore bring important ethical considerations to bear on a modernist understanding of the relationship between emancipation and reason.

It is important to underscore, however, that if we do not clarify Lyotard's very broad definition of "postmodernity," we risk overlooking that few continental philosophers dismiss the modern narrative of emancipation outright. On the contrary, as I will demonstrate with reference to the modern ideal of "critical reason," the philosophical "decentring" of the transcendental subject does *not* ensue from an outright dismissal of the "metanarrative" of modernity; the subject is decentred, rather, as a logical consequence of the attempt *to account for* (or, to render reason to) the very legitimacy on which modern discourses of philosophy, education and politics are based. Indeed, I have characterized deconstruction as a mode of reading that illuminates the groundlessness *of* these discourses' very grounds. What I want to clarify now, however, is that this groundlessness is revealed as a direct outcome of the modern, philosophical imperative *to* provide grounds, or *to* legitimate, in the first place. Since modernity is thus already "constitutionally and ceaselessly pregnant with its postmodernity," as Lyotard puts it in the epigraph to this chapter, the charge that "postmodernists" negate the modern ethos of reason or displace it with unreason cannot be sustained.

Unfortunately, Lyotard's own characterization of the "condition of postmodernity" in terms of "incredulity" tends to elide this very point. For the word "incredulity" signals "an inability to believe" (Burbules 1996, 40), what one might call an attitudinal problem; it thus reduces substantially diverse philosophical interrogations to a generalized mood of distrust or scepticism. On such a view, to be sure, the analyses just briefly outlined can be seen as a variety of rhetorical expressions of an overriding, cultural ethos endemic to late-capitalist, Western society. Patti Lather, for example, writes that "poststructuralism is not so much about a seismic cultural shift as it is about the Academy catching up with one. Poststructuralism is part of the *Zeitgeist*, the culture and ethics of its time," and this time is one characterized by a "crisis of confidence in Western conceptual systems" (1991, 89, 159). Similarly, Wilfred Carr characterizes the "postmodern" condition as the "gradual erosion of the self-confidence and self-understanding of those who have embraced Enlightenment ideals" (1995, 79). In contrast to these claims, I argue that the analyses under discussion are rigorous interventions *into* the philosophical discourse of modernity, not merely cultural expressions that bemoan its diminishment, and that this is why they should be taken seriously by critical theorists of education.

Specifically, this work bears on the fact that the ethico-political narrative of emancipation through Enlightenment was originally authorized by the tacit endorsement of logic's priority within the classical "sciences of language" (*trivium*). As I showed, this priority was not discarded in the discourses of modernity; on the contrary, logic remained the linchpin of the Kantian architectonic as a whole. More precisely, I proposed that two premises are necessary for Kant's original inclusion of "practical reason" within the metaphysical system of knowledge and, hence, for the notion of "criticality" that he inaugurated.[2] In analytical order these premises are, a) the *autonomy* of the categories of logic and rhetoric – that is, the premise that logic can be definitively distinguished from rhetoric – and b) the *primacy* of language's logical function (and, or as, grammar) over and above its rhetorical function (and, or as, the sublime or the apocalyptic, for example) – that is, the premise that logic can decide or determine (in effect, can "master") rhetorical ambiguity. These two assumptions are implicit in the claim that a given (ethical *or* epistemological) judgement is scientific (neutral) rather than dogmatic (politically-interested), philosophical rather than literary or aesthetic, and universal rather than contingent. Together, they are necessary for the legitimation of the Enlightenment ideal of critical reason and are thus foundational to the emancipatory "metanarrative" of modernity.

If deconstructive strategies of reading really do undermine the priority of logic entrenched in the Kantian architectonic by showing that such a system is constitutively incapable of mastering the sublime, the apocalyptic or the mystagogical dimensions of theoretical discourse, therefore, then this does far more than simply cast a "mood" of doubt on the educational ideal while leaving its legitimacy intact. Indeed, we have seen that just as rhetoric cannot be finally subjugated to logic within the *trivium* because "literariness" (theory$_2$) can neither be assimilated to nor circumvented by a "science" (theory$_1$) of language, and just as the sublime can neither be included in nor excluded by the critique of aesthetic judgement, so the apocalyptic cannot either be absorbed by *or* fully expelled from the philosophical delimitation of mystagogy. But to appreciate fully the implications of these analyses is to realize that what is at stake in the deconstructive interrogation of philosophy is the very legitimacy *of* the procedures for (or standards of) legitimacy – procedures or standards among which Kantian practical reason is only one instance. Or, to put this differently, what is at issue in the "modernism–postmodernism" debate is the actual normative sense, the ethico-political *promise*, of "enlightenment" as a vehicle of social and political betterment.

In this chapter, therefore, my purpose is to show that just as the problem at hand is not best understood as a "crisis of faith," so the question for educational theorists is not how to uphold a traditional emancipatory educational agenda in the face of postmodern "doubt" (Burbules 1996). Such an effort to come to terms with the "postmodernist" challenge entails the very assumptions that "postmodernism" puts into question. That is to say, to leave the ideal itself intact while reflecting only upon our "postmodern" reluctance to embrace it is tacitly to accept the autonomy and primacy of logic that grants that ideal its original legitimacy. For this reason, Burbules can be grouped with unabashed defenders of the discourses of modernity; he does not provide an alternative to those who *accept* the autonomy and primacy of logic, and who thus dismiss "postmodernism" on the grounds that it "aestheticizes" philosophy.

In contrast to both sorts of views, the normative point I shall elaborate throughout the course of this book is this: the conception of "critical" reason that numerous educational theorists wish to retain or reformulate – the capacity to decide between justice and injustice, legitimacy and illegitimacy, or truth and ideology – can only ever figure as an educational 'good' by virtue of an *illegitimate* (an ideological) occlusion of its impossible conditions of possibility. But this is an occlusion we cannot do without; it is the question that *must* be begged for the sake of the very emancipation that contemporary critical theorists wish to uphold. In other words, paradoxically, the erasure of the uncontainable excess is required in order for the Kantian notion of critical reason to assume its undeniable, political force. And what this means, as I shall go on to argue in Chapter Four, is that a certain "violence" is always already embedded in the very notion of critical reason that theorists hope to mobilize against ideology, injustice and harm.

In order to substantiate this claim, it is necessary to begin by refining a number of key terms that, thus far, have been used only in their broadest senses. They are "critique," "legitimation" and, relatedly, "critical." Most importantly, the terms "critique" and "legitimation" denote two analytically distinct levels of discourse – what one might call a "meta" and a "micro" level of argumentation – that, although linked, must be carefully delineated if the emancipatory sense of "reason" is to be properly understood. If the term "critical," in contrast, cannot be analyzed in this way, this is exactly what is so interesting about it; as I will show, "critical reason" necessarily denotes both of these levels of at once.

With these distinctions in view, I then turn to Lyotard's analysis of the meaning of "postmodernity." What I will show is that, although he elaborates the "postmodern condition" in a much more nuanced way than Burbules and others suggest, Lyotard ultimately misconstrues the analytical difference between what I am calling the "meta" and the "micro" sense of "critique." Specifically, Lyotard sees these moments as symmetrical, and is led to characterize two equivalent but distinct metanarratives of legitimation that are said to be undergoing separate processes of delegitimation: a scientific one and an emancipatory one. When the difference between the "meta" and the "micro" levels of "critique" is taken in the asymmetrical sense that I propose, on the other hand, it becomes clear that only one broad "metanarrative of legitimation" is actually at stake in Lyotard's account, and it is neither exclusively scientific nor strictly emancipatory. In fact, it partakes of both of these discourses at once. And what this means, I will submit, is that the internal resistance *to* theory_1 that takes the form of the rhetorical, the sublime or the apocalyptic, for example – the theory_2 or "delegitimation" that is at issue *in* the European Enlightenment metanarrative of legitimation – must be formulated anew.

Before this point can be developed, however, it is necessary to begin by refining the definition of "critique." As is well known, this term was first employed by Kant to designate the transcendental investigation into the legitimate scope (or reach) of human knowledge. Not only is its task, as Lewis White Beck explains, to "rescue those principles that constitute metaphysics 'as science'" (in Kant 1993a, ix), but what Kant entitles the "Critique of Pure Reason" (1929, 58) *itself* takes the form of a "special science." As Kant writes,

> [R]eason is the faculty which supplies the principles of *a priori* knowledge. Pure reason is, therefore, that which contains the principles whereby we know anything absolutely *a priori* … [W]e can regard a science of the mere examination of pure reason, of its sources and limits, as the *propaedeutic* to the system of pure reason. As such, it should be called a critique, not a doctrine, of pure reason. Its utility, in speculation, ought properly to be only negative, not to extend, but only to clarify our reason, and keep it free from errors – which is already a very great gain. I entitle *transcendental* all knowledge which is occupied not so much with objects as with the mode of our knowledge of objects in so far as this mode of knowledge is to be possible *a priori*. (1929, 58–9; emphases his)

As the transcendental "examination of pure reason, of its sources and limits," "critique" thus denotes the knowledge (or science) *of* knowledge.

It is specifically aimed at determining what Kant calls "all the interests of my reason" as these are 'combined' in three decisive questions: "What can I know?"; "What ought I to do?" and "What may I hope?" (1929, 635).

In attempting to answer these questions in his three *Critiques*, Kant thus understood his task in terms of a preparation (propaedeutic) *for* a complete system or "doctrine" of knowledge, but not *as* that doctrine itself. Significantly, however, the difference is by no means clear. For the purpose of the critique of pure reason[3] is specifically "to lay down the complete architectonic plan" for the "idea of a science," or "transcendental philosophy" (1929, 60), and an architectonic plan, in turn, is that "systematic unity" that "first raises ordinary knowledge to the rank of science, that is, makes a system out of a mere aggregate of knowledge" (1929, 653). As such, "architectonic" is, according to Kant, none other than "the *doctrine* of the scientific *in* our knowledge" (1929, 653; emphasis added).

The difference between a propaedeutic (that critique which provides a unified, "scientific" explication of the a priori conditions of all knowledge), and a *doctrine* (a complete, unified system or "science" of knowledge) thus begins immediately to blur. This is because, in Kant's view, a "philosophy of pure reason" – alternatively called "speculation" or "metaphysics" – appears to entail both meanings at once. On one hand, he says, the

> title "metaphysics" may … be given to the whole of pure philosophy, *inclusive of criticism*, and so as comprehending the investigation of all that can ever be known *a priori* as well as the exposition of that which constitutes a system of the pure philosophical modes of knowledge of this type. (1929, 659)

On the other hand, however, Kant also claims that, together with metaphysics, "*especially* that *criticism* of our adventurous and self-reliant reason which serves as an introduction or propaedeutic to metaphysics, alone *properly constitutes what may be entitled philosophy*" (1929, 665; emphases added). The critique of pure reason (i.e., the overarching *critical* project) is thus itself conceived as a scientific *doctrine* or philosophy – it lays down a unified plan – *of* the philosophy of pure reason, that is, of metaphysics, or a unified theory of knowledge as a whole (i.e., *inclusive* of its overall plan). Critique is thus, impossibly, the philosophical doctrine of a doctrine of philosophy that includes it.

Now, this transcendental or speculative investigation into the conditions for knowledge as a whole, understood provisionally as an overarching "doctrine" of knowledge (of its possibility), is what I will call "Critique" at the "meta" level (hereafter, with the upper case). I discuss later the problematic nature of "Critique" in this doctrinal sense. For the moment, however, what is important is merely this: by systematically establishing the logical grounds of knowledge in terms of a priori principles, Kant ensures the coherence and, hence the scienticity, of the architectonic as a whole. This is how reason in both its theoretical *and* its practical employment is granted philosophical legitimacy (hereafter "Legitimacy" in the upper case).

"Critique" in this broad sense thus corresponds well to the concept of theory ($theory_1$) discussed in Chapter One. "*Theõria*" (or 'contemplation'), it must be recalled, was already for Boethius that stable and universal system of knowledge, based on the logical correspondence of the *trivium* and the *quadrivium*, through which the reliability of scientific and humanistic understanding was ensured. Interestingly, the term Boethius used for this was "*speculatio*" (Inwood 1992, 271). Thus, Rodolphe Gasché writes, "speculation, or *speculatio* … together with *contemplatio* makes up the Latin translation of the Greek concept of *theõria*" (1986, 42). This is what Kant was later to call "speculation." For "*Spekulation*," in Kant's work, is "linked to *Metaphysik*" (Inwood 1992, 272) – and metaphysics, we have seen, is for Kant a complete philosophy of pure reason. Insofar as it qualifies as *theõria* ($theory_1$), then, Kantian "Critique" corresponds with speculative philosophy as such. Like any speculative philosophy, Kantian Critique represents,

> a form of theorizing that goes beyond verifiable observation; specifically, a philosophical approach informed by the impulse to construct a grand narrative of a worldview that encompasses the whole of reality … It sets for its goal a unifying matrix and an overarching system wherewith to comprehend the considered judgments of cosmology, psychology, and theology … [S]peculative philosophy aspires to a comprehensive understanding and explanation of the structural interrelations of the culture spheres of science, morality, art, and religion. (Schrag 1995, 758)

As a speculative "theory" of knowledge, then, Kantian Critique is the condition of possibility for – and the Legitimation of – all the "interests of my reason," including the possibility of the moral interest, which takes the form of Kant's second question: "what ought I to do?" But only the particular knowledge of reason in its practical employment may be entitled "critique" and, accordingly, be said to give rise to "legitimation," in the narrow sense of both terms. For Kant is very clear, particularly in the second *Critique*, that the maxims of practical reason which follow from the a priori condition of "freedom" in no way extend our *theoretical* knowledge as speculation (1993a, 4, esp. 141–2). They do, however, provide a procedure (in the form of a categorical imperative or a moral "law") by virtue of which *knowledge* of the difference between legitimate (lower case) and illegitimate moral norms can be gained. The moral law thus expresses a standard of "critique" in a narrow, quite common, sense of the word: it allows us to make *reasoned* judgements concerning justice.

As James Ellington says, the categorical imperative is a "precise formulation" of "*a consistent standard according to which everyday actions are judged* as being moral or not" (in Kant 1993b, vi; emphasis mine). Moreover, as Seyla Benhabib reminds us, "critique," together with "crisis," is etymologically connected to the Greek word κρίσις – "which means dividing, choosing, judging and deciding." Benhabib writes,

> *Krisis* refers to dissent and controversy, but also to a decision that is reached and to a judgment that is passed. "Critique" is the subjective evaluation or decision concerning a conflictual and controversial process – a crisis. The connection between a process of social and natural disturbance and subjective judgment upon this process is even more striking in medical terminology, to which the terms were restricted in the Middle Ages. In this context, "crisis" designates a stage in the development of a disease that is a turning point and during which the decisive diagnosis concerning the healing or worsening of the patient is reached. (1986, 19)

Practical reason is "critique" in that it entails the use of reason to resolve a "controversy" or a "crisis" by providing the criterion for a moral *decision*. On the basis of the moral law, a turning point with respect to moral uncertainty can be achieved.

As I have suggested, Kantian "critique" (i.e., reason in its practical employment alone) represents a momentous change with regard to prior moral theory. Most notably, it entails for the first time a fully epistemological explication of moral legitimacy. Because the categorical imperative is logically founded on a principle of reason, Kant claims, we can have determinate knowledge of – not merely a traditional, dogmatic or religious prescription for – "what [we] ought to do." This is because the pure practical distinction between justice and injustice gains its Legitimacy as a particular kind of knowledge insofar as it is positioned within an overarching architectonic (a unified matrix of reason in its totality). Therefore, "critique" in the micro sense depends first and foremost on "Critique" in the meta sense. In the Kantian text, "Critique" furnishes the Legitimation *of* legitimation, or of "critique."

Critical political and educational theorists cannot simply do away with a speculative theory of knowledge – what Lyotard calls a "grand narrative" of Legitimation[4] – therefore, even if they do consider it "untrustworthy." For, without some version of the narrative in place, there is no way to establish a *rational* standard for normative critique nor, consequently, is there a basis for the ideal of "critical" consciousness that educational theorists wish to retain. Indeed, it should be recalled, "critical" consciousness is the *epistemological* perspective from which an understanding of the requirements for justice, a *moral* decision, can be reached. If this "critical" notion of reason is everywhere at play in current theories of pedagogy, this is hardly surprising; the normative project of education has long been understood as the attempt to inculcate a spirit of "critique." Importantly, however, this means that "Critique" in the meta sense cannot be discarded, because it is the condition of possibility for such standards and ideals.

It is precisely the 'meta' status of Critique with regard to critique that deconstruction exposes as troubled. As I have said, the normative consequence of a deconstructive reading is the exposure of the problem that the necessary condition *for* critical reason cannot be recovered *by* reason. This insight does not issue from a "postmodern mood" of scepticism that is brought to bear on the philosophical discourses of modernity. It stems, rather, from a rigorous exposition of the impossibility of grounding criticality, that is, of Legitimating "critique," in the first place. In Lyotard's analysis, for example, what is often overlooked is that the process of delegitimation symptomized by "the postmodern condition" is not simply imposed from without as though it were extrinsic to scientific thought – as if, for example, "postmodernism" were merely a politically-motivated attack *on* scientific 'objectivity.' Rather, Lyotard argues, the inability to believe in *les grands récits* is "fueled by the demand for legitimation itself" (1984, 39). Here is the passage in its entirety that was only partially cited earlier.

> The "crisis" of scientific knowledge, signs of which have been accumulating since the end of the nineteenth century, is not born of a chance proliferation of sciences, itself an effect of progress in technology and the expansion of capitalism. It represents, rather, *an internal erosion of the legitimacy principle of knowledge.* There is erosion at work *inside* the speculative game, and by loosening the weave of the encyclopedic net in which each science was to find its place, it eventually sets them free. (1984, 39; emphases mine)

What Lyotard here calls the "speculative game," it should be noted, refers specifically to "the discourse on the [L]egitimation of scientific discourse" (1984, 33). This "language game" of Legitimation, on his view, is only one of two. It is "not state-political, but philosophical," and it is linked to the politics of the high school and the university (1984, 33, 31). He writes, "the University is speculative, that is to say, philosophical." And the role of philosophy, in turn, is to

> restore unity to learning, which has been scattered into separate sciences in laboratories and in pre-university education; it can only achieve this in a language game that links the sciences together as moments in the becoming of spirit, in other words, which links them in a rational narration, or rather a metanarration. (1984, 33)

Significantly, although Lyotard has in mind the Hegelian model in particular, the meta notion of Kantian Critique discussed above corresponds quite directly to the speculative narrative of Legitimation as well. Lyotard's explication of Legitimation is particularly telling:

> German idealism has recourse to a metaprinciple that simultaneously grounds the development of learning, of society, and of the State in the realization of the "life" of a Subject, called "divine Life" by Fichte and "Life of the spirit" by Hegel. In this perspective, knowledge first finds legitimacy within itself, and it is knowledge that is entitled to say what the State and what Society are. But it can only play this role *by changing levels*, by ceasing to be simply the positive knowledge of its referent (nature, society, the State, etc.), *becoming in addition to that the knowledge of the knowledge of the referent – that is, by becoming speculative.* In the names "Life" and "Spirit," knowledge names itself.
> (1984, 34–5; emphases mine)

Insofar as Kantian Critique (the scientific knowledge *of* knowledge) has been seen as precisely that 'change of levels' Lyotard describes, we can add Kantian "reason" to the list of names by which speculative knowledge "names itself."

Interestingly, however, Lyotard characterizes Kantian philosophy in terms of a fundamentally different narrative of Legitimation. For he distinguishes the "speculative" narrative with its scientific principle of unity and its insistence on the self-legitimating capacity of knowledge from another discourse: the "narrative of emancipation," or "freedom." This other narrative, which is linked to the politics of primary education rather than to the university, is described as follows:

> According to this version, knowledge finds its validity not within itself, not in a subject that develops by actualizing its learning possibilities, but in a practical subject – humanity. The principle of the movement animating the people is not the self-legitimation of knowledge, but the self-grounding of freedom or, if preferred, its self is the story of its emancipation from everything that prevents it from governing itself. (1984, 35)

"Clearly," he continues, "this mode of [L]egitimation through the autonomy of the will gives priority to a totally different language game, which Kant called imperative and is known today as prescriptive" (1984, 36).

Just as each of these narratives solves the problem of Legitimacy in a different way – one by virtue of the speculative principle of knowledge, the other by virtue of the emancipatory principle of freedom – so the inherent potential for erosion is different in each. In the scientific narrative, erosion is due to the demand for Legitimacy itself, which concerns the possibility of "proof." Specifically, Lyotard argues that science demands that its fundamental axioms must themselves be Legitimated or 'proved' as justifiable.

In order to Legitimate the axiomatic itself, therefore, a "metalanguage" is required, and that "metalanguage" is logic (1984, 42).

This is where scientific Legitimacy begins to falter. For if we then ask, with Lyotard, "by what criteria does the logician define the properties required of an axiomatic?" (1984, 42), we are led to the general criteria for a logical mathematical system. These criteria are consistency, syntactic completeness, decidability and independence (i.e., "of the axioms in relation to one another" [1984, 42]). Yet, as Lyotard remarks, Kurt Gödel established that mathematical systems are themselves unable to meet these requirements. As Rodolphe Gasché elaborates,

> Gödel demonstrated that metalogical statements concerning the completeness and consistency of systems any more complex than logical systems of the first order cannot be demonstrated within these systems. Derrida, in *Dissemination*, transcribes Gödel's theorem in the following terms: "An undecidable proposition, as Gödel demonstrated in 1931, is a proposition which, given a system of axioms governing a multiplicity, is neither an analytical nor deductive consequence of those axioms, nor in contradiction with them, neither true nor false with respect to those axioms. *Tertium datur*, without synthesis." (Gasché 1987, 9; internal references omitted)

Moreover, Lyotard proposes, undecidable propositions are found not only in mathematical systems; rather, the situation can be generalized (1984, 43). Consequently, complex formal systems are necessarily incomplete and thus internally limited. Or, to put this in slightly different terms, they all are open to (in a state of) deconstruction. The recognition of this complication gave rise not only to the mathematics of the Bourbaki group, Lyotard says, but to analogous developments in other sciences as well: "they owe their status to the existence of a language whose rules of functioning cannot themselves be demonstrated but are the object of a consensus among experts" (1984, 43).

This insight has a number of consequences. The first is that the goal of the production of scientific proof changes from truth to "performativity" (1984, esp. 46–53). Another result, Lyotard says, is that knowledge may now be seen to "progress" in two distinct ways: "one corresponds to a new move (a new argument) within the established rules; the other, to the invention of new rules, in other words, a change to a new game" (1984, 43). What is most directly relevant here, however, is that regardless of the form that any new "game" may take, "what never fails to come and come again … is the question of [L]egitimacy. For it is not philosophy that asks this question of science, but science that asks it of itself" (1984, 54).

The problem of the erosion at work inside the "speculative game" corresponds to the relationship between theory$_1$ (a unified system of knowledge) and theory$_2$ (theory's inherent "resistance" to systematization) that was treated previously. But before I return to it, it is necessary to linger over Lyotard's distinction between the scientific principle of self-Legitimating knowledge, and the "metanarrative of emancipation" with its "self-grounding" principle of freedom, because this distinction is misleadingly formulated. Specifically, the metanarrative of emancipation cannot be said to prioritize "a *totally different* language game" – that is, that of the "imperative" or the "prescriptive" *rather than* that of the "truth" (cited above, my emphasis). To say this is to forget that the discursive "games" of prescription and truth (of "critique" and "Critique") are fundamentally entwined from the start. Consequently, the "erosion" (or "resistance") at work in the discourses of science and emancipation will necessarily be common to them both.

Lyotard overlooks the entwinement of the principle of emancipation with the principle of science, however, because he treats the Kantian explication of practical reason independently, without regard for its placement within the Critical system as a whole. Lyotard says that the "distinguishing characteristic" of the "emancipation apparatus flowing from the *Aufklärung*," is that, "it grounds the [L]egitimation of science and truth *in the autonomy of interlocutors* involved in ethical, social, and political praxis" (1984, 39–40, my emphasis). So it does, to be sure. This does not mean, however, that the principle of "freedom" is vulnerable *as such*, or that it embodies its *own* form of delegitimation.

On Lyotard's view, the metanarrative of emancipation is subject to erosion insofar as it entails an unbridgeable divide between the theoretical and the practical employments of reason. He says, "There is nothing to prove that if a statement describing a real situation is true, it follows that a prescriptive statement based upon it (the effect of which will necessarily be a modification of that reality) will be just" (1984, 41, 81). Not only is this difficulty insoluble, Lyotard avers, but the distinction between descriptive and prescriptive statements effectively places science on a par with morality, which is an altogether different discourse and, in so doing, delegitimizes the former. This has implications for the Legitimacy of the metanarrative of emancipation as well. Once science loses its status as a master discourse, Lyotard contends, the road is paved for a dissolution of the social subject altogether, who becomes lost in a veritable multiplicity of (equally relative) language games. If the potential for erosion inherent in the scientific (philosophical/speculative) metanarrative is that it cannot satisfy its own conditions for Legitimacy, then, the problem with the metanarrative of freedom, in contrast, is that it supposedly entails the introduction of a language game that *competes* with science, and thereby opens the door to a multiplicity of discourses, none of which can be finally established as supreme.

Now, this discussion may give rise to some confusion given that I argued earlier that reason qualifies as scientific or "speculative" for Kant insofar as it encompasses both theory *and* practice. Indeed, Kant is explicit on the point. In the *Critique of Practical Reason* he asserts that,

> if pure reason of itself can be and really is practical, as the consciousness of the moral law shows it to be, it is only one and the same reason which judges *a priori* by principles, whether for theoretical or for practical purposes. Then it is clear that, if its capacity in the former is not sufficient to establish certain propositions positively (which however do not contradict it), it must assume these propositions just as soon as they are sufficiently certified as belonging imprescriptibly to the practical interest of pure reason. It must assume them indeed as something offered from the outside and not grown on its own soil, and *it must seek to compare and connect them with everything which it has in its power as speculative reason*. (1993a, 127–8; emphasis mine; compare 1993b, 4)

This is for Kant the "path to wisdom"; it "must for us men unavoidably *pass through science*" (1993a, 149; my emphasis). This is why I suggested earlier that Lyotard's description of a unifying philosophy that 'changes levels' (such as Hegelian speculation) applies to Kantian Critique as well. The confusion can be cleared up, however, once it is noticed that Lyotard's understanding of the metanarrative of emancipation does not implicate the Critique of pure reason as a whole. It is based, rather, on his consideration of practical reason alone. Lyotard specifies, for example, that the emancipatory discourse is one in which knowledge is conceived not as an end in itself, but merely as a means to determine legitimate moral action, or the knowledge of what we are to *do* (1984, 36). This corresponds with Kant's contention that in practical reason the understanding is in the service of reason, rather than the other way around. The practical knowledge Lyotard describes, therefore, is what I have called a standard or process of "critique" – the means of "legitimation" – in the narrow sense of both terms.

Once this is understood, it becomes obvious that there is only one metanarrative of modernity. To suggest there are two is to lose sight of the fact that practical reason *qua* critique is not a metanarrative at all, but merely legitimation in the lower case. Taken out of its Critical context, to be sure, practical reason can be distinguished quite sharply from theoretical reason. Thus, Kantian philosophy, entailing as it does a substantial explication of the difference between freedom and nature, is commonly thought to inaugurate a decisive distinction between ethics and epistemology – the distinction no doubt at work in Lyotard's dualistic characterization of modern Legitimacy (see Bernard 2011). But what Lyotard calls the "emancipation apparatus flowing from the *Aufklärung*" depends crucially on the scientific status of the Critical system as a whole; it cannot be confined to the moral sphere as such. Indeed, the epistemological role of the Critical architectonic (of the scientific plan) is that it Legitimates all forms of knowledge, *including* the specifically practical knowledge of (the prescription for) what we "ought" (morally) to do. What Lyotard does not notice, in short, is the necessary relationship between critique and Critique.

Once the asymmetrical nature of this relationship is taken into account, it emerges that what Lyotard sees as a problem for moral legitimacy (as such) is not really one: by virtue of the Critical project as a whole, the "freedom" of the interlocutors is itself *scientifically* authorized as a Legitimate principle of moral action – provided, that is to say, that logic's priority over rhetoric is retained from the *trivium*, thereby ensuring the scienticity of the system itself. Thus, to put it more simply, the narrative of emancipation that Lyotard wants to separate out as a different and competing discourse turns out to be itself Legitimated by the *speculative* unity characteristic of *theõria* (theory$_1$) since Boethius and defined by Kant as "science."

In distinguishing between the metanarratives of science and freedom as he does, Lyotard thus misrecognizes the precise nature of the internal erosion or "resistance" (theory$_2$) that threatens them both, and so ultimately misdiagnoses the root of the "postmodern condition." Specifically, insofar as emancipation and science (prescription and description) are for the Enlightenment both entwined "*inside* the speculative game," they share the requirement for "self-legitimation" that science demands and that logic is intended to provide. But Enlightenment speculation is neither purely scientific nor purely emancipatory; on the contrary, its distinguishing characteristic is precisely that it is both. By this token, the potential for erosion that inheres in the grand narrative of the modern European Enlightenment will necessarily touch on both aspects. In contrast to Lyotard, I therefore want to suggest, the delegitimation in question concerns *neither* (simply) the impossibility of logically establishing the completeness of a mathematical system, *nor* (simply) the impossibility of relating prescriptive to descriptive claims. It has to do, more precisely, with the impossibility of establishing the self-Legitimating principle of science (with its unifying, systematic *telos) as* the normative "end" of the subject in his, her or their *freedom*. What is at risk in the postmodern delegitimation of knowledge, more simply, is the unconditional status of a *normative* principle of reason. It is this possibility on which the ethico-political good of "critical" reason depends.

Kant's Critical philosophy can be seen as an attempt to make good on precisely this aim. As we have seen, his systematization of theoretical and moral knowledge within a unifying architectonic is a Critical formulation of the speculative philosophical project *as* an ethico-political, emancipatory enterprise. This is the modern project *par excellence*: it is the educative enterprise of "Enlightenment." If the rational status of moral critique depends upon its inclusion in a systematic Critique of reason, however, and if the Critical system as a whole, in turn, can only Legitimate the moral law by virtue of its *logical* systematicity (its character as "science"), then moral legitimacy is (always already) vulnerable to the "erosion" that is "fueled by the demand for [L]egitimation itself" (cited above). It is this deconstructive potential, rather than a mood of scepticism, that constitutes the "postmodern condition."

Here we might turn to a second definition that Lyotard offers for this phrase – one that is certainly less famous than the first but is arguably more apt:

> The postmodern would be that which, in the modern, puts forward the unpresentable in presentation itself; that which denies the solace of good forms, the consensus of a taste which would make it possible to share collectively the nostalgia for the unattainable ... The [postmodern] artist and the writer ... are working without rules in order to formulate the rules of *what will have been done.* Hence the fact that the work and text have the characters of an *event*; hence also, they always come too late for their author, or, what amounts to the same thing, their being put into work, their realization (*mise en oeuvre*) always begins too soon. *Post modern* would have to be understood according to the paradox of the future (*post*) anterior (*modo*). (1984, 81; emphases his)

Similarly, we might say, the "postmodern" delegitimation of knowledge is, in a phrase, what modern Legitimacy *will (always already) have been about.* For "Critique" itself, we shall now see, inherently resists (or deconstructs) its own claim as "science" and, thus, fails to establish the Legitimation (in the "meta" sense) it was intended to provide.

Notes

1 The alternative phrasings are based on Misgeld's modifications (1985, 81).

2 Here the term "metaphysical" should be understood in its Kantian sense; as he explains, "the system of pure reason, that is, the science which exhibits in systematic connection the whole body (true as well as illusory) of philosophical knowledge arising out of pure reason ... is entitled metaphysics." Kant continues, "Metaphysics is divided into that of the *speculative* and that of the *practical* employment of pure reason, and is therefore either *metaphysics of nature* or *metaphysics of morals.* The former contains all the principles of pure reason that are derived from mere concepts (therefore excluding mathematics), and employed in the *theoretical* knowledge of all things; the latter, the principles which in *a priori* fashion determine and make necessary *all our actions.*" (1929, 659).

3 Unless otherwise specified, the phrase, "the critique of pure reason" refers to Kant's entire critical project, which includes his investigation of all three forms of judgement (theoretical, practical, and aesthetic or reflective). The phrase does not refer merely to the first of the three *Critiques* (which is always identified with italics, as it indicates the title of a text).

4 For the sake of clarity, I will use the upper case to indicate "Legitimation" in the meta sense. While Lyotard does not distinguish graphically between a meta and a micro level of legitimation, he is clearly working with the same distinction, as I explain below.

4 Deconstructing Kantian Critique

> The question of this [Leibnizian interpretation of] reason cannot be separated from a question about the modal verb "must" and the phrase "must be rendered." The "must" seems to cover the essence of our relationship to principle, it seems to mark out for us requirement, debt, duty, request, command, obligation, law, the imperative. Whenever reason can be rendered (*reddi potest*), it must. Can we, without further precautions, call this a moral imperative, in the Kantian sense of pure practical reason? It is not clear that the sense of "practical," as it is determined by a critique of pure practical reason, gets to the bottom of the "must," or reveals its origin, although such a critique has to presuppose such a "must."
>
> (Derrida 1983b, 8)

The potential for erosion that inheres in the modern metanarrative of Legitimation, according to Lyotard, is a consequence of the undecidability (in the precise Gödelian sense) that afflicts all formal logical systems of sufficient complexity. If Lyotard is correct it will afflict the Kantian architectonic as well. And, insofar as the critical system as a whole is what establishes in turn the Legitimation of practical reason ("critique" in the narrow sense), this erosion directly compromises the emancipatory Enlightenment project. In this chapter, I show how the analysis is borne out in the Kantian text. Undecidability or "*différance*" does play at the heart of the Kantian system; it concerns nothing less than the inside and the outside – the "meta" and the "micro" levels of "critique" – on which the concept of critical reason depends. On one hand, as I hope to make clear, the *difference* between the critical system and its epistemological objects is necessary, because it is the only basis on which an ethico-political standard of critique with its corresponding vision of justice can be philosophically justified. *Différance* at the heart of the Kantian system thus potentially deconstructs the very architectonic through which the ideal of "critical reason" first came to be known.

On the other hand, however, *différance* remains a logically necessary condition for this particular understanding of criticality as well. Most importantly, without an undecidable "play" between the system's inside and its outside – a play within the very meaning of "critique," so to speak – Kant cannot establish both a scientific justification of moral knowledge and a moral justification of science. As I shall demonstrate, the politico-educational ideal ultimately requires no less. The consequence of this analysis is thus not only that the condition of possibility for ethico-political "critique" is impossible (indeed, is critique's own impossibility), but that the impossible determination of the undecidable must itself be covered over through the violent institution of a transcendental subject if the critical Enlightenment ideal is to continue to stand. I conclude the first Part of this study by enumerating the consequences of this deconstruction for emancipatory political and educational thought. These consequences are taken up directly in Part Two.

In order to demonstrate how the scientific demand for Legitimacy 'fuels' its own delegitimation, it is necessary to return to Kant's discussion of the relationship between a propaedeutic "Critique" and a metaphysical "doctrine" of pure philosophy. I drew attention earlier to a veritable möebius strip with respect to that relationship. In particular, I showed that Kant equivocates between the sense of "Critique" as a doctrine of knowledge, and its sense as the determination of the a priori principles on which a scientific doctrine is based. The formulation I suggested was that Critique is (impossibly) the (all-inclusive) doctrine of a doctrine that includes it. Paradoxically, "doctrine" and "Critique" are each the condition of possibility for one another. Another way to formulate this would be to say that the idea of science as a unified system of knowledge (a "doctrine" of pure philosophy) and the idea of Critique as a speculative systematization of the a priori conditions *of* that doctrine, cut across one another in the form of a chiasmus.[1]

In itself, this had no immediate bearing on the previous argument, since in that context it was merely the status of Critique as a unified theory or "system" that it was necessary to highlight. Moral knowledge can only be Legitimated, I argued, by virtue of the Critique's systematicity (its doctrinal quality). Significantly, however, Kantian "Critique" is not reducible to what Kant understands as a "doctrine of pure philosophy" notwithstanding its doctrinal character, because the term "Critique" as Kant employs it is *also* in a chiasmic relation with the meaning of "critique" (i.e., with the explication of reason in its practical employment alone). In effect, as I will establish shortly, it is only because it is *not* possible to differentiate clearly between a scientific "Critique" of the a priori conditions of knowledge in general, and a moral "critique" of ethico-political legitimacy in particular (i.e., the difference between Legitimacy and legitimacy) that it *is* possible to distinguish between a propaedeutic "Critique" – the scientific knowledge *of* knowledge – and a metaphysical "doctrine" that denotes the "whole of pure philosophy" and therefore includes its Critique (i.e., an encyclopaedia *of* that knowledge itself). Because Critique becomes critique, in short, "Critique" can be distinguished from "doctrine."

Conversely, insofar as a Critique *shares* with a doctrine of pure philosophy the scientific quality of logical systematicity, Critique can be distinguished from critique. As I elaborate in Part Two, this "play" on the signifier "critique" has direct consequences for the ideal of "criticality" that theorists on both sides of the modernism–postmodernism debate tend to uphold.

What is important now, however, is that neither of these distinctions can be relinquished. What is at stake in the first distinction – between a doctrine of pure philosophy and a propaedeutic "Critique" – is the scientific (meta-)Legitimacy of "pure (transcendental) philosophy." Critique guarantees this Legitimacy by virtue of the fact that, precisely *qua* the propaedeutic determination of the a priori principles of reason and not *qua* "doctrine," it grounds the systematic doctrine, thus confirming its scienticity. But the second distinction, between "Critique" and "critique," is just as significant as the first. For on the second distinction hinges the very possibility at which Kantian Critique, as a speculative *system* of knowledge, aims: the establishment of an overarching "theory" (a unified *doctrine* of knowledge) *within which* a critical standard of moral legitimation can be established. *Qua* "doctrine," Kantian "Critique" is differentiated from merely moral "critique," and thereby confirms the Legitimacy of reason in its practical employment (in its morality) as well.

It is only when "critique" is mobilized in both of these senses at once, therefore, that Kant actually instantiates the politico-educational ideal of *critical* reason; that is, an ideal of reason that is simultaneously scientifically Legitimate *and* practically normative. This simultaneity is the logical condition of possibility for such an ideal. Taken together, these distinctions entail a play on the term "Critique," whereby it oscillates between the meaning of "doctrine" and that of "critique." This equivocation is not immediately apparent as long as only one of the distinctions is being put to work at a time. But when they are mobilized simultaneously, it emerges that "Critique" is *both-neither* "doctrine" *and-nor* "critique."

In this sense, the equivocation of Kantian "Critique" signifies a structural "undecidability" (in Gödel's sense) – what Derrida calls "*différance*" – at work *in* the very difference between the inside and the outside (legitimacy and Legitimacy) of the Kantian architectonic. For, as I now want to show, "Critique" signifies not only a unified "doctrine" of pure philosophy, or the 'outside' of the Kantian architectonic, but also its 'inside'; as "critique," (meta-)Critique also indicates the standard for moral legitimacy alone. Something we might designate as "C/critique," thus, is to the difference between "doctrine" and "critique" just what the "sublime" is to the difference between the aesthetic and the teleological judgement: C/critique is that 'critical' 'something' that is neither scientifically doctrinal (Critique), nor strictly moral (critique) but which, impossibly, partakes of both.

In order to see how "Critique" slides from its doctrinal meaning of a comprehensive, epistemological system into "critique" as a rational standard of moral judgement more narrowly, let us begin with "Critique." As the propaedeutic for a doctrine of pure philosophy, the Critique of pure reason is intended to uncover all the a priori conditions of knowledge. Among these, however, none is as important as the unconditioned condition of *freedom*: the a priori principle of reason in its purely practical employment. As Kant writes in the second *Critique*, "every interest is ultimately practical, even that of *speculative reason being only conditional* and reaching perfection only in *practical use*" (1993a, 128; my emphasis). If the speculative dimension of metaphysical philosophy is "only conditional" upon its practical use rather than an end in itself, then it would seem that "pure" philosophy (the *knowledge* of the unconditioned) is ultimately Legitimated by the Critique of practical reason alone. In other words, if speculation itself reaches perfection only when it is used for moral ends, then we must be able to determine what our unconditioned moral ends actually are, and this requires the Critique or Legitimation of reason in its pure practicality. And indeed, immediately following the description of metaphysics provided in the *Critique of Pure Reason*, Kant writes,

> Now, morality is the only code of laws applying to our actions which can be derived completely *a priori* from principles. Accordingly, the metaphysics of morals is really pure moral philosophy, with no underlying basis of anthropology or of other empirical conditions. (1929, 659)

Not only does the Critique of practical reason provide the (scientific) ground for the only "pure moral philosophy," moreover, but Kant also insists that pure moral philosophy is in turn "superior" to "all other occupations of reason" (1929, 658). For, "moral philosophy" is the philosophy which "deals with the whole vocation of man" – what he otherwise calls 'man's' "ultimate" or "highest ends." These, together with the "subordinate ends" of reason (the means by which the ultimate ends are achieved), are what Kant calls the "*essential* ends of human reason" (1929, 658, 657, my emphasis). The essential ends of 'man' thus represent, in a phrase, the "practical interest" of reason as reflected in the question "What ought I to do?" Within Critique *qua* a unified "doctrine of the scientific in our knowledge" (1929, 653), then, the Critique of practical reason – providing as it does the only "completely" a priori principle and thus scientifically Legitimating the "highest occupation of reason" – sits at the apex.

The pre-eminence of the moral law over the natural law of causality within the Critical architectonic emerges quite clearly in the *Critique of Practical Reason* as well. As Kant announces in the Preface, "The concept of freedom, in so far as its reality is proved by an *apodictic* law of practical reason, is the *keystone* of the whole *architecture* of the system of pure reason and even of speculative reason" (1993a, 3; emphases mine). Again,

Kant here explicitly acknowledges that, precisely because it alone is "apodictic" (necessarily certain), the moral law is the primary element of the Critical architectonic. As such, it is the "keystone" (or the final stone of an arch, for example [*Schlussstein*]) of the scientific *doctrine* of philosophy (i.e., of "the whole architecture" [*Gebaeude*]).[2] In light of the explication offered in the second *Critique* as well, then, it is clear that the a priori principle of practical reason (the moral law) constitutes the apex of the Critical system, and is thus the *sine qua non* of its preparatory (or *propaedeutic*) work for a complete metaphysical doctrine of philosophy.[3]

I have drawn attention to the pre-eminence of the Critique of practical reason within the Critical system as a whole (and to the pre-eminence of practical reason itself above all other employments of reason), in order to highlight the following point: although the Kantian distinction I have been discussing concerns a doctrine and a Critique of pure reason in general, the primacy of practical reason within the system alerts us to the fact that the Critique that is especially at issue is the Critique of pure practical reason. Notwithstanding the difference in its subject matter, however, it is important to recall that the Critique of practical reason is intended as no less of a "scientific" investigation into a priori conditions for all that. It is therefore especially significant that this particular Critical investigation can be distinguished from a doctrine not so much by virtue of the scienticity of the principle it discovers (as was the case with theoretical reason), but by virtue of its morality. In other words, the scientific verification of the a priori condition of pure *practical* reason is the very investigation in which "Critique" slides inexorably away from its link to a scientific "doctrine" of pure philosophy, and into the moral meaning of "critique."

The principle of freedom, to be sure, does appear at the outset to qualify as the "scientific" or a priori ground of pure practical knowledge (the "law" of its possibility), just as the a priori principle or law of natural causality was shown to ground pure theoretical knowledge (e.g., 1993a, 49). However, this parallel does not actually hold up. For, as Kant explains, the possibility of practical reason is merely the possibility of the will not being sensibly conditioned; that is, the possibility of "autonomous" action (1993b, 34). Hence: "An absolutely good will, whose principle must be a categorical imperative, will therefore be indeterminate as regards all objects and will contain *merely the form of willing*; and indeed that form is autonomy" (1993b, 48, my emphasis). In the *Grounding for the Metaphysics of Morals* it thus already becomes apparent that, as Kant will insist throughout the second *Critique*, the principle of freedom is "inseparable" from the moral law to legislate universally and, hence, 'freely' (1993a, 58, 98; also 29, 47, 73, 124).

In fact, they are fundamentally the same. For the moral law is itself named as "causality through freedom" (1993a, 51), insofar as it expresses the imperative to "[s]o act that the maxim of your will could always hold at the same time as the principle giving universal law." Because this imperative to legislate for oneself universally (i.e. 'lawfully') thus expresses "nothing else than the autonomy of pure practical reason, i.e., freedom," (1993a, 34), Kant maintains that the moral law "*is itself demonstrated to be a principle* of the deduction of freedom as causality of pure reason," and that this "is a sufficient substitute for any *a priori* justification" (1993a, 49; my emphasis). This point is later confirmed: "the causality [of freedom] is determinable only through the moral law" (1993a, 82).

The question at stake in the *Critique of Practical Reason* is thus not how to determine that freedom is the principle of moral causality. This "principle" is already given by virtue of an awareness of the moral law which immediately expresses it (1993a, 29, 30). Indeed, Kant often refers to "freedom" as a "postulate" rather than as a principle (1993a, 138–9; see also 129, 149–50). "Freedom" is also described as a "faculty" (1993a, 110), a "concept" (1993a, 111), the "autonomy" inhering in the moral principle (1993a, 33–4), and as the moral law itself (1993a, 51). The question, rather, is how do we *know* the moral law itself, as the mere form of lawfulness, to be inherently binding on or imperative for us? In Kant's formulation, "how is the *consciousness* of the moral law possible?" (1993a, 29; emphasis added). Kant's answer to this question reveals why the a priori determination of freedom and the a priori determination of natural causality are far from strictly analogous. For Kant's "Critique" of the way in which reason "prescribes" its laws is significantly different from his "Critique" of the way in which "nature" does so: the *Critique of Practical Reason* uncovers the moral law only insofar as "Critique" becomes "critique."

Kant begins his investigation by remarking that the practical law, the rule that "One ought absolutely to act in a certain way," enjoins the subject categorically because, by virtue of it, the will is determined by the "mere form of the law" completely independently of all empirical conditions (1993a, 31). The concept of "autonomy" is first introduced here: "The sole principle of morality," Kant says, "consists in independence from all material of the law (i.e., a desired object), and in the accompanying determination of a choice by the mere form of giving universal law which a maxim must be capable of having" (1993a, 33). Autonomy or freedom thus entails what Kant calls both a "positive" and a "negative" sense: the will can be said to be determined by a "negative" autonomy insofar as it is free from all sensible conditions (that it is objective) and hence is *contra* to natural causality. At the same time, the will is also "positively" determined insofar as it does (positively) legislate solely to itself, without any "heteronomous" influence from sensibility (1993a, 33–4).

Now this self-legislating capacity or "positive autonomy" – like the moral law itself – is said to be a "fact of reason," not an empirical fact; by virtue of the consciousness of the law, reason "*proclaims* itself as originating law," or, "*shows* itself actually to be practical" (1993a, 31–2, 43; my emphases). Thus, Kant says, the "fact" of the moral law is "inextricably bound up with the consciousness of freedom" – that is, it is bound up with the "fact" of our consciousness of reason's self-legislating capacity (1993a, 43). This means, however, that the *consciousness* of the moral law is itself intrinsically related to the "positive" sense of autonomy as this capacity for self-legislation. Yet this consciousness is merely the result of logical reflection. As Kant explains, the idea of freedom as an unconditioned cause first arises for speculative reason by virtue of the logical assumption that "for every series of conditions there must be something unconditioned, and consequently a causality which is entirely self-determining" (1993a, 50; compare Kant 1929, 409–15). Kant's speculative postulation of an intelligible world, along with the principle of freedom as causality it is said to entail, thus merely expresses the desire for *logical* coherence: "speculative reason had to assume [the faculty of the will] as at least possible (*in order not to contradict itself* in finding among its cosmological Ideas something unconditional in its causality)" (1993a, 49; emphasis added). Thus, the question remains as to why the mere capacity for self-legislation may be said to exhibit not simply a speculative but indeed a uniquely "moral" interest as reflected in the question, what 'ought' I to do?

In the *Grounding for the Metaphysics of Morals*, Kant forgoes any attempt to answer the question; "Here then is the extreme limit of all moral inquiry," he says (1993b, 61). In the *Critique of Practical Reason*, in contrast, he cannot again leave the question merely at that. For, as James Ellington comments, the purpose the second *Critique* is not only to show that moral philosophy falls under the province of a single principle, but to justify that principle as the a priori ground of moral action (in Kant 1993b, v–vi; viii, ix). Kant must therefore explain exactly how it is that "the certainty of a disposition which agrees with the law is the first condition of any worth of the person" (1993a, 75–92, esp. 76). He does so, moreover, with a specific view to elaborating the claim first made in the *Grounding*; namely, that "a mere thought which itself contains nothing sensuous can produce a sensation of pleasure or displeasure" (1993b, 59–60). This is what provokes his well-known assertion concerning our necessary "respect" for the moral law. Specifically, his argument is that the "positive" and "negative" senses of the term "autonomy" each entail a special kind of non-sensuous "feeling." On one hand, we can see a priori (negatively) that the constraints of sensuous impulses and inclinations that the moral law demands "produce a feeling which can be called pain" (1993a, 76). On the other hand, the moral law has a positive "feeling" associated with it as well. The consciousness of a capacity for self-legitimation is itself "an object of respect," Kant says, because the moral law 'strikes down' or "humiliates" self-conceit (1993a, 77). "Respect for the moral law, therefore, is a feeling produced by an intellectual cause, and this *feeling* is the only one which we can know completely *a priori* and the necessity of which we can discern" (1993a, 77; emphasis mine). As he elaborates,

> If anything checks our self-conceit in our own judgment, it humiliates. Therefore, the moral law inevitably humbles every man when he compares the sensuous propensity of his nature with the law. Now if the idea of something as the motive of the will humiliates us in our self-consciousness, it awakens respect for itself so far as it is a positive motive. The moral law, therefore, is even subjectively a positive motive. (1993a, 78)

Most significantly, this is not to say that the moral law *has* a subjective motive; in fact, it does not, for this would make it heteronomous. It is to say that the moral law *is* a subjective motive. As Kant writes, "*Thus respect for the moral law is not the drive to morality; it is morality itself*" (1993a, 79; emphasis mine).

It is by virtue of this "drive," then, that the subjective effect of the moral law is to inscribe the moral "interest" (1993a, 83). Kant explains,

> Since the law itself must be the drive in a morally good will, the moral interest must be a purely nonsensuous interest of practical reason alone … But it is a feeling which is concerned only with the practical, and with the representation of a law simply as to its form and not on any account of any object of the law; thus it cannot be reckoned either as enjoyment or as pain, yet it *produces an interest in obedience* to the law, and this we call moral interest. And the capacity of taking such an interest in the law (or of having respect for the moral law itself) is really moral feeling. (1993a, 83, my emphasis)

This moral "feeling" alone – this feeling of respect for the moral law which, we have seen, is the positive sense of "autonomy" as self-legislation and also the only feeling "we can know completely *a priori* and the necessity of which we can discern" – is the true ground of practical reason on Kant's account. Hence, the "apodictic law of practical reason" through which the reality of freedom is "proved" (1993a, 3) turns out to be not the principle of freedom as such, not the moral law which expresses it, and not even the mere consciousness of the moral law. What alone is "apodictic," rather, is the specific experience of the "sublime" feeling (1993a, 8) of "respect" *for* the law.

In fact, Kant writes, the concept of respect "can never have other than a moral ground"; "we use the term to pay attention to the *mysterious and wonderful*, but frequent, regard which human judgment does have for the moral law" (1993a, 85, nt.; emphasis mine). Kant writes,

> Duty! Thou sublime and mighty name that dost embrace nothing charming or insinuating but requirest submission and yet seekest not to move the will by threatening aught that would arouse natural aversion or terror, but only holdest forth a law which itself finds

> entrance into the mind and yet gains reluctant reverence (though not always obedience) – a law before which all inclinations are mute even though they secretly work against it; what origin is worthy of thee, and where is the root of thy noble descent which proudly rejects all kinship with the inclinations and *from which to be descended is the indispensable condition of the only worth which men alone can give themselves*? (1993a, 90; emphasis added)

The "root" of its "noble descent, Kant answers, is "man's" "own personality" as an intelligible being; because of 'man's' sublime, supersensible nature, Kant argues, the moral law is "holy" and thus exacts unconditional respect.

It is, then, the "sublime," "mysterious and wonderful," moral 'feeling,' not the logical idea of freedom, that provides the "indispensable condition" of moral worth and thereby allows us to *decide* whether the will has been solely determined by practical reason and whether an action is, consequently, truly just. The "supreme norm" or a priori principle of practical reason is the *moral* feeling of *respect for the moral law* of universalization. This feeling alone determines what is "morally good" and, hence, alone provides a "standard of critique." This means, however, that the meta Critique of practical reason – the scientific determination of its principle – and the critical standard for moral legitimacy in particular (the basis for the knowledge of what we 'ought' to do) are ultimately indistinguishable. For, on the one hand, the function of the (meta) Critique was the determination of an a priori law for practical reason that can be apodictically known and, as such, incorporated into an architectonic – a (scientific) doctrine "of the scientific in our knowledge." In the course of this Critical investigation, however, it emerges not only that the knowledge of the principle of freedom follows from the knowledge of the moral law rather than the other way around, but that the knowledge of the moral law, in turn, stems from the sublime *moral* 'feeling' of intellectual "respect." This is what the Critique of practical reason, *qua* Critique, establishes.

Once put thus, critique emerges as the condition of possibility for Critique. For on the other hand, "critique" – the standard with which we determine what *is* morally legitimate – is nothing but the injunction *to respect the law* by legislating lawfully. That is to say, the standard for moral legitimacy is a "categorical imperative": legislate in such a way that your maxim can become a universal law. To "will" (to legislate) in such a way is nothing more and nothing less than to act morally: it is to base an action on the (necessary) respect for the moral law (for the sake of it, and not merely in accordance with it). To act responsibly, in effect, is to enact a *response-ability* to the law.

Now, if this moral imperative *to* respect the law (to respond to it) is itself the only thing that can be apodictically known *as* the law and, as such, is the epistemological condition of possibility *for* the practical law of causality as freedom – if, in other words, what alone is "apodictic" and thus known a priori is merely the moral feeling of respect – then "critique" (with its rational principle of strictly *moral* legitimacy in particular) is the condition of possibility for "Critique." In other words, we cannot know how moral knowledge is possible (what its condition is and, thus, why it is Legitimate) unless we already know what *is* morally legitimate to begin with. Since to have the latter (the moral feeling of respect) is at once to establish the former (the logical principle of freedom), critique in this case precedes Critique, and provides *its* ground.

Yet this does not mean the relationship between an epistemological Critique and an ethico-political critique can be reversed. For even though the principles of nature and of freedom are by no means strictly analogous (because natural causality is logically determined, whereas causality as freedom is morally determined), the Critique of practical reason does still ensue in an a priori determination of "freedom." As Critique, in other words, this investigation does establish an a priori moral "interest" in the logical principle of freedom. The principle of morality therefore qualifies for inclusion in the scientific architectonic as a whole. By virtue of its inclusion, the moral knowledge of what one ought to do in a given case is deemed to be possible. Thus, a meta-account (an overarching, speculative theory *of* knowledge) is still the condition by virtue of which critique in the micro sense – the rational distinction between just and unjust norms – may be considered to be a Legitimate form of knowledge. In short, Critique is *also* the epistemological condition for "critique." Again, therefore, we encounter the paradoxical figure of the chiasmus. The Critique of practical reason (the apex of the Critical "doctrine" of Legitimation), and the moral procedure itself (the "critical" standard by virtue of which a moral crisis is resolved), cut across each other in such a way that each is the condition of possibility for the other.

Yet it is precisely because of this second chiasmus regarding critique and Critique that the *difference* between a doctrine of pure philosophy and a Critique can be made clear. Recall, first, that the Critique of practical reason is the linchpin of the Critical architectonic because it provides the "only completely" a priori principle, and thus scientifically Legitimizes the "highest occupation of reason." This occupation, second, is the realization of the "essential ends" of 'man' as these are reflected in the purely practical "interest" of reason. What the Critical investigation actually shows, however, is that this practical "interest" is first known as an inescapable *feeling* of moral respect – that is, as "the *certainty of a disposition* which agrees with the law" (Kant 1993a, 76; my emphasis). Consequently, we saw in the third place, the law *of* the practical interest that was uncovered by its Critique turned out to be an inescapable interest *in* the moral law; namely, a *response-ability* that instantiates moral legitimacy as such, and that thereby establishes a rational standard of "critique." On this basis, I claimed, the moral interest of practical reason is established by Critique in its role as critique. Significantly, however, it is just *because* "Critique" in its quintessential moment – that is, in the investigation of the only pure a priori there is (that of practical reason) – can be re-signified as (micro) "critique" (as the determination of moral legitimacy), that "Critique" is *not* reducible to a scientific system (or "doctrine") of pure philosophy.

Specifically, a "Critique" is different from a "doctrine" proper because Critique *qua* critique provides the normative L/legitimation *of* the philosophical doctrine. Indeed, according to Kant, practical reason's "interest" in 'man's "essential ends" provides the fundamental ground (the "real basis") of doctrinal "philosophy":

> Hitherto the concept of philosophy has been merely a scholastic concept – a concept of a system of knowledge which is sought solely in its character as a science, and which has therefore in view only the systematic unity appropriate to science, and consequently no more than the *logical* perfection of knowledge. But there is likewise another concept of philosophy, a *conceptus cosmicus*, which has always formed the real basis of the term "philosophy" ... On this view, philosophy is the science of the relation of all knowledge to the essential ends of human reason (*teleologia rationis humanae*), and the philosopher is not an artificer in the field of reason, but himself the lawgiver of human reason. (1929, 657, 658)

Now, "knowledge solely in its character as science" provides the condition and hence the epistemological Legitimation of the moral concept of "freedom." That "scientific" conception of philosophical knowledge, we have seen, confirmed an irreducible difference between a "Critical" doctrine of metaphysics in its entirety (an epistemological doctrine) and a strictly moral "critique." What here becomes clear, however, is that "freedom" itself – the essential "interest" of reason *qua* the sublime feeling of moral respect – provides the L/legitimation *for* philosophy in its very scienticity. In other words, the above citation reveals that the very autonomy that is known as the moral respect for the law is itself the ground (the "basis") *of* that "science" *through which* practical reason was supposed to be scientifically Legitimized in the first place. This was, after all, the very purpose of the transcendental Critique. Yet Kant explicitly states that the real basis of philosophy (as metaphysical speculation, or as *theõria*) concerns its relation to 'man's' ends (the subject's moral "interest," or object). And this means that *the scientific concept of reason* (1929, 653) is underwritten by *pure practical reason's concept of science*, that is, by "critique" in the lower case.

Thus, just as it was first established that, Critique could be *distinguished* from "critique" by virtue of its identity with a "doctrine of pure philosophy," so it now becomes clear that "Critique" can be differentiated from a doctrine by virtue of its *identity* with "critique." Critique as the determination of the ultimate a priori condition *for* a doctrine of philosophy thus loses its doctrinal status precisely when it becomes critique: the moral principle of practical reason alone (the principle instantiated by "respect"). The scientific doctrine of philosophy is grounded on this ultimate "apodictic" law.

There is a third chiasmus, then, that underwrites the other two: the standard of "critique" is (impossibly) the legitimating ground for a doctrine of philosophy that Legitimates it. "Critique" is not only the scientific (doctrinal) determination of normativity, but it is also, *qua* "critique," the normative determination of scienticity – which means that it is neither. Or, conversely, C/critique signifies neither scientific Legitimacy as such, nor normative legitimacy more narrowly within this particular speculative "game," precisely because it means both. Morality and scienticity are *both* founded, in one and the same move, on the rhetorical sublimity entailed by our "respect" for the moral law. As such, C/critique is the ungrounded ground, the *différantial* and thus non- or illegitimate 'basis,' of the specific *difference* between a Legitimating, epistemological doctrine and a legitimate, moral critique.

Thus, Lyotard is not wrong at least in this: there is indeed a sense in which the principle of "freedom" grounds "the [L]egitimation of science and truth" within the grand narrative of emancipation (1984, 39). Insofar as this is true, however, it is a serious problem with regard to the necessarily asymmetrical relationship – between an epistemological Critique and a moral critique (a standard of moral judgement) – that was shown to be essential for the educative ideal of critical reason. Specifically, the Kantian determination of a *rational* standard for normative critique depends upon (meta)narrative authority, or Critique, because the latter establishes the logical boundaries of Legitimate knowledge. These boundaries blur, however, if the moral law grounds the scientific doctrine at one and the same time that the doctrine grounds or Legitimates the moral law. For this means that the crucial difference between the inside and its outside of the Critical architectonic is indeterminable; the possibility of an epistemological doctrine cannot be clearly demarcated from the epistemological objects the doctrine is said to contain. Instead, the systematic unity or logical coherence of the whole architectonic is itself (in)determined rhetorically as C/critique.

Thus, to return to the argument presented in Chapter Two, the Kantian explication of the "sublime" feeling of moral respect can be shown to parallel precisely that "apocalyptic" gesture that is inscribed in philosophy, according to Derrida, as its perpetual opening. For not only is the a priori "feeling of respect" the 'revelation' of a "moral" response that is itself "mysterious and wonderful," but this sublime feeling is also an indispensable condition of scientific Legitimacy. What is "sublime" *in* us reveals *for* us (unveils) the 'true' meaning of philosophy and opens us to its "scientific" path. As Kant writes, "science (critically sought and methodically directed) is the narrow gate that leads to the doctrine of wisdom" (1993a, 169–70). So understood, the sublime 'feeling' inaugurates critical emancipatory thought, but it comes from one 'knows not where.'

It is this unmasterable moment of "deconstruction" inside the Enlightenment, speculative "game" to which Lyotard's understanding of the potential for erosion properly refers. Moreover, this deconstruction can be said to be "fueled by the demand for legitimation itself" because it occurs by virtue of the attempt to account for, or to legitimize, the Enlightenment metanarrative of Legitimacy. The attempt itself results in a logical "undecidable" in precisely Derrida's sense. Specifically, Kantian C/critique cannot be restricted to either the (meta) doctrinal or to the (micro) moral sense of the term, because it exceeds the meaning, and is ultimately constitutive, of both. As such, "C/critique" is what Derrida might call an "arche" notion (as in, "arche-critique") that corresponds directly to his description of "arche-writing" or "*différance*" (1982, 3–27, esp. 12). As Derrida explains,

> What is written *différance*, then, will be the playing movement that "produces" – by means of something that is not simply an activity – these differences, these effects of difference. This does not mean that the *différance* that produces differences is somehow before them, in a simple and unmodified – in-different – present. *Différance* is the non-full, non-simple, structured and differentiating origin of differences. Thus, the name "origin" no longer suits it. (1982, 11)

On Derrida's account, *différance* is a "generalization" of difference, in that it marks the moment of an irreducible, structural condition that is neither strictly active nor passive, that cannot itself be determined as such, and that is necessary for the determination of any particular *difference.*[4] *Différance* 'determines' difference in the sense that it is the differing/deferring *process* through which signification becomes meaningful (see Derrida 1982, esp. 13). It thus corresponds to what I described before as an "apocalyptic gesture" of speech: the gesture "come" opens discourse by naming an 'us' (and, concomitantly, a 'them') *into* being, but cannot (itself) be recovered *by* it.

The undecidable term "critique" functions in the Kantian text in just this way: "C/critique" marks in the critical philosophy of pure reason a logically-unmasterable or undecidable "trace" that both preserves and negates (is "the playing movement" of) the logical relationship between doctrine (system) and critique (object), thereby instituting (non-originally) their *difference.* "C/critique" *qua* "arche-critique" is a (non) 'originary' *différance*, then, precisely insofar as it is the sublime "supplement" to the logical system of philosophy; that is, at once both necessary and unassimilable. Within/without the Critical system, archi-critique "itself" (but this is exactly what is in question) is not an *is* but a *trace*; it brings forth infinitely (Gasché 1995, 116) the difference between the outside (doctrine) and the inside (critique) by virtue of remaining hidden. It is indeed, in Derrida's sense, an abyss. He writes,

> The principle of reason installs its empire only to the extent that the abyssal question of the being that is hiding within it remains hidden, and with it the question of the grounding of the ground itself, of grounding as *grunden* (to ground, to give or take ground: *Boden-nehmen*), as *begrunden* (to motivate, justify, authorize) or especially as *stiften* (to erect or institute, a meaning to which Heidegger accords a certain pre-eminence). (1983b, 10)

Clearly, this apocalyptic moment within modern philosophy has not simply been imposed on the basis of "postmodern" incredulity, nor has logic been refused or replaced with literariness. On the contrary, the discovery of a certain "unmasterable polytonality" at the heart of the political project of Enlightenment emerged through a logical inquiry into the structure of the Kantian Critique of pure reason. This "Critique," it must be underlined, is lauded for establishing legitimate, moral knowledge, and so marking the difference between the ethical and epistemological domains. Yet the undecidability in question – the *différance* from which derives the very *difference* between epistemological Legitimation and moral legitimacy (doctrine and critique) – imposed itself strictly by virtue of the fact that the possibility of Legitimacy has been taken entirely seriously. In the attempt to honour the classical principle of reason by 'going to the root' (Derrida 1983b, 8) *of* the normative principle of reason, we arrive at an uncircumventable breach in the speculative system itself. Therefore, it can be seen that it is precisely by paying heed to theory$_1$'s own "loftiest aims" (to borrow again the terms of Paul de Man's analysis) that we arrive at a knowledge (a theory$_2$) of the "resistance" to theory – a deconstructive potential for erosion – that inheres *in* the logical unity itself.

*

The consequences of this analysis for emancipatory political thought are profound and far-reaching. First and foremost, "critical" reason *qua* the emancipatory aim of Enlightenment is necessarily instituted violently. For critical consciousness is established by virtue of restricting the subject's logically undecidable, *excessive* imperative to respect the law (whichever one) – to a determinable object of its consciousness (*a* moral 'good') – and this means an illegitimate and unwarranted reduction has occurred. Regardless of the moral good that is at stake, in other words, the occlusion of the epistemological metanarrative's "hidden" (unrevealable) opening is what enables the possibility of critique.

Recall, in the first place, that the moral "interest" must be grounded or Legitimized – the reason for it must be rendered – since it is only in this way that the moral standard can be said to be rationally rather than arbitrarily based. As I elaborate in Part Two, this remains true whenever "critical reason" is at issue: the Legitimation of the legitimacy of moral knowledge is the epistemological role of a meta- Critique. Indeed, the relationship is maintained even in some versions of pragmatism. For example, if knowledge is said to be contingent in nature (Rorty 1989), then the moral "good" is deemed contingent as well, for precisely that reason. Thus, the relationship between what I am calling "Critique" and "critique" is not severed even if philosophy takes "post-foundational" form. This relationship has been particularly important for the historical development of philosophical reflection on education, moreover, because of the way in which it establishes the normative character of reason as critique. By incorporating morality into a logically coherent *system* (or "theory") of grounded knowledge, Kant turned ethico-political judgement into something we can know. A critical or emphatic conception of reason thereby became the normative ethos of the emancipatory, educative project of the modern "Enlightenment," and it remains much in evidence today.

Yet, in the second place, I have shown that the epistemological grounding or Legitimation of moral legitimacy only obtains by virtue of what I have called "arche-critique": the *différantial* "bringing forth" of the presentational system that Kant calls our inescapable, "sublime" response to the moral law of universalization. Thus, the moral "interest" of the modern subject is only knowable *as* that subject's transcendental essence by virtue of (a) *différance*. Otherwise understood, *différance* (is) the apocalyptic gesture that issues "come" or, alternatively, the sublime response that incites the philosophical investigation in the first place. What this means, however, is that the epistemological ground of the moral interest depends upon the occlusion of a philosophical *unknown*. Not only is the undecidable *différance* "hidden," it must remain so, in order for the *difference* between the moral subject and its epistemological object to be instituted or erected. This is why Kant's move is clearly illegitimate; logic can only be determined as primary with regard to language's rhetorical excess by virtue of the occlusion of *différance*.

Thus, moral legitimacy entails an ideological moment, and it is *inescapable*: the determination of a moral standard of critique entails a decision about the undecidable essence of the subject and, hence, depends upon the ideological erasure of the subject's "sublime," excess. The judgement which 'cuts' or decides the *différance* of "arche-critique" by instituting a *difference* between "Critique" and "critique" is thus itself not a "critical" judgement at all. It is, rather, a mystifying, *political* move whereby structural undecidablity is ideologically erased. It is specifically by virtue of this erasure that reason can be said to give rise to a standard of responsibility, to a basis for an emancipatory "critique."

As we shall see shortly, contemporary critical theorists of education do not leave the Kantian problematic of Legitimation behind because, in fact, they cannot. For, the ethico-political "freedom" said to ensue from "critique" is necessarily founded on an occlusion of the *différantial* (non) grounding of the difference between the subject and its moral object whenever the moral good is said to be rationally determinable – in effect, whenever social and political emancipation is associated with epistemological "enlightenment." A certain violence thus attends "critique" wherever and whenever it is invoked in the name of a determinate 'good' such as "freedom." It entails the illegitimate restriction of the subject to a particular essence, and it is not circumvented simply because one no longer determines the subject precisely as Kant did. In other words, we need not call our essence "freedom," nor need we name the subject as "supersensible man." On the contrary, although the Kantian approach is still undeniably appealing, there has been a veritable explosion of debate over the last few decades over the question of how to name the subject in a more politically progressive way; some alternatives to "Man" include, for example, woman, human, Black, worker and queer.

Yet this response to deconstruction is misguided. To be sure, the deconstructive exposure of "arche-critique" as an inherent resistance *to* theory from within it does decentre the transcendental subject. But in so doing, it puts into question the very notion of "responsibility" or "agency" that gains its *critical* force in precisely that way, and thereby destabilizes the critical ideal (as it has been understood traditionally) itself. In other words, a deconstructive interrogation of "critique" does not simply celebrate "difference" by shifting the site of moral agency – the root of ethico-political knowledge – from one kind of subject to a different one: from the transcendental to the empirical, from Man to Woman to the transexually-gendered, from White to Black, from the colonizer to the colonized, from the heterosexual to the gay, lesbian, bisexual or queer, from the able-bodied to the disabled or from the bourgeois individual to the working class as a group. It reveals, rather, that a (certain) subject(s) is *necessarily* inscribed as the transcendental site of unconditioned moral knowledge as soon as the emancipatory possibility of a rational standard for "critique" is invoked at all. This is a logical effect of the appeal to so-called "critical consciousness" *no matter which* subject(s) come to occupy the centre of the political–theoretical discourse.

To mobilize a rational standard of critique in the name of emancipation is to suppose there can be such a thing as a Legitimating meta-Critique (a metanarrative), by virtue of which the conditions for and the limits of knowledge can be established. Therefore, even in various contemporary versions of ideology critique (Marxist, feminist or multicultural, for example), a form of meta-Critique can be found at work in its original, speculative role; the meta-Critique is an overarching doctrine or "theory" within which the knowledge of moral legitimacy can emerge in demystified form (i.e., as unconditioned), and can thus be *known* as a standard of ethico-political "critique." The positing of a determinate standard of critique necessarily brings the Kantian formulation of the relationship between morality (or ethics) and epistemology into play, in other words, because the possibility of (re)presenting "freedom" as a transcendental *object* of the consciousness of the subject (as moral *knowledge*) requires epistemological justification, and this justification, in turn, entails that an unthematizable, sublime "response-ability" *to* the moral law is restricted (or, as it were, is "violently" object-ified) *as* the transcendental essence (as the unconditioned "as such") of the subject in its supersensibility. The "critical" consciousness by virtue of which moral legitimacy is objectified and thus known is, therefore (by definition) always already the consciousness *of* the transcendental subject, and this is true for Habermas no less than for Kant.[5]

As Derrida says,

> The modern dominance of the principle of reason had to go hand in hand with the interpretation of the essence of being as objects, an object present as representation [*Vorstellung*], an object placed and positioned *before* a subject. This latter, a man who says I, an ego certain of itself, thus ensures his own technical mastery over the totality of what is. The "re-" of *repraesentatio* also expresses the movement that accounts for – "renders reason to" – a thing whose presence is encountered by rendering it present, by bringing it to the subject of representation, to the knowing self. (1983b, 9–10)

Kant inscribes this relation of logical grounding and subjective "essence" when he determines the principle of morality as the "freedom" or the self-legislation of the subject. Indeed, we have seen, the universality or lawfulness of the moral law is "an object of our respect" and as such interests us a priori (as 'ground'), which is to say, transcendentally. Thus "respect" for the moral law can be determined as the epistemological object of pure practical reason and can be mastered, as such, *by* the transcendental subject who so determines it. To mobilize the notion of self-legislation (the subject's capacity for his, her or their self-determined "freedom") as a normative ideal, then, is simultaneously to 'name "Man" *into* being' – to transcendentalize the subject even in its specificity (as concretely embodied) – as well.

Significantly, therefore, the second consequence of the present analysis is that the violence is structural and, consequently, uncircumventable; it inheres in *any* naming whereby an unthematizable moral response is determined as what "we" *are* in order to establish what is legitimately 'good.' In other words, no matter how the subject is essentially determined, it cannot serve as the source or "cause" of a moral "imperative" unless it is first reduced to its own "mysterious" desire *for* moral legitimacy. For this desire, we have seen, can only be qualified as a moral imperative by virtue of a restriction of the "generalized" or the strictly unthematizable (e.g., "sublime") character of the subject to its purported *essence.* (This is why the question of "essentialism" continues to plague political movements based on identity.) Consequently, a claim made on the basis of a rational standard of critique – on the basis of a moral legitimacy that is known (and indeed taught as a politically progressive critical "consciousness") – is a claim that violently institutes a particular subject (one that is exclusive of other subjective possibilities) *as* the ground of the moral "good." It thereby repeats the Kantian manoeuvre. Insofar as a critical political theory assumes the possibility of a rational standard by which to determine moral legitimacy, in short, the critical reason at which it aims will still entail the occlusion of "C/critique."

Third and finally, since this "violence" is not imposed *on* the emancipatory ideal of "enlightenment" but emerges, instead, from within it, the imposition in question remains (almost) ineradicable *by* enlightenment. As I shall elaborate below, it is unavoidable precisely for we who, "in the daylight of today … cannot not have become the heirs of these *Lumières*" (Derrida 1983a, 22). Arche-critique *must* be occluded in the critical discourses of politics and education alike, in other words, as long as the political aim is entwined with the normative ethos of Enlightenment, which is to say, with the emancipatory promise of a legitimate, ethico-political critique. Exactly what is the normative status of this insight, of course, still remains to be seen. This is the focus of Part Three, where I offer a psychoanalytic explication of deconstruction as critique. But regardless of how deconstruction's critical status is understood, it remains that insofar as critical theorists presuppose that legitimate knowledge of a rational standard of critique is both achievable and teachable, they cannot leave the Enlightenment legacy behind. At the same time, if violence and mystification are inherent in critical reason itself, then deconstruction exposes an ideology we cannot do without.

In effect, what "we" (here, now, today) cannot do without is the possibility of *knowing* the difference between just and unjust norms. Not only must we be able to determine what is 'good,' but these determinations must themselves be decidable in terms of their justice. Thus, to represent deconstruction simply as anti-Enlightenment discourse – either as a nihilistic denial of "agency" (as "modernists" say), or as the replacement of the world-disclosing, logical capacity of language with language's aesthetic dimension (as "postmodernists" say)[6] – is not only to overlook the original co-implication of these categories. More importantly, it is to fail to understand that the emancipatory, critical pedagogical ideal cannot be retained if one discards the primacy of logic over rhetoric on which it depends. Consequently, I show, modernists cannot *but* have the upper argumentative hand.

For, even though the defenders of a certain "post"-modernity do not want to occlude the "sublime" or apocalyptic opening of the logical, philosophical discourse of Enlightenment, and even though they try to avoid enacting the "violence" that such an occlusion entails, they ultimately support the same "critical" reason that modernists themselves embrace. Indeed, theorists of critical, radical and feminist pedagogy attempt to think through the possibility of a teaching practice that explicitly aims to inculcate a capacity for "critical reason." Clearly, therefore, such theories can never be said to aim at less "enlightenment" rather than more. This "enlightenment" may now be seen to be based on an epistemological metanarrative that does not hold up, because it illegitimately reduces the subject in an unwarranted way to an arguable essence. But without this reduction, a rational standard of critique cannot be said to stand at all. Thus, radical political theorists (pedagogical or otherwise) cannot appeal to a fragmented, partial or ungrounded subject in the name of "postmodernism," except at the cost of an outright incoherence in the political–theoretical project itself.

Yet, at the same time, neither can those who would defend the emancipatory discourse of modernity dismiss deconstruction. To do so is to reinstate the ideological dimension of modern philosophy they explicitly hope to remove. In other words, as I show next, the paradoxical 'un-doing' or delegitimation of Enlightenment Legitimation imposes itself inescapably on theorists on both sides of the modernism–postmodernism divide. For, without the risk of its deconstruction, there is no "critical reason" to speak of at all. It is directly to the theoretical literature in education, therefore, that I now want to turn.

Notes

1 As Robert Bernasconi and Simon Critchley explain, "the figure of the chiasmus [is] etymologically constituted by the two lines of the Greek letter χ" (Bernasconi and Critchley, eds. 1991, xiii). Here perhaps a brief clarification is in order. "Critique" and "doctrine" can be said to form a möebius strip with regard to the simple question of their *difference*. The figure of the chiasmus represents the specific question of their *priority*.

2 I am indebted to Dieter Misgeld for these translations. The usage to which these have been put is my responsibility alone. Interestingly, in another context Derrida interprets a "keystone" as "a central, commanding point" (cited in Wortham 1999, 174).

3 On this point, see also the section entitled "On the Primacy of Pure Practical Reason in its Association with Speculative Reason" in the second *Critique* (1993a, 126–8). See also Lewis White Beck (in Kant 1993a, xv–xvi).

4 The most well-known version of this argument is the "generalization" of textuality, which Derrida calls "arche-writing." Derrida has similarly "generalized" the concept of "friendship" in his analysis of the distinction between politics and friendship, wherein he shows that the concept of "friendship," properly understood, must be both excluded from the political domain, and yet remain as its necessary condition of possibility (1988c). For a good explanation of Derrida's usage of the terms "restricted" and "generalized," see Alan Bass (in Derrida 1982 19, nt.23).

5 I develop this point in Chapter Eight.

6 Notable exceptions within the educational literature include Britzman (1998), Felman (1982) Flax (1992), Mohanty (1986) and Readings (1996).

Part II

The Ends of Education

5 From "Neo" to "Post"

Strategies in Theory

> [T]he "de-" of *de*construction signifies not the demolition of what is constructing itself, but rather what remains to be thought beyond the constructivist or destructionist scheme. What is at stake here is the entire debate, for instance, on the curriculum, literacy, etc.
>
> (Derrida 1988a, 147)

Contrary to what numerous political philosophers have assumed, "postmodernism" – at least in its deconstructive mode – does not spell the end of any kind of normative or political engagement whatsoever because deconstruction *is* a normative engagement in the classical philosophical sense. A deconstructive reading such as the one undertaken in the previous chapter honours the principle of reason by 'going to the root of' (by "radicalizing") the Kantian concept of "Critique." In particular, the above investigation into the conditions of possibility for "Legitimation" in its quintessential, modern sense (i.e., as the determination of grounds, or "Critique") reflects the attempt to bring reason to bear on (to render the reason *for*) reason's *own* ethico-political force. Ironically, if that investigation revealed the impossibility of the primacy of logic over rhetoric that modern political discourse seems to require for its very insistence *on* reason's ethico-political force, it remains that the result of this analysis is (it was always already) consequent upon the demand for Legitimation itself. For, the deconstructive investigation of epistemological Legitimacy can only destabilize the philosophical ethos of grounding action on reason to the extent that it heeds the classical philosophical imperative to render reason – to provide grounds and so to Legitimate – in the first place.

One way to understand this enigma, however, is to recall that the normative demand to which deconstruction responds – the demand that whenever reason can be "rendered" it *must* – did not originate at the onset of modernity, even though this demand takes its particular, contemporary meaning from Leibniz, who thematized it only then. For notwithstanding its modern articulation, the imperative to "render reason" by determining 'roots,' 'principles' and 'causes' was already deemed by Aristotle to be the paramount obligation of "metaphysics" or "primary philosophy"

(Derrida 1983b, 8). Thus, the primacy of logic that emancipatory thought reflects in its demand *for* legitimate "grounds," along with its "postmodern" deconstruction, can both be traced to a classical philosophical requirement that can be brought to bear, quasi-legitimately as it were, on the Enlightenment ethos of critical reason itself. It is for just this reason that I have suggested that deconstructive strategies of reading are properly characterized as "quasi-responsible" rather than as nihilistic – a claim to which I shall return again.

To be sure, such a "quasi-responsibility" *for* the principle of reason yields a number of paradoxical effects, the most important of which is arguably the emergence of that *différance* here called "C/critique." Specifically, I showed that *différance* – a structural necessity whereby "Critique" both must be and cannot be "critique" – (is) the logical condition of possibility for the specific *difference* between the (epistemo-) logical "meta" project of the transcendental Critique, and the micro standard of moral critique to which critical political theory appeals in the name of emancipatory ends.

It is only on the basis of an abyssal difference that it is logically impossible and yet politically necessary to bridge, then, that Kant can Legitimate (that he can logically ground) the moral standard he variously calls "freedom," "autonomy" or "self-legislation." As we have seen, this standard serves as the rational basis for ethico-political judgement and is therefore the minimal condition of possibility whereby a legitimate decision concerning justice can be said to obtain. What a deconstructive reading reveals, however, is that such a standard can only be established as epistemologically Legitimate (as properly "rational") insofar as Kant covers over the radical impossibility of its logical, a priori ground. He does so by determining the subject ideologically: the subject's unrepresentable, mysterious, sublime, response-ability or "respect" in the face of the strictly *theoretical* law of universalization is rendered *as* the subject's true essence and, as such, as the subject's *moral* end. The subject's "response-ability" to the law of universalization is thereby restricted as the objective, logical ground that Legitimates the transcendental, moral principle of freedom. Insofar as the subject in its transcendentality *is* morality's unconditioned ground, moreover, the philosophical discourse of modernity represents the original form of identity politics.

As I have explained, deconstructive strategies of reading decentre the subject on which this Enlightenment discourse, this very identity politics, is based. For this reason, deconstruction has been variously characterized as nihilistic, as morally reprehensible, or even as politically-pernicious nonsense (i.e., as a discourse that is said to "deconstruct itself" and thus to lie beyond the bounds of reasonable debate altogether). It is important to recall, however, that deconstruction merely reveals an ideological gesture that is *there*: a certain "mystagogy" inheres in the Kantian determination of a rational procedure for ethico-political critique. To say that deconstruction exposes the illegitimacy of an inescapable epistemological gesture that restricts the subject's "sublime" feeling of response-ability *as* its representable essence (and, as such, as a determinable object of transcendental knowledge), therefore, is also to say that the logical condition of Kantian critique *is* its (own) deconstruction. In effect, "critique" reveals itself as premised upon an ideological or mystagogical "centring" of the transcendental subject; critique reveals itself (self-deconstructs) insofar as a mystagogical move is the very condition of possibility *for* the meta-Critical determination of a non-ideological, demystifying, rational standard of ethico-political critique. Ironically, therefore, the *normative* outcome of deconstruction is the recognition that ideology is just what a political theory aimed at an emancipatory notion of reason – at the end of ideology and at the horizon of Enlightenment – needs.

It is in the context of this particular paradox that what I have called deconstruction's own "quasi-responsibility" comes into view. That is, if a deconstruction of the term "critique" reveals the rhetorical, the mystagogical, the apocalyptic, or what Kant himself calls the "sublime" opening of logical, philosophical thought on which the possibility of ethico-political legitimacy depends, and if it does so by respecting even more rigorously the normative principle of reason that impels us to seek after grounds (that is, to undertake a procedure of epistemological "Critique" or "Legitimation") than did the Kantian explication of ethico-political legitimacy in the first place, then this means that normative political thought will necessarily take on a significantly different aspect. As I will show, instead of being grounded on a determinate standard of critique, critical political theory must assume the manner of a "certain critique." This reformulation of critical theory in terms of *quasi* ethico-politico-philosophical form of responsibility is precisely what I undertake to explain in Part Three.

Before I do so, however, it is important to remark that the result of "critique's" (self) deconstruction is not only that critical political thought requires reformulation in terms of a "certain" critique. In addition to this, the above demonstration has another equally paradoxical result – one that is especially important for critical political theorists of education. It is that the ethico-political *ends* of educational theory require reformulation as well. For what follows from the analysis presented here is that a progressive pedagogical theory can either be aimed at inculcating a spirit of (quasi-) "critique," or it can be aimed at inculcating a determinate epistemological standard, but it cannot be coherently directed at both.

With regard to this second result, recall that the exposure of the (self) deconstruction of "Critique" is simply what happens if we look for the grounds of (if we undertake a meta-Critical investigation into) reason's ethico-political force. As we have seen, an investigation into the logical grounds of practical reason cannot be shown to issue in a determinate standard for "critique" without an ideological move that distinguishes Critique from critique. This move is the one which occludes a *différance* here called "C/critique" and thus effectively halts the meta-Critical investigation before it deconstructs (itself). In this sense, a meta-Critique reveals that the very achievement of a rational standard for micro critique signals an illegitimate closure of the responsibility *to* reason. Critical reason in the sense that Kant understood the term thus undoes itself; it always already de-legitimates the possibility of its own Legitimacy. It follows, therefore, that reason can give rise to (a "certain") critique, but it can do so only at the expense of a Legitimate (epistemologically grounded) ethico-political purchase on the question of what is legitimate (or 'good').

More significant still, this argument also holds the other way around. Just as a (quasi) *critical* theory of education that adheres rigorously to the protocols of Enlightenment Critique forgoes the political decision, so a *political* theory of education aimed at emancipation is won at the cost of denying the very critical impulse that gave rise to that project in the first place. For it is important to recall as well that it is by virtue of the achievement of a rational standard for critique that it was deemed possible to make a legitimate judgement about justice – a moral judgement, that is to say, about what 'ought' to be the case as compared to a merely theoretical judgement about what 'is.' Specifically, the practical knowledge of what one 'ought' to do was thought to be given by virtue of the rational standard for moral judgement that reason provides for itself (namely, autonomy as self-legislation). On this basis, Kant thought he had ensured a link between philosophy and politics – the very link, that is to say, that was first promised by the emancipatory idea of "Enlightenment." It is this political promise (said to be) inherent in philosophy that is inscribed in the modern, emancipatory discourse of education.

Now if, in the first place, the socio-political emancipation (said to be) consequent upon Enlightenment is based on a rational standard of critique by virtue of which the difference between justice and injustice can be known, and if, in the second place, the determination of such a standard depends upon a decision regarding the logical status of that rhetorical undecidable here called "C/critique," and if, in the third place, the primacy of logic over rhetoric that this decision (this 'cut' between Critique and critique) requires can only be accomplished by virtue of an illegitimate restriction of the subject to its ostensible essence – a restriction that halts the Critical investigation midway – then the illegitimate *closure* of Critique is just what a political educational theory aimed at emancipation needs. The second result of the above analysis, in other words – it follows from the meta-Critical exposure of the *différantial* structure of C/critique – is that if the knowledge of a rational, determinate standard for critique is *still* said to be possible notwithstanding its undecidable ground, then such knowledge is acquired only at the expense of the very (meta) Criticality that ostensibly lent practical reason its Legitimacy to begin with. This is why I maintain that the ethico-political end of education, its emancipatory promise, requires reformulation as well. Once the undecidable nature of

C/critique is exposed, it emerges that progressive theorists of education are faced with a choice. They can either advocate the inculcation of a capacity for "critical" reason (which will issue in deconstruction), *or* they can promote the knowledge of a politically emancipatory standard of critique (which will occlude *différance*). They cannot coherently do both of these at once.

This, at any rate, is the conclusion that follows from a deconstructive reading of the Kantian elucidation of "critique." The consideration at hand now, however, is the extent to which this conclusion can be generalized. For philosophical reflections on the social and political ends of education draw on a variety of different approaches, among which Kant's critical philosophy is only one. In addition to the Kantian formulation of transcendental "reason," for example, noted philosophical resources for educational theory include Freirean critical pedagogy, Deweyan pragmatism and Marxist, feminist and anti-racist critiques of ideology. These alternative theoretical resources are often mobilized (in various combinations) as bases for emancipatory theories of education and pedagogy and, without a doubt, each of them issues in an educational project that is significantly different from Kant's. It would seem perfectly plausible, therefore, to object that one can formulate a politically emancipatory, critical theory of education that explicitly denounces the modern metaphysical tradition, and that therefore evades the problems inherent in theories that draw on Kant. It is this objection that the present part of this study is intended to address.

Specifically, I argue that the Kantian formulation of "critical reason" does not warrant the intense focus to which I have submitted it merely because, as Wilfred Carr puts it, "the Enlightenment conceptions of reason and the rational subject … received their clearest expression in the philosophy of Kant" (1995, 79). More importantly, Kant's formulation warrants this focus because, notwithstanding the fact that contemporary theorists and philosophers of education mobilize just such alternative philosophical resources as those identified above in order to develop a "postmetaphysical" standard of critique, they do so without fully appreciating that the idea of critical inquiry at work in emancipatory theories of education is *already* dependent on Kant. At the deepest level of analysis to which these attempts can be put, in short, there is no alternative to the Kantian philosophical paradigm.

In particular, I submit, what is peculiarly Kantian (as well as, more generally, quintessentially modern) is not the specific procedure for (or the standard of) legitimacy that Kant himself upheld. More fundamentally, it is the assumption that underlies that procedure or standard; namely, that a principle of ethico-political judgement is something we can teach because it is something we can establish legitimately, without recourse to ideology, mere opinion, or culturally-contingent mores. Insofar as this basic, meta-epistemological claim is implied, there is an assumed relationship between epistemological grounds (Critique) and ethical judgement (critique) – the assumption obtains, in other words, that there can and must be such a thing as moral *legitimacy* in the first place. This is the core of the idea of Enlightenment as emancipation that Kant was the first to elaborate, and its continued political significance is precisely why debates within philosophy about the legacy of 'pure' reason carry so much political weight.

Theorists and philosophers of education who believe (whether happily or unhappily) that a deconstructive reading of philosophy reverses the logic–rhetoric dualism – that it celebrates the aesthetic or rhetorical dimension of literature and narrative as an alternative 'good' over the logical, world-disclosing, problem-solving capacity of philosophy and science – are thus fundamentally misguided, certainly with regard to the problem that Derrida's work actually poses for the political ideal of emancipation through education, possibly with regard to the nature of that emancipatory ideal itself, and sometimes with regard to both. For they fail to appreciate that deconstruction demonstrates the irresolvable *co-implication* of the two sets of categories (logic and rhetoric) rather than the epistemological primacy of either one and, thus, that deconstruction has implications for the very possibility of moral legitimacy as such.

When focused on the concept of "critique," for example, deconstruction reveals a bond between the epistemological and the ethical levels of legitimation that is *both* inescapable for political theory (logically necessary and, hence, ineliminable by a "postmodern" theory of emancipation) *and*, yet, ideologically established (i.e., rhetorically or "mystically founded" [Derrida 1992a] and, hence, irredeemable by a modernist theory as well). That both of these characteristics apply has been shown by the previous analysis. The bond between ethics and epistemology is inescapable in the sense that a rational standard of ethico-political critique necessarily mobilizes the epistemological metanarrative or Critique; it does so because it is the theoretical metanarrative (the doctrinal meta-Critique) that grounds moral knowledge in logical terms, and thereby determines its specificity as a distinct epistemological object. Only in this way is the possibility of a rational standard for critique both logically confirmed and epistemologically known. But the bond between epistemology and ethics is ideologically established as well. For moral legitimacy requires – for its very specificity as a moral rather than an epistemological 'object' – that a restricted, logical difference between meta "Critique" and micro "critique" can be said to obtain. And, as we have seen, the condition of possibility for this difference is a generalized and hence a logically undecidable *différance*: the notion of "arche-critique" (or "C/critique"). Since this undecidable is covered over (it is mystified) as soon as the difference is established, there is an ideological moment inherent in the very determination of an epistemologically legitimate standard of moral critique. The corollary of the deconstruction of the concept of "critique," therefore – and thus the precise problem that a certain "postmodernism" poses for educational theory – is that *the possibility of moral legitimacy in particular cannot be coherently separated from a meta-Critical, epistemological, "metanarrative" of Legitimation in general, but nor can it be finally cleansed.* To attempt either of these moves is to reinstate rather than resolve Kant's dilemma. This is the problem (it is one of them, at any rate) that a *critical* theory of education must seek to address.

If this problem is underappreciated, however, it may be because so many theorists have followed Lyotard, who himself misrepresents the nature of the "postmodern condition" with regard to this point. Specifically, Lyotard fails to underline the ways in which practical and theoretical reason (or ethics and epistemology) are necessarily co-implicated for modernity. As a result, he characterizes the discourse of emancipation erroneously: as equivalent to, and as separate from, the scientific metanarrative of Legitimation.

In response to Lyotard's characterization of two distinct metanarratives, it was therefore important to underscore that the emancipatory, *political* end of Enlightenment was only ever thought to be guaranteed by virtue of the inclusion of ethical reasoning into a philosophical, speculative, *scientific* system of Critique. Indeed, we have seen, reason can be said to embody the specific emancipatory interest that Kant described only insofar as the three "faculties" of reason (theoretical, practical and aesthetic) are each logically grounded and systematized together in a scientific doctrine (a metanarrative) of pure philosophy. As I have explained, the Legitimacy of practical reason thus depends entirely on the primacy of scientific logic that Kant borrowed from the classical model of the *trivium*. That is to say, it is by virtue of the very subjugation of rhetoric by logic and its isotope grammar within the *trivium* – or, analogously in the Kantian architectonic, by virtue of the epistemological primacy of the purely aesthetic judgement of taste with its logical principle of "subjective purposiveness" over the potential irruption of the sublime – that it was possible to establish the coherence of that scientific system (*theōria*) within which moral knowledge could be enclosed as one of reason's objective "interests." The primacy of logic over rhetoric that was based on the classical *trivium* and later fully realized in the Kantian architectonic, therefore, is what guaranteed the coherence of a system that is the *sine qua non* of a legitimate, non-relative knowledge of the moral world. And the possibility of this practical knowledge, in turn, is what promises emancipation.

It is perhaps unsurprising, then, that Derrida, de Man and other "deconstructionists" are taken to task by political and educational philosophers alike; they are seen as advocating (with Lyotard) a reversal of the very relationship between logic and rhetoric that "critical" reason requires. Yet even if the case against (or, indeed, for) deconstruction is not nearly so clear, its threat to the Enlightenment conception of emancipation stands; as critics of deconstruction well know, a challenge to the primacy and autonomy of logic is at once a challenge to the scientific or systematic coherence that grants a standard of ethico-political "critique" its duly rational (and, hence, its *non*-relative, and *non*-ideological) status.

Critical theorists of education who believe that a "postmodern" interrogation of reason entails reversing logic and rhetoric as though these are equivalent *values* and, relatedly, that it is possible to uphold a discourse of emancipation in distinction from a scientific one, are thus mobilizing the modern belief in moral legitimacy (in an ethico-political standard that is epistemologically justified) even while they discard Kant's Critique (the justificatory apparatus). As a result, they are faced with a particular burden that those who would defend a modern conception of reason are quick to point out. It is that if an ethico-political notion of the 'good' such as "voice," self-legislation or self-determination is taken out of Kant's meta-Critical (transcendental) system but is still understood to serve as a political standard in any meaningful sense (as a fixed measure), the 'good' must be otherwise authorized. Thus, unless some "metanarrative" other than Kant's is provided for the specification and Legitimation of a standard of critique, unless some generalized account of the moral 'ends' of 'man' *qua* "Man," or, alternatively, *qua* "human," *qua* "Woman," *qua* "Black" or *qua* "queer" (for example) is provided to serve the same meta-Legitimating role as the Kantian Critique, the risk at hand – even as it is identified by "postmodern" critical theorists of education themselves – is that of an arguably relative political 'good.'

The point here is not that one can avoid mobilizing a determinate notion of the 'good' in any given moment of political contest; on the contrary, one always fights for, resists, defends or upholds some*thing* in particular. Whenever one is taking a stand on justice one necessarily (inescapably) engages in just this kind of rhetoric. The point, rather, is that such claims will have politically exclusionary effects, because they will have to entail an unjustifiable 'restriction' of what is 'generally' undecidable – namely, the political subject's moral 'end' – in order to establish the basis for a determinate notion of justice that can be brought to bear against what is considered unjust. A theory of education or of politics that purports to be *critical*, therefore, must take responsibility for, must render reason to, the ideological nature of this restriction.

I return to the question of this necessary responsibility, this moral "must," below. For now I want only to underline that what follows from the very nature of moral legitimacy is this: to dismiss the Enlightenment "metanarrative" as hopelessly metaphysical, as "fictional" or as based on a "literary" narrative instead of on pure science, is necessarily to cede the possibility of a determinate standard for (micro) critique as well, regardless of where (in which alternative philosophical tradition) this standard is said to be found. The one theoretical option that is not available, in other words, is that of maintaining that critical consciousness can issue in or can be based upon a determinate, knowable and legitimately generalizable political 'good' (such as "freedom," "autonomy," "self-legislation" or "voice") notwithstanding our "incredulity" in the face of the Enlightenment metanarrative of Legitimation. Once we have rendered the "postmodern" condition more accurately in terms of a potential for internal deconstruction (or "erosion") that inheres in the Enlightenment metanarrative of emancipation as a whole, in short, it is possible to see how the Kantian problematic bears on contemporary progressive pedagogical theory, and by extension on critical theory more generally, even in the context of an explicit rejection or reformulation of Kant's emphasis on the scientific dimension of moral philosophy. For, theorists of education who adopt a Lyotardian rejection of Enlightenment speculation but still view education in its quintessentially political sense – as a vehicle of social emancipation – find themselves caught on the horns of a dilemma.

On one hand, insofar as one wishes to maintain the possibility of a critical standard by virtue of which the difference between justice and injustice can be legitimately established, one will necessarily invoke some version of the Kantian apparatus of (epistemological) Critique along with it. Those who opt for the strategy of endorsing a determinate standard of critique can thus be shown to reinscribe (albeit inadvertently) the very transcendentalism that the proposed, "post-metaphysical" alternative is intended to displace, even while they purport to have left the Enlightenment metanarrative of speculative philosophy behind. On the other hand, insofar as one gives up on the possibility of modern "reason" (the scientific metanarrative of Legitimation) in view of its exclusionary effects, one must discard its attendant standard of rational critique as well. In this case, one would be left with a purely ethical or political understanding of the 'good' that is essentially singular; such an understanding is thus strictly unrepresentable in or by a *theory* of educational aims. A genuinely contingent and indeterminate political 'good' that makes no epistemological claims whatsoever, in other words, can be neither generalized legitimately nor even specified adequately.

Thus, for instance, norms such as "responsibility," "solidarity," "tolerance" or the imperative to alleviate "suffering" may well be rhetorically powerful and even politically effective, and any of these might conceivably forgo epistemological Legitimation.[1] It remains, however, that these norms are not only highly contestable, as numerous critics rightly suggest; in addition, they are impossible to pin down epistemologically, and therefore serve strangely as the substance of an emancipatory educational project that purports to inculcate a determinate and hence knowable standard of critique. As I shall demonstrate, theorists who adopt the strategy of dismissing Enlightenment philosophy *tout court* in the name of an emancipatory politics aimed at such goods as social tolerance or collective solidarity are therefore regularly (and indeed rightly) accused of explaining the educational dimension of the proposed political practice on grounds that are logically nonsensical. The reason that Kant's critical philosophy may be said to be centrally implicated even in educational theories that differ significantly from it, in short, is that the very idea of "criticality" that various progressive theorists of education support – and, indeed, that they need to support if the educative practice they espouse is to be both epistemologically sound and politically emancipatory as many insist that it must – already embodies Kant's philosophical legacy.

In order to substantiate this claim, that the political purchase of progressive educational theory is bought at the cost of metaphysically 'centring' or transcendentalizing the subject (and, thus, at the cost of the persistence of C/critique), I investigate in the three chapters that follow the three strategic responses to "postmodernism" that are most prevalent in critical pedagogical and educational theory. These strategies are designated in what follows as "neomodernist," "anti-modernist" and "anti-postmodernist" respectively. They entail the attempt to *separate* or decouple ethico-political critique from its epistemological framework (from Kant's Critique) while trying to retain critical legitimacy (neomodernism); the attempt to formulate a political educational theory and practice that entirely *takes the place of* the philosophical discourse of modernity – that is, to do without rational critique and the Legitimating framework of Critique alike (anti-modernism) – and, finally, the attempt to *counter* contemporary interrogations of the Enlightenment metanarrative and the moral legitimacy that goes with it by Legitimating moral universalism in terms of a contingent and fallible notion of reason that is ostensibly non- or only quasi-transcendental (anti-postmodernism).

This third strategy, which I call the "Habermasian gambit," entails the attempt to reformulate the Critical metanarrative such that it no longer suffers from Kantian metaphysics, but still serves as a quasi-transcendental, epistemological Legitimation of critique.[2] Specifically, as I demonstrate in Chapter Eight with regard to the anti-postmodernist approach, theorists such as Nigel Blake, Helmut Peukert, Wendy Kohli, Les Burwood and Harvey Siegel depend on Jürgen Habermas's theory of communicative ethics to counter the "postmodern" critique of Enlightenment. I show, however, that Habermas fails to ground critique non-metaphysically. Before I develop that case, however, it is important to stress that the Kantian problematic – the impossible but necessary co-implication of Critique and critique – is not simply bypassed in either the "neo"- or the "anti"- modernist case either.

On the contrary, with regard to those who adopt the "neomodernist" strategy of maintaining a morally legitimate standard of critique while (ostensibly) eschewing the metaphysics of Kantian "reason," the tension between transcendentalism and relativism is plainly in view in the work of those such as Peter McLaren, Henry Giroux, Peter Roberts, William Carr, Paul Smeyers, and Willem Wardekker and Siebren Miedema. This approach to educational theory is treated in Chapter Six. With regard to those who lean more heavily in the direction of the second ("anti-modernist") strategy, on the other hand – those who advocate displacing the philosophical apparatus of "Critique" altogether by reversing the categories of logic and rhetoric with a view to endorsing the latter – the work of those such as

Elizabeth Ellsworth, Suzanne de Castell, Patti Lather, Vincent Arcilla, Cameron McCarthy and Patrick McGee will be shown to be especially relevant. As I recall in Chapter Seven, the sublime can no more be promoted to a place of total primacy within the Kantian system that produces it than can rhetoric within the *trivium*. For, we have seen, "*nothing* can overcome the [logical] resistance to theory [*qua* rhetorical reading]," because "theory *is* itself this resistance" (de Man 1982, 20; first emphasis mine). Consequently, the proposal to replace traditional philosophical categories based on reason with such categories as rhetoric, sublimity, partiality or difference emerges as both theoretically misguided and as practically impossible. Thus, we shall see that problems that attend the concept of "critique" – problems revealed in contemporary continental analyses of modern philosophy but misdiagnosed in "modern" and so-called "postmodern" social theory alike – lead to irresolvable difficulties in the first two cases as well.

Notes

1 One might cite numerous examples. Regarding "responsibility," for instance, Emmanuel Levinas offers a phenomenological rather than a strictly epistemological justificatory frame (Levinas 1989, 1991). Analogously, Charles Taylor attempts to make a communitarian argument for "tolerance" based on the inherent value of certain traditions (in Gutmann, ed., 1994). Compare Richard Rorty (1989), who follows John Dewey in supporting the good of "solidarity" on the explicitly political grounds of democratic forms of social organization.

2 While views that cannot be included in this rough framework undoubtedly exist, my purpose in this section is not to be exhaustive; rather, it is to illustrate the most general tendencies among, and the most common difficulties that attend, critical theories that are engaged with "postmodernism." This analysis of a series of critical educational theoretical strategies is directly applicable to the field of critical political theory more broadly, insofar as I treat what are arguably still the most common and influential approaches to "postmodernism."

6 Neomodernist Critical Pedagogy

Among the three strategic approaches to "postmodernism" listed in the previous chapter, "neomodernism" is problematic in a way that other responses to "postmodernism" are not. For unlike either the anti-modernists or the outright anti-postmodernists, neomodernists try to have it both ways. Neomodernists both reject *and* mobilize modern Enlightenment principles, even while they refuse *and* embrace, simultaneously, various critiques of modernity. The distinct problem with this approach is therefore that either it offers no real alternative because it is surreptitiously based on an illegitimate centring of the subject (on Kant's transcendental manoeuvre) – or else it entails forgoing the ethico-political legitimacy which neomodernists nonetheless claim. And what this means is that "neomodernism" is not only marred by difficulties that attend every attempt to mobilize the concept of "critique" for emancipatory political ends; it is theoretically incoherent as well.

Consider, for example, John and Jean Comaroff's description of the "neomodern" response to the "postmodern condition," from whom critical educational theorist Peter McLaren borrows the term "neomodernism" (McLaren and Giarelli 1995, 13). According to McLaren, the Comaroffs say that this is a method of social scientific inquiry into ideology that,

> takes seriously the message of critical postmodernism yet does not lose the possibility of social science; that takes to heart the lessons of cultural Marxism, seeking a conception of culture that recognizes the reality of power, yet does not reduce meaning to either utility or domination; that builds on the techniques of cultural history, pursuing the dialectic of fragment and totality without succumbing to brute empiricism; that, above all, proceeds, as it must, by grappling with the contradictions of its own legacy, seeking to transcend them – if only provisionally and for the moment. (Qtd. in McLaren 1995, 278)

What I distinguish as "neomodern" is exactly this: the strategic assumption of the legitimacy of modern ethical and epistemological norms in the face of a "critical postmodernism" that subjects those norms to epistemological and political contest.[1]

McLaren claims, for instance, that

> Critical ethnographers need to develop the will and the competence to reposition their sites of enunciation and narrative authority and to make choices outside the comfort and danger of an *a priori* standard based on Western, monocultural and universal constructions of identity and difference. (1995, 291)

Just as this claim explicitly refuses the metaphysics of Kant's conception of "Enlightenment," so McLaren elsewhere endorses "a postcolonial pedagogy and research practice [that] avoids a collusion with the antimonies of essential oppositions such as self/other by refusing the Hegelian foundationalism of positing the self-identical ground of all difference" (McLaren and Giarelli 1995, 14). On the one hand, we thus find throughout McLaren's work a clear rejection of the "impartial universal absolutism or foundationalism" (McLaren and Giarelli 1995, 7) that epitomize the modern philosophical tradition. Even in an early piece in which he announced his own "ambivalence toward postmodernity" (1988, 66, and 77 nt.1, 79 nt.5), McLaren maintained that

> [t]he project of placing desire into critical and self-conscious circulation ... needs a *non-totalizing language* that refuses to strip experience from its contingency and open-endedness, that refuses to textualize oppression, and that refuses to dehistoricize or desexualize or degender the body, or to smooth over difference in the name of justice or equality. (1988, 67; emphasis added, internal reference omitted)

Because McLaren objects to "the Enlightenment ideal of a unified human subject" and "the conventions of teleological closure" (Lankshear and McLaren 1993, 47), he rejects the orthodox Marxist perspective from which "the concept of ideology must be defended as something to be logically unveiled according to a defensible criterion rooted in objective reality" (1989b, 176) and which emphasizes "the primary determinants of distortion and false consciousness" (1989b, 200). This understanding of ideology as "false consciousness," he maintains, is based on "claims of science to universality, scientificity, and normativity," and is "grounded in an *essentialist* conception of society and social agency" (1989b, 180, 179; 180 emphasis his). According to McLaren, these conceptions have been seriously weakened by (among others) Ernesto Laclau's post-structural adaptation of Gramsci and Althusser, insofar as Laclau sees the social as indeterminate in nature and as fundamentally exceeding any structuralist constraint. As McLaren writes,

> This perspective highlights the relational character of identity and at the same time clearly renounces the fixation of those identities in a

> system. Instead, Laclau links the social with *an infinite play of discursive differences.* Thus the meaning of the social becomes impossible to fix because it no longer takes the form of an underlying essence. (1989b, 180; his emphasis)

McLaren therefore proposes to replace the epistemological categories of "true" and "false" (consciousness) with the ethico-political categories of "emancipation" and "domination." Drawing on Ernst Bloch, he argues that although we cannot distinguish between ideological and non-ideological representations of reality on the basis of a criterion of "truth" – because, as Foucault argued, the "'effects of truth' are produced within discourses that are neither true nor false" (1989b, 183) – we *can* distinguish, *within* those discursive frameworks, between "good" and "bad" ideology (1989b, 185).

"Good" ideology, for McLaren, is ideology in its "positive," or enabling function (1989b, 188, 189). As he explains,

> although particular discourses considered in isolation may indeed be structured in dominance within capitalist productive relations, nevertheless, through particular intersections, forms of reversal, and combinations with other discourses they may also be … capable of generating forms of knowledge which effectively escape assimilation into the dominated contents of capital accumulation. (1989b, 185)

"Bad" ideology, in contrast, refers to the way in which the discourses, narratives and symbolic frameworks that allow us to make sense of and to act meaningfully in the world will inevitably be selective and thus distorting to some extent. Because the negative function of ideology therefore goes hand in hand with its positive function, McLaren speaks of ideology as a "double-sided process" (1989b, 187).

But McLaren's eschewal of Enlightenment scientism with its stress on objective truth is not at all consistent. For just as Bloch links good and bad ideology to "*true* false consciousness" and "false consciousness" respectively, according to McLaren (1989b, 185; my emphasis), so McLaren himself stresses that understanding ideology requires "investigating *which* concepts, values and meanings mystify our understanding of the social world and our place within the networks of power–knowledge relations, and which clarify such an understanding" (1989b, 188; emphasis his). McLaren cites Henry Giroux on this point as well, noting that "Giroux defines ideology as generic with 'the production, consumption, and representation of ideas and behaviour, which can *either distort or illuminate* the nature of reality'" (1989b, 188; emphasis mine).

Given that McLaren's own understanding of ideology as simultaneously enabling and constraining logically precludes the existence of a non-mystifying concept *per se*, this seems an odd claim to make. More importantly, however, these comments indicate that McLaren is mobilizing the classic Enlightenment view: the purchase of critique hinges on its capacity to "illuminate" the nature of reality. The fact that McLaren defines ideology in the ethico-political terms of "domination" and "emancipation" rather than in terms of truth and falsehood does nothing to displace this assumption. McLaren's protestations notwithstanding, therefore, "critique" as it is explicated here does not diverge substantially from the sense it already had for Kant: an epistemological lever by virtue of which a legitimate moral decision can be reached (cf. Lankshear and McLaren 1993, 21, 42). To the extent that McLaren does not contest the epistemological status of "critique," he has not actually decoupled moral legitimacy from the epistemological (or meta-Critical) framework on which that legitimacy depends.

One might of course object, here, that the reference to clarifying *rather than* mystifying concepts and values is merely a moment of awkwardness in McLaren's thinking. This awkwardness does not implicate the broader argument that social relations are contingently, discursively and only ever incompletely structured. As a result, ideologies need not be conceived in exclusively negative terms; arguably, they can mobilize people for social change even though they may also have constraining or dominating effects. For example, as McLaren goes on to argue, political–theoretical analysis should aim at determining the "various *degrees* of an emancipatory or dominating logic" that social relations and practices represent, and this analysis should be based on "a set of core ethical principles" rather than on empirical criteria (1989b, 199; emphasis added). He writes,

> At this point I would assert that it matters less that any test for the "truth" of an idea is incontrovertible than that the idea can be linked to a praxis of emancipation. Although political praxis cannot be the criterion for theoretical truth, it is politics, not philosophy or science, which seems the more appropriate site for understanding the rules of justice and social transformation. (1989b, 199)

On its face, the claim seems persuasive enough. It does not address the challenge that deconstruction poses to emancipatory political thought, however, because it fails to account for the necessity of grounding political principles epistemologically. In other words, the claim that an analysis is propelled by ethical principles rather than by empirical or speculative "truth" does not alter in any way the strictly logical function such principles must serve; namely, as the basis for an epistemological cut between emancipation and domination, by virtue of which we can know the difference between them. And, once they are seen to perform this irreducible epistemological role, the principle(s) of critique themselves must be rationally determinable. First, therefore, one would need to know what *are* the "core ethical principles" that allow one to gauge the 'degree of emancipatory logic' a given set of social relations entails. Second, the objection still persists: by virtue of what are one's "rules of justice" legitimately generalizable and determinate *principles* of critique that can be brought to bear on a contingent political situation in the service of illuminating or clarifying what is (truly) 'just'? In the absence of a *knowledge* of the 'good', how can any specific ethical principles escape the charge that they represent a politically-interested, dogmatic and purely strategic attempt to get what "we" want now? Does this charge not apply precisely when "politics" is given as the "site for understanding the rules of justice and social transformation"?

It was exactly this question, 'how do we *know* what we ought to do,' that provoked Kant's analysis in the first place. The question is not rendered irrelevant simply because one calls for a "non-totalizing language" that eschews the "impartial universal absolutism and foundationalism" of modern philosophy. On the contrary, McLaren recognizes the need to universalize his claims if they are to bear the political purchase he intends. He says, "Somewhere between the essentialism of the orthodox position and the voluntarism of the ultrarelativists, *a common ground for discussing ideology* must be sought by both Marxists and nonMarxists alike" (1989b, 200; emphasis mine). Similarly, he writes elsewhere,

> We need to understand, as critical educators, that we are living in an epochal transition to an era of multiple feminisms, liberalisms, Marxisms which, on the one hand, hold the enabling promise of liberation, while on the other hand threaten to splinter the Left irrevocably in a maze of often mutually antagonistic micro-politics. This calls for some form of *totalizing vision* – what I want to call an arch of social dreaming – that spans the current divisiveness we are witnessing within the field. (1988, 74; my emphasis)

It follows on the basis of McLaren's own view, therefore, that unless some form of "metanarrative" of the political subject's moral ends *other than* Kant's is provided for the Legitimation of a standard of critique, the risk at hand is that of a relative and indeterminate political principle. As McLaren and Giarelli say,

> Unless we have some provisional narrative of liberation, we can easily and unknowingly establish . . . practices that fall prey to the very error that critical educators seek to correct, that duplicate the original silencing of the Other, that replicate the concepts and systems of power they seek to revoke, that relegitimate the very terms they seek to reject. (McLaren and Giarelli 1995, 9–10)

This metanarrative need not take the form of Kant's or Hegel's in order to embody the illegitimate primacy of logic over rhetoric that a deconstructive analysis reveals. Indeed, in this case the illegitimately-determined 'good' McLaren wants to avoid *is* the one contained in the "Eurocentric, patriarchal, and colonialist narratives" (McLaren and Giarelli 1995, 10) derived from the Enlightenment. Nonetheless, it makes no difference which metanarrative one espouses with regard to the way in which the argument structurally demands what I have called the occlusion of C/critique. For what McLaren and James Giarelli are here emphasizing is that, unless the ethical principles underlying critique are grounded on a broader vision of *human* emancipation, the liberating promise will be lost in antagonistic, micro-political battles. To this end, the principle guiding critique must be robust enough, compelling enough and firmly enough grounded on what is *universally* true to bridge the political divisiveness McLaren identifies and to point towards a broadly acceptable "common good" (see McLaren 1988, 73). This is why a "metanarrative" or "totalizing vision" is required, however "provisional" it is said to be (McLaren and Giarelli 1995, 8, 9).

As McLaren well knows, however, whatever is said to be true about our moral "ends" will be vulnerable to a deconstructive critique, because any determination of *the* universal human interest will entail restricting the subject to an essence that is constitutively undecidable and that, consequently, will have been violently reduced in order to be known (i.e., to be representable by a subject as an object of its consciousness). In other words, *if* all "representation is re-presentation within particular ideological configurations" and "every signification constitutes a mask" (McLaren 1995, 281) – *if*, so to say, rhetorical undecidability is a constitutive feature of logical determination – then any representation of the subject's "ends" will "constrain" *as well as* "enable" human liberation, because it will exclude other features of human experience or social action that need to be revealed (i.e., the representation will also take the pernicious form of "negative" ideology). In effect, then, McLaren's "neomodern" response to the postmodern condition is that ideology critique both does and does not illuminate what is really 'true' because it both is and is not based on legitimate knowledge (on an undistorted epistemological perspective) at the same time.

McLaren fares no better in the attempt to provide an alternative to Kant's transcendental principle of moral "autonomy" than he does in the attempt to overcome the need for a Legitimating, epistemological frame. On the contrary, the "core ethical principles" of critical pedagogy that he calls for are virtually impossible to pin down. Certainly, it is as true for him as for first generation critical theorists that the ultimate target of political theory is "the reality of human suffering and struggle in a world rife with pain and suffering" (McLaren and Lankshear 1993, 412). McLaren speaks of "a new ethics [or ethos] of compassion and solidarity" (1988, 70, 74), for example, and of "relations of cooperation, mutuality, and reciprocity" (1995, 273). But these claims are only meaningful contextually; unless compassion and suffering are conceived as all or nothing propositions (i.e., as absolute categories whereby they are said to obtain either purely, or not at all), the moral line between "justice" and "injustice" will have to be determined within particular socio-political contexts and with regard to particular, political claims. This is precisely where a *logical* principle of ethico-political critique will come into play, a principle by virtue of which the *difference* between oppression and liberation can be logically established.

McLaren makes a number of gestures in this direction, but they are either inconsistent or ambiguous. Most notable are his arguments concerning bodily authenticity (McLaren 1988, 70, and 1995, 280) and the "hermeneutical privilege" or "prominence" he urges on behalf of marginalized "Others" (McLaren 1988, 75, and 1995, 289; McLaren and Lankshear 1993, 406). To be sure, either the "body" or the "voice" of the oppressed can function as the critical lever McLaren requires, but they can only do so at the cost of (re)essentializing the subject, that is, by signifying an ontological 'real' that speaks simply for itself in a transparent and undistorted way. Perhaps in recognition of this, McLaren tends to undercut his claims at the very moment that he makes them. In so doing, however, he unwittingly undercuts the standard of critique by virtue of which the 'degree of emancipatory logic' can be gauged.

With reference to the body as a category of political–theoretical analysis, for example, McLaren writes,

> The ethical project known as critical ethnography is one that does not emerge transcendentally in textual forms detached from perception, bodily experience, and the friction of social reality. It is an ethics that emerges concretely *from the body, is situated in the materiality and historicity of discourse, in the call of the flesh, in the folds of desire.* (1995, 280; emphasis his, internal reference omitted)

On first consideration, this seems significantly different than the transcendental principle of autonomy theorized by Kant. Unlike the category of "pure reason," bodily experience is said to be socially, historically, politically and discursively produced. Specifically, "the body" is for McLaren "an effect of power/knowledge relations and … a site of their articulation" just as, conversely, knowledge can be understood as "a typography of embodiment" (1995, 279) by virtue of which "culture is somatized" or "incarnated in and through our bodily acts and gestures" (1989b, 191). In McLaren's concept of "enfleshment," then, we seem to encounter a thoroughly constructivist notion of bodily experience: there is virtually nothing "essential" about it. Thus, the category of "the body" apparently obviates the entire Critical apparatus of the Kantian architectonic; it is posited as an alternative, non-transcendental standard of ethico-political critique that is politically rather than epistemologically based.

Significantly, however, a closer examination of the way in which the body serves as a critical category reveals the same choice that emerged from the deconstruction of Kant's "Critique": one can aim at inculcating a (certain) spirit of "critique," or one can aim at inculcating ethical–political knowledge of the good (a determinate epistemological standard), but one cannot coherently do both. Similarly, McLaren's critical category of bodily experience can *either* impel the delegitimation of traditional socio-political norms, *or* it can serve as a legitimate standard of critique by virtue of which the difference between justice and injustice can be known. But the second possibility depends on a metaphysical and hence illegitimate determination of the subject's transcendental essence, and therefore forecloses the possibility of the first.

That bodily experience can inform a certain (deconstructive) form of critique is clear from McLaren's remarks. He suggests that,

> it is imperative that as educators for the postmodern age we begin to examine issues such as the feminization and masculinization of the body and the reification of the body politic. We need to study how our needs and desires as educators have been shaped in contradictory ways through dominant cultural forms, modes of subjectivity, and circuits of power. A critical pedagogy must grapple with the ways in which youth resist the dominant culture *at the level of their bodies* because in so doing the utopian moments to which such resistance points can be transformed pedagogically into strategies of empowerment. (1988, 69–70; his emphasis, internal reference omitted)

However, this understanding of "critique" as the critical interrogation of Western culture based on contingent bodily experience or desire does not deliver what McLaren promises: a "totalizing vision" of liberation that "transcends" the contradictions of the modernist legacy (1995, 278), or a "pedagogy of hope" that leads to a concrete political "praxis" (1988, 71, 72). It can reveal those contradictions, but it cannot resolve them, because it does not contain (nor is it said to contain) a legitimate ethico-political purchase on the question of what is 'good.'

On the contrary, McLaren argues that bodily experience only becomes meaningful insofar as it is discursively representable – through, that is to say, symbolic frameworks of representation that are themselves locally, historically, socio-politically and contradictorily structured. Such experiences are given as subsequent effects of discourse, in short, rather than pre-existing, ontological facts. Understood in this way, they cannot be said to ground an alternative vision of the 'good', because any experience or desire that would be posited as a ground for critique would be as contestable as whatever is displaced. Nonetheless, a resistance rooted in the body might well be mobilized to contest prevailing ethical or political norms and, thereby, to give rise to a "certain" critique.

It should be stressed, of course, that to say bodily experience is an effect of discourse is not to say that such experience *is* discourse and, therefore, textual rather than "real." This common objection to "postmodernism," as I have shown, misconstrues the deconstructive analysis of the *co-implication* of various traditional categories – such as logic and rhetoric, philosophy and literature, "politics" and "aesthetics" or, in this case, materiality and textuality – *as* a justification for their reversal. Thus, just as the demonstration that "apocalyptic" crosses through philosophy as its perpetual opening does not elevate the apocalyptic over the philosophical but rather complicates philosophical discourse as such, so the claim that "the" body is not meaningful *prior* to signification does not mean it is not real (see Butler 1992, esp. 21 nt.13). It means, rather, that only what is signified *as* "matter" can be *experienced* as real; thus, our "real," authentic, bodily experiences, such as they are, are socially, culturally and politically contingent rather than ontologically necessary. This means, in turn, that experience – what we know as "real" – is an ideological effect and, as such, open to political contestation and reinterpretation.

If this understanding of bodily experience is given, however, then McLaren's claim that it can inform a "totalizing vision of liberation" falls apart. For, in order to establish the "arch of social dreaming" that he promotes, McLaren would have to appeal to an incontrovertible essence in or of the body that an ideology critique (based on "*true* false consciousness") is in a privileged position to reveal. And, indeed, McLaren wants and promises more than an analytic category that can be mobilized to reveal the illegitimacy of given norms and values. He explicitly advocates a notion of "critique" that entails "*going beyond* the structure of oppositions and sanctioned negations that [a discourse] supplies," and thereby *escaping* "the still invisible logic of domination" that underwrites political struggles (McLaren and Giarelli 1995, 8–9, 10; emphases added). For this purpose, however, bodily experience must also serve, contradictorily, as a legitimate and categorical basis of critique. Something incontrovertible is required, in other words, to establish when "resistance" serves as a form of "lived critique" and when it does not (1989b, 196). McLaren suggests this second possibility when he says that,

> even in these postmodern times we are capable of seizing the stage of history in the unity of our thinking and doing, and bringing forth a new world at the command of our own voices and with the strength of our own hands. The prerequisite for such an enterprise lies in *reclaiming the authenticity of the body* and in formulating strategies of opposition whose primary referent consists of new ways of thematizing knowledge and subjectivity. (1988, 70; emphasis mine)

The view that authentic bodily experience provides an alternative standard of the 'good' appears in his later text as well. There we find that, despite his insistence that "an ethics grounded in the body" cannot be understood as "objective," McLaren nonetheless maintains that "projections of embodied image schemata" that take the form of understanding and knowledge "can form the basis of mutual understanding, since *bodily experience is shared*" (1995, 281, 280; my emphasis).

To be sure, if something about bodily experience is to serve as the ground or "core ethical principle" of McLaren's pedagogical project, it cannot be viewed as an a posteriori effect of discursive representation. For unless we can tell *which* experience, desire or bodily pleasure (or which dimension of these) among an infinite variety of possible choices is actually an "authentic" one, we do not have any ground (bodily-based or otherwise) for a critical vision of liberation that "transcends" the contradictions of the modernist legacy. In this context, the appeal to shared bodily experience provides a basis on which to determine the difference between, for instance, "our *real* needs and those of our students from fantasies in pursuit of *artificial* needs" (1988, 70; emphases mine). The problem here, however, is that McLaren's narrative of liberation logically requires that he *abstract* what is ontologically prior to discourse from the cultural contingency of experience – that he make a transcendental or quasi-transcendental, a priori claim about what "authentic" bodily experience or "real needs" truly are. Only on this basis can a given bodily experience serve as a standard which demystifies or clarifies the difference between what is liberating ("*true* false ideology") and what is oppressive and, thus, merely "false."

By treating the body as a source of authenticity, McLaren can establish the standard of critique he requires. But he can only do so at the cost of illegitimately essentializing and transcendentalizing the subject and, thus, at the expense of his own understanding of the effects of power/knowledge *on* the body. Conversely, if McLaren accepts that "we cannot peel away the flesh to yield an unobstructed view to some irreducible urge or desire" (1989b, 201), then he can no longer lay claim to the epistemological lever he needs to gauge the ethico-political difference between "emancipation" and "domination," and to ground his alternative conception (his "totalizing vision") of what is 'good.' As long as this problem remains, Kant's legacy has not been left behind. On the contrary, the transcendentalism that McLaren risks when he tries to overcome relativism is not something he can do without. For McLaren, at least, the progressive pedagogical ideal of "criticality" still embodies the necessary yet impossible co-implication of epistemological grounds and ethical norms – of "Critique" and "critique" – that the neomodernist response to "postmodernism" purports to undo. This ideological dimension of critique is what his critical determination of "justice" demands. For just this reason, I have claimed, the political purchase of the theory is bought – it is *necessarily* bought – at the cost of a "certain" critique.

Insofar as it involves decoupling a standard of ethico-political critique from Enlightenment foundationalism and scientism, neomodernism is this contradiction writ large: neomodernists reject and embrace critical legitimacy simultaneously. The difficulty that this entails takes a different form depending upon the philosophical context from which the alternative standard of critique originates, but in each case the structural problem is the same. Thus, just as McLaren's (and Lankshear's and Giarelli's) pedagogical theory leads both to the assertion and to the rejection of such ontological grounds as the "body," or the "voice" of the oppressed,[2] so Henry Giroux's attempts to mobilize Freire's thought (in particular) in response to the "postmodern condition" manifests a crucial equivocation as well. Consequently, we can find in Giroux's work, as in McLaren's, an ambivalence regarding the grounds for a determinate standard of critique, even while Giroux would agree that a critical theory of society must embody a vision in which social justice rather than injustice prevails.

Giroux's equivocation takes the form of a refusal to decide whether the phrase "literacy and voice" signifies the ground for a legitimate moral distinction between justice and injustice – whether it *is* a standard for critique – or whether the phrase signifies an epistemological framework or metanarrative (a doctrinal meta-Critique) through which the possibility of all knowledge, including a knowledge of what is just, can be (quasi-) transcendentally established. This difference is significant, given that Giroux's "postmodern" reformulation of Freire's "critical literacy" takes into account (as does McLaren's) the power/knowledge nexus elucidated by Foucault (1980). If it is understood as a meta-Critical appraisal of the epistemological possibilities and limits of critique rather than as a legitimate critical standard, however, Giroux's pedagogy of "literacy and voice" would *preclude* the possibility of a rational or determinate moral standard based on what is purely 'true.'

The difficulty can be elucidated as follows. On the view that Giroux is positing "literacy and voice" as a standard of critique, it could be said that Giroux's vision of a just society is based on a Freirean understanding of "critical literacy," an understanding that is offered as a theoretical *ground* for ethico-political critique. "Critical literacy" takes its meaning, on this view, in contrast to a conventional theory of "literacy" that tacitly keeps unequal relations of power and privilege in place. Thus, for example, Giroux regularly evokes the categories of "voice" (Giroux 1988b, 68, 71), self-determination (1988b, 70) and individuals' own "experiences and commonsense perceptions" (1988b, 63) as critical lenses through which students can interrogate "the history they are told" (1988b, 68). Here the emphasis is clearly on the way in which "literacy" (in the Freirean sense) provides a standard of critique by virtue of which ideologically-structured forms of knowledge and subjectivity can be both identified and combatted by actors who become increasingly self-aware and self-determining as a result of their critical political praxis (e.g., 1988b, 70).

At the same time, however, Giroux is not unaware of the problems attached to the Enlightenment conception of autonomous agency he evokes. For instance, he directly urges that "the culture that such students [from subordinate groups] bring to the schools may be in dire need of critical interrogation and analysis" (1988b, 63). Thus, it could equally be argued that the phrase "critical literacy and voice" does not signify for Giroux a standard for critique *per se*, but rather an epistemological framework that delimits the conditions of possibility for knowledge in general. This second view follows from claims such as the following:

> As a narrative for agency and a referent for critique, *literacy provides an essential precondition for organizing and understanding the socially constructed nature of subjectivity and experience and for assessing how knowledge, power, and social practice can be collectively forged* in the service of making decisions instrumental to a democratic society rather than merely consenting to the wishes of the rich and the powerful. (1988b, 65–6, emphasis mine; cf. 1988b, 70 and 1993)

and,

> *a critical pedagogy of literacy and voice must be attentive to the contradictory nature of student experience and voice and therefore establish the grounds whereby such experience can be interrogated and analyzed* with respect to both its strengths and weaknesses. Voice in this case not only provides a theoretical framework for recognizing the cultural logic that anchors subjectivity and learning, it also provides a referent for criticizing the kind of romantic celebration of student experience that characterized much of the radical pedagogy of the 1960s. (1988b, 72; emphasis mine)

As an epistemological metanarrative, to be sure, "a critical pedagogy of literacy and voice" may well provide "a referent for criticizing" a "romantic celebration of student experience" (i.e., of "voice"). Clearly, however, such a referent cannot *be* the 'voice' of the oppressed, since what is to be criticized *is* the voice of the oppressed (e.g., "students from subordinate groups," as above). As a "framework for critique," in other words, "critical literacy" can perhaps illuminate the contradictory nature of the cultural logic through which subjectivity and experience are socially constructed and 'anchored.' Consequently, Giroux could be said to be describing a theory that offers real insight into the ideological dimensions of every student's and every teacher's "voice." On this view of Giroux's formulation of critical pedagogy as a "certain" critique, however, he could not be said to have delineated a standard by virtue of which we can know (can make a logical determination as to) *when* student voices are in "dire need of critical interrogation and analysis" and when they are not.

Of course, one might well go with the first interpretation instead, in which case student experience/voice would itself be "the referent" or standard for an ethico-political critique of social injustice and oppression. Significantly, however, if the phrase "literacy and voice" is taken as signifying a "referent for critique" rather than a theoretical framework which outlines the discursive (and thus ideological) grounds of all forms of self-representations (of all "voices"), then it is again being assumed that there is something that is ontologically basic or prior to ideology in the voice of the oppressed that can be represented as "true." In other words, insofar as the "voice" and experience of those who have been oppressed *is* the principle that does the interrogating, so to speak, and insofar as individuals' own "experiences and commonsense perceptions" (their own "voices") are intended to serve as a critical lens through which to interrogate "the history they are told," these voices are not themselves available *to* ethico-political interrogation. On the contrary, to exactly this extent they must be taken as fixed for the purposes of the critique. Consequently, a critical inquiry into the social and political constitution of those voices and experiences will have been foreclosed.

In effect, then, what Giroux is advocating is a "pedagogy of literacy and voice" that both celebrates and interrogates "voice" at the same time. It does so because "literacy and voice" is *both* a "theoretical framework" and a "referent" *for* the critical interrogation and analysis *of* "student experience and voice." Insofar as "literacy and voice" is the "theoretical framework" for the interrogation of the "referent" "voice," however, Giroux has emptied the term "critique" of its analytical meaning. In other words, if the Kantian imperative that the "referent" for (or standard of) critique must be "grounded" in a meta-Critical doctrine (in a "theoretical framework") here appears to be satisfied, this is because both levels of legitimation have been collapsed into the same thing: "voice" appears to fulfil both the epistemological and the moral function of "critique" (*qua* C/critique) at once – which means that it fulfils neither. As with the category of bodily experience in McLaren's theory, then, "voice" is said to be both ontologically basic and discursively-constituted at the same time. Where Giroux equivocates, specifically, is on the question of whether "literacy and voice" describes a moral principle (of "critique"), or whether it represents an epistemological framework (a "Critique") through which knowledge can be revealed as ideologically structured and constituted.

In both cases, the result is the same. For Giroux and McLaren alike "voice" both *is and is not* a legitimate ground for an ethico-political vision of a democratic "human community" – a community in which "*all voices in their differences become unified*," and which is "developed around a *shared conception of social justice*, rights, and entitlement" (Giroux 1988b, 72 and 1991, 56; emphases mine). That is to say, since "difference" *per se* is not "a basis for solidarity and unity" (Giroux 1988a, 174), Giroux's vision of global unity would have to be premised upon a unifying principle such as an essentialist conception of "voice" that *transcends differences*, just as McLaren's would. For it is only as an ontological concept – only if the category of difference is turned *into* a ground for sameness – that "voice" can be said to unify legitimately (rather than merely to be itself implicated in) "the socially constructed nature of subjectivity and experience." On the basis of an essentialist conception of "voice" Giroux could indeed ground his political vision; ironically, he would also have reinstated the Hegelian trope of the "self-identical ground of all difference" (McLaren and Giarelli 1995, 14; cited above).

On the other hand, I have argued, Giroux could forgo, and indeed he does frequently seem to wish to forgo, the essentialism that his political thought logically demands. In this case, however, critical literacy would not provide a basis on which to distinguish between emancipatory and oppressive expressions of "voice," nor would it offer any insight into what "social justice, equality, and democratic community" (1988b, 68) might concretely entail. Paul Smith makes the same point in response to another text by Giroux (i.e., Giroux 1983). He writes,

> [E]ven though he certainly recognizes that all oppositional behaviour is not necessarily to be defined as resistance, he [Giroux] offers very few real clues as to how such a distinction could be made or to what end. What is at stake here is a question of the *reach* of ideology, or a question of whether resistance to ideology can itself be described as ideologically determined, and this is a matter that is clearly tied to the definition of human agency. (1988, 67; emphasis his)

As this comment indicates, insofar as Giroux adopts a "neomodern" approach to social scientific inquiry – an approach that mobilizes the modern belief in an ethico-political standard that is epistemologically justified even while it discards (with "postmodernism") the transcendental, justificatory apparatus of Critique – his pedagogical theory is fundamentally flawed as well. For, when taken as a *theoretical framework*, Giroux's modified version of Freirean "literacy" fails to provide the critical standard needed for the interrogation of student "experience and voice." Conversely, when taken as a legitimate *principle or standard of critique* that can be brought to bear on the ideological occlusion of injustice and suffering, the category of "literacy and voice" mobilizes an implicit essentialism that contradicts Giroux's own insistence on the socially constructed nature of subjectivity.

If Giroux's "neomodern" elaboration of Freirean pedagogical theory is no more successful than McLaren's, however, this might well be expected. To be sure, in Giroux's theory C/critique persists by virtue of the peculiar fact that "literacy and voice" is said to signify both a meta-Critical "theoretical framework" for the critique of essentialism, and an ontologically-basic or essential "referent" of ethico-political critique. But this attempt to have it both ways is contradictory. It is a form of the incoherence that lies at the heart of any neomodernist attempt to reconcile a modernist understanding of the emancipatory potential of schooling – the school as the democratic site of the development of a critical and hence *non*-ideological consciousness, as per Freire, for example – with radical "postmodern" interrogations of such categories as authenticity and subjectivity, and their roles in the ethico-epistemological metanarrative of modernity.

This incoherence will obtain in one way or another as long as the "postmodern condition" is understood as a process of delegitimation that pertains to scientific "truth" alone – leaving the modern metanarrative of emancipation untouched – rather than as an insight into the ideological nature of their entwinement. In other words, critical theoretical approaches to education aimed at emancipation will necessarily occlude that logically undecidable (or rhetorically-based) difference between epistemology and ethics that Kant's Critical philosophy first instantiated, as long as it overlooks the ways in which ethico-political legitimacy (and the metanarrative of emancipation it supports) is part and parcel of modern, scientific–epistemological ideals, not distinct from them.

In both McLaren's and Giroux's theories, for example, moral legitimacy is not and cannot be formulated as independent of modern epistemological assumptions, because their standards of critique already embody those assumptions; the theories gain political purchase only to the extent that they entail epistemological *Legitimacy* – which is to say, only insofar as a meta-Critical, transcendental or essentialist characterization of the subject is implicitly being made. Thus, even though McLaren and Giroux purport to be taking "postmodernism" into account, their "neomodern" solutions are fundamentally incompatible with "postmodern" insights concerning the (self) deconstruction of critique that I have described. Moreover, insofar as this incompatibility between modernist political ideals and deconstructive insights gives rise to inescapable contradictions within the theory, it is possible to reveal the limitations of any progressive pedagogical theory that is based on the neomodernist approach – the 'both/and' approach to the modernism–postmodernism debate – that was profiled above.

It makes no difference, in other words, whether one relies on Freirean praxis or whether one turns instead to Dewey's educational theory, Wittgenstein's conception of "forms of life" or Vygotsky's developmental psychology for an alternative to Kantian metaphysics. Regardless of these specifics, theories aimed at the modernist, ethico-political goal of emancipation need to establish the difference between oppression and liberation in a generalizable way, and this determination can only be bought at the cost of the "postmodern" principles the theory sets out to adopt. Freire himself, apparently, seemed to understand this quite well. He characterized critical consciousness in terms of,

> depth in the interpretation of problems; by the substitution of causal principles for magical explanations, by the testing of one's "findings" and by openness to revision; by the attempt to avoid distortion when

> perceiving problems and to avoid preconceived notions when analyzing; by refusing to transfer responsibility; by rejecting passive positions; by soundness of argumentation; by the practice of dialogue rather than polemics; by receptivity to the new for reasons beyond mere novelty and by the good sense not to reject the old just because it is old – by accepting what is valid in both old and new. (Qtd. in Roberts 1996, 180)

On Freire's view, the "critical consciousness" that sits at the apex of conscientization (the process through which we aspire to our 'ontological vocation' to become more human) reflects the epistemological values of modern, Western scientism. The critical subject is proficient at generating both deductive and inductive forms of proof; aspires to interpretations that are non-ideological and legitimately grounded rather than dogmatic or politically-interested in kind; displays the virtue of autonomy; and is an active subject rather than a passive object. However contestable these dualisms may be, they nonetheless provide a clear guide with which to gauge criticality. "Critical" reflection (so understood) can thus be brought to bear on the "conditions of oppression" and, for just this reason, can clearly be seen to embody a "political character and liberatory intent" (Roberts 1996, 195).

For Freire no less than for Kant, however, that criticality obtains by virtue of an ineluctable reference to something about the subject that transcends the contingencies of given political and social determinations; something about the subject must be seen as ontologically and thus necessarily (rather than only contingently) 'true' if the *logical* difference between justice and injustice is to stand. Accordingly, in both Kant and Freire we find a metanarrative of emancipation that is premised on what we essentially 'are,' and this is why both philosophical frameworks, although different in so many significant respects, can issue in a determinate standard of critique. On the other hand, if one replaces Freire's subject-centred, modernist epistemological frame with a "postmodern" understanding that *all* modes of consciousness and all levels of knowing are "partial, incomplete, and possibly contradictory," as Peter Roberts suggests (1996, 195), then it is no longer clear on what basis the achievement of critical consciousness can be claimed. Most importantly, if we deny the ideally autonomous subject (individual or collective) its role as the epistemological ground of the political–theoretical analysis, we are left with a view of conscientization as praxis that essentially has nowhere to go. To reformulate Roberts's claim, "particular emphasis" *cannot* "be placed on enhancing possibilities for moments of dialogical, critical reflection on conditions of oppression" (1996, 195), since the theory does not provide a basis on which to determine when such reflection is actually occurring and when it is not.

The problem that underlies the characterization of critical consciousness in terms of Freirean "conscientization" also attends Deweyan "social intelligence" (Carr 1995), the responsibility inherent in 'our' (Wittgensteinian) "form of life" (Smeyers 1995a, 1995b) and Vygotskyian "openness" and "change" (Wardekker and Miedema 1997). In the case of Deweyan pragmatism, for instance, democratic engagement is given as open-ended, non-essentialist, contingently-structured and experimental in nature. This is because, according to William Carr, Dewey saw

> the effort of Enlightenment philosophers to ground their vision of society in some timeless philosophical truths [as] really nothing other than a rhetorical device to present this vision as something more than a historical project designed to promote the development of a more secularised and humanistic European culture. (Carr 1995, 81).

In place of Enlightenment philosophy, therefore, Dewey proposed an open-ended conception of the 'growth of social intelligence' (Carr 1995, 86–7). For Dewey, this involved a form of reasoning that evolves socially rather than strictly on an individual basis, that is the contingent result of solving practical problems rather than the realization of a transcendental subjective essence, and that entails the elaboration and application not of rationally grounded 'truths,' but merely of historically-situated practical belief (Carr 1995, 88; cf. Rockefeller 1992, 180).

So understood, "social intelligence" serves neither as an epistemological lever for the appraisal of "timeless truths," nor as a determinate standard of ethical–political critique. Significantly, therefore, the Deweyan reconstruction of philosophy might give rise to a "certain critique," whereby the ethico-political values of the modern philosophical tradition are interrogated. It cannot however, issue in the "*principled* view of education" that Carr advocates (1995, 78; 1997, 323, 325). To rectify the problem this poses for a neomodern approach to educational theory – an approach that insists on moral legitimacy but eschews the Kantian Critique – one would have to conceive of "social intelligence" teleologically, for example, or endorse "cooperation" as a privileged feature of human nature rather than as a contingent social practice. Carr's attempt to mobilize Deweyan theory in support of "the emancipatory aim of rational autonomy" (1995, 87, 76–7), in other words involves inscribing in Dewey's thought the very essentialism that Carr wishes it to escape. Alternatively, if one concedes that social intelligence is a relative rather than a rational principle of judgement, then it is not clear why its development should be seen as an improvement over, or indeed as *legitimately* better than, any previous state of affairs. The most that might be said is that the Deweyan perspective supports a relative 'good' that is historically and culturally specific.[3]

Contrary to Carr's suggestion that it is possible to formulate an emancipatory educational ideal that does not reproduce the metaphysics of Kantian philosophy, therefore, it is clear that in the case of Deweyan pragmatism the link between ethics and epistemology that is accomplished through an illicit transcendentalizing of the subject is one which Carr cannot logically avoid – not if he is to provide the "principled" view of education on which he insists. For the problem attending moral legitimacy is that the very attempt to establish a logical principle of critique entails an ideological restriction of the subject to one particular essence; it requires, that is to say, an (impossible) logical decision about what is rhetorically undecidable. This means that the problem is not bypassed when a different essence is posited in the place of Kantian reason, but nor can the essentializing move be avoided altogether, except at the cost of a standard for critique itself.

By just this token, Paul Smeyers's Wittgensteinian attempt to discover "something non-relativistic, something non-contingent … about what the educator should or ought to do … in an ethical sense" and to explain "how his actions can be justified" (Smeyers 1995a, 110) exemplifies yet again the untenability of the neomodernist approach. Unlike Carr, Smeyers does not seek a principled view of education in the wake of "postmodernism." For, while he does favour a form of "postmodernism" that "tries to rescue fragments of the past," Smeyers insists that his preferred "postmodernism" advocates a "justification of education …[that] is of a looser (weaker) type than within the Kantian framework" (1995b, 412). Specifically, Smeyers replaces the Kantian metanarrative (with its attendant transcendentalism) with a justificatory framework that he calls, following the later Wittgenstein, a "form of life." As Smeyers explains,

> With the concept of the 'form of life', Wittgenstein indicates what he considers to be the bedrock of our 'language-games'. This … comprises all of the most fundamental propositions on the ethical, epistemological, metaphysical and religious level. They are *given*. Precisely because of their givenness, justification comes to an end. (1995b, 402; his emphasis)

This framework differs from the Kantian metanarrative of Critique in at least two important ways. First, a "form of life" is not a *justificatory* framework. Rather it is "the complex network of the constituent rules of social life and of the language which we use" (1995b, 402). So understood, a form of life is merely the "boundary" which determines "what we call objective and true" (1995b, 402) – the frame, as it were, within which our justifications and arguments are meaningful. Second, because the bedrock of our "language games" is not a rationally established speculative theory in the Kantian sense but rather an intersubjective structure into which we are initiated and which constitutes for "us" our "common world" (1995b, 407), any claims about "what the educator should or ought to do … in an ethical sense" must be understood as strictly relative to the culture that is "ours." On this view, ethical claims are necessarily contingent upon particular forms of life. To this extent, the possibility of moral *legitimacy* has not only been decoupled from the meta-Critique; it has been denied altogether.

It is intriguing, therefore, that Smeyers hopes to base "something non-relativistic, something non-contingent" on his Wittgensteinian account. For a form of life constitutes *a* culture rather than the human condition *per se*, and culture (in this broad sense) is multiply-determined, heterogeneous and irreducible to a unified essence. Thus, although one may indeed provide "many many reasons" (1995b, 412) for a given educational goal, someone else may offer many many *other* reasons to reject that goal. These other reasons may well be based strictly upon one's different position in, or one's different relation to, the same indeterminate "form of life." For just this reason, Smeyers acknowledges "there can and has to be a discussion concerning who is the 'we', in the expression 'what *we* care for', and even this will have to be decided, at least to a certain extent, politically" (1995b, 411; his emphasis).

The question of what culture *is* is thus hardly an unimportant or peripheral matter, as Smeyers suggests (1995b, 410, 411). For what is lost in the theoretical shift of frameworks that Smeyers proposes – from a Kantian meta-Critique with its universalist pretensions to a Wittgensteinian form of life understood in its local and contingent sense – is precisely the question of the "*criteria* to be used in working out what should be studied" (1995b, 410; my emphasis). What is sacrificed, in effect, is a non-relativistic, and non-contingent standard of critique by virtue of which we can "reveal what is unjust in society" (1995b, 408) and what, concomitantly, an educator ought to do. For this, "a *different* inspiration has to be looked for" (Smeyers 1995b, 408; my emphasis). Indeed, Smeyers acknowledges, if it is taken as presented, the Wittgensteinian account leads to the conclusion that the educative task is merely "to initiate people into a conservative blend of 'what is'" (1995b, 407); it does not provide a way to determine how what 'is' should be changed. Thus Smeyers's rejection of the Enlightenment metanarrative in favour of a decidedly non-metaphysical conception of "form of life" does not deliver the theoretical results he promises; namely, the resource with which "to speak to a human culture, or more generally to discuss and criticize its content" in the wake of "postmodernism" (1995b, 401). It merely offers the broad notion of responsibility (as an intrinsic caring about what is worthwhile) which, while by no mean entirely "random," is nonetheless directly vulnerable to political contestation in the name of a different 'good.'

Willem Wardekker and Siebren Miedema's Vygotskyian strategy leaves us in much the same boat. Just as McLaren's "metanarrative" or "totalizing vision," Giroux's "framework" of "literacy and voice," Roberts' evocation of 'our' "ontological vocation" to become increasingly critical, Carr's insistence on the epistemological–ethical category of "rational autonomy" and Smeyers's search for something non-relativistic and non-contingent all tacitly reinstate the (epistemological) metanarrative their particular 'goods' are said to stand without, so Wardekker and Miedema call for a "*theory* of the historical genesis of rationality" (1997, 59; emphasis mine) that can support a standard of critique of society, while they simultaneously criticize the continual reintroduction of "ahistorical and even transcendent principles" into the critical pedagogy tradition (1997, 52). These approaches all *explicitly* reject the epistemological support required to legitimize the modernist ideals they evoke, and this in the name of a putative "postmodern" fragmenting, decentring or shattering of the subject, even while support for Legitimacy is *implicitly* slipped in from behind.

In the Vygotsky-inspired approach proposed by Wardekker and Miedema, the incoherence that characterizes neomodernism in general is perhaps at its most stark. Here "openness" is given as a fixed educational "aim" and as the principle of ideology critique (1997, 59), while the validity of ahistorical, universalist and transcendental principles is denied (1997, 52, 56). Here it is said that an overarching theory of the historical genesis and development of rationality is needed to account for how human beings can become (at least) partially independent of social and political structures and can thus develop into rationally autonomous agents (1997, 59, 60, 56; compare Cherryholmes 1988, 149), while it is equally urged that the development of personal identity is a "thoroughly *political*" result of the partial internalization of external expectations that are mutually contradictory (1997, 59, 57; emphasis theirs). And here it is argued that a 'postmodernism that denies history and replaces it with mere social change' is one which loses sight of the standard of critique by virtue of which to know which 'direction of development is desirable' (1997, 59), even while it is simultaneously maintained that the term "history" signifies nothing other than that 'development has taken place,' and that the only ideal is "change" (1997, 58).

The basis of these contradictory claims appears to be Wardekker and Miedema's rejection of the modernist assumption that "a *consistent* and *uncontradictory* identity is a necessary condition for being an adequate subject as a source of 'agency'" (1997, 56; their emphases). Against this view, they argue that in the current "postmodern era" it has become clear that "a fixed and stable identity has always been an ideological illusion" (1997, 57). Indeed, they insist, identity is better understood as an intersubjective "activity" that "is always only a local stability" rather than a permanent essence. For, "within every person there are different voices, which can be, and usually are, contradictory" (1997, 57). Thus, identity is not only "produced dialogically," but it "always retains a dialogical character" (1997, 57; emphasis omitted). Once the nature of identity is understood in these terms, they continue, education would be better served by Vygotsky's developmental model of subjectivity rather than by the Enlightenment's transcendental one. This is because a Vygotskian-inspired theory begins from the premises that no "authentic" human subject exists and that identity cannot be understood apart from its rootedness in the contingencies of social life (1997, 58).

If the merit of the Vygotskian approach to education is thus that it decentres, de-transcendentalizes and de-essentializes the subject, however, the problem is that it is no longer clear why the idea of human agency ought to be embraced as an educational aim at all (1997, 49). Indeed, as the authors themselves specify, "postmodern theories" demonstrate that there can be no knowledge that is untainted by power. Consequently, one cannot appeal to a notion of authentic human subjectivity that escapes, transcends, and ultimately masters contingent determinants of subjectivity that are social and political in kind (1997, 56–8). And, if this is so, then it becomes difficult to sustain the goal of agency – "the idea of a free and self-aware humanity" that has "[emancipated itself] from the coercion of nature and of tradition" (1997, 56) – as the standard of critique which provides a "point of reference for values and norms," and which thereby legitimates the educational project (1997, 59). How, in short, can one sustain the educational aim of "rational activity" through the inculcation of an awareness of oneself "as a continuously judging and acting person" (1997, 56) – that is, as one who *gives* meaning for oneself in a continuous way – without a transcendental conception of the subject, of its moral end *of* agency, that is epistemologically secure?

The answer, of course, is that one cannot. For, insofar as it is agreed that Wardekker and Miedema do *not* put the rational, coherent subject at the centre of their theory – as, for example, a driving force of history – insofar as they do see identity as radically unfixed, they have no basis on which to determine why or when change is good. As in Roberts's account, the problem with rejecting Kant's implicit essentialism is that we are left without a logical criterion on which to base the crucial ethico-political decision that the concept of education as emancipation requires. In other words, much like Roberts's open-ended understanding of "critical consciousness" – or, for that matter, the concept of "voice" that McLaren and Giroux espouse, Carr's ideal of undetermined "growth" and Smeyers's notion of education as initiation into an unfixed and unfixable form of life – the Vygotskian concept of "openness" cannot itself serve as "a point of reference for values and norms" as the authors propose (1997, 59). For if openness itself is what is lauded, the authors will have effectively foreclosed the possibility of establishing which subjective and social formations are ethically just, and which are not.

It is at just this moment that Wardekker and Miedema introduce the need for an epistemological meta-Critique, a "*theory* of the historical genesis of rationality" (1997, 59; emphasis added). By virtue of such a theory, it emerges, the moral principle of "continuous change" can be imbued with a teleological end; namely, the presupposed 'good' of enhancing one's historically-evolved capacity for 'managing *one's own* development' (1997, 58). Indeed, the role of a theory that makes reference to social, political and historical categories is to "speak to the relationship between the private and the public sphere between the development of the person and that of society," and so to account for the way in which "the child learns to *give meaning and act socially in an autonomous way according to her own judgment*" (1997, 56; emphasis mine). What a theory of the historical genesis of rationality implicitly provides, therefore, is an epistemological (or meta-Critical) basis on which to specify what is "a desirable direction to the development of society and of rationality" (1997, 59) – or, in other words, on which to specify a standard for critique. That standard is, in a word, 'autonomy.' Significantly, Wardekker and Miedema uphold this standard notwithstanding the fact that they agree that the subject should not be ideologically restricted to this or any other essence. This puts the onus on them to explain why *this* is the moral principle that one necessarily will, or necessarily ought to, respect.

Behind the non-teleological conception of "continuous change," then, there rests a tacit endorsement of the moral principle of autonomy or self-determination that is epistemologically-grounded. An historical account (or metanarrative) of the genesis and development of rationality (of enlightenment) is thus essential to the argument that the brute, ontological "openness" that characterizes the human subject on Vygotsky's developmental account can serve as a principle of ideology critique, just as Kant's epistemological, doctrinal Critique was essential to the argument that the logical principle of freedom can give rise Legitimately to moral knowledge as such.

As in other neomodernist arguments considered here, therefore, Wardekker and Miedema evoke the Enlightenment ideals of autonomous judgement, agency and authorship – which is to say, they evoke the transcendental subject – as the logical ground of ethico-political critique at the very moment that they call for a "theory of the *historical* genesis of rationality" (1997, 59; emphasis mine) that is intended to circumvent the reintroduction of "ahistorical and even transcendent principles" into the critical pedagogy tradition (1997, 52). If this contradiction seems like a problematic response to the condition of "postmodernity," however, it must be recalled that Wardekker and Miedema are merely varying on a theme. This particular contradiction reflects the general, constitutively-irresolvable problem that inheres in any attempt to produce a Legitimate standard of ethico-political critique: these attempts will either issue in relativism, or they will reinstate just the kind of transcendental metanarrative that neomodernists purport to renounce. While the theories reviewed in this chapter appear to issue in both outcomes at the same time, anti-modernist theoretical strategies, we shall see next, result in a different set of concerns.

Notes

1 What I call "neomodern" is what Nicholas Burbules and Suzanne Rice call "postmodern," namely, an approach that is "fundamentally continuous with the

modernist tradition, although it seeks to challenge and redefine it" (1991, 397). Burbules and Rice distinguish this from "antimodernism" by virtue of the middle ground between metaphysics and relativism the former manages to secure. "The view we have termed postmodernism," they write, "has sought to turn these critiques [of knowledge, authority and traditional educational aims and practices] toward an alternative conception of education *based partly on the reformulation of selected modernist principles* such as democracy or self-determination, *but without sharing modernist assumptions*, such as a belief in progress or the rational rule of law" (1991, 399; my emphasis). Their "postmodernism" is thus my "neomodernism."

2 Insofar as the contradictions that emerge in McLaren's discussion of the body emerge with respect to his appeals to the "voice of the oppressed" as well, the same analysis applies.

3 This reading of Dewey as offering a politically relative rather than a rationally-grounded conception of critique is offered by Blake (1996, esp. 217), who suggests that Dewey does not attempt to substantiate a rational or universal principle that is morally "legitimate." The implication of this is that Dewey is more properly identified as "anti-modernist" than as "neomodernist" since, as I explain in Chapter Seven, anti-modernism is a theoretical strategy that understands itself as grounded in a politically contingent rather than in a logically necessary way. I return to Blake's own "anti-postmodernism" directly in Chapter Eight.

7 Pedagogy without Foundations

Feminism and Anti-Racism

> Henceforth, it must be recognized that all the determinations of such a trace – all the names it is given – belong as such to the text of metaphysics that shelters the trace, and not to the trace itself. There is no trace *itself*, no *proper* trace. Heidegger indeed says the difference could not appear as such. ("Illumination of the distinction therefore cannot mean that the distinction appears as a distinction.") The trace of the trace which (is) difference above all could not appear or be named *as such*, that is, in its presence. It is the *as such* which precisely, and as such, evades us forever. Thereby the determinations which name difference always come from the metaphysical order.
>
> (Derrida 1982, 66)

No matter to what extent neomodernists embrace the "postmodern" turn, they tend not to leave the ideal of self-legislation – the moral righteousness of "voice" – very far behind. On the contrary, an appeal to the rational principle of self-determination or autonomy still undergirds the neomodernist, pedagogical–theoretical enterprise, even though neomodernist theorists appreciate that, in the wake of "postmodernism," it is no longer possible to lay claim to that very "reason" which, in purportedly producing a "sublime" feeling of intellectual respect grounds or determines itself, and thereby gives rise to a moral standard of critique. Nonetheless, neomodernists appeal to some version of self-determination as a logical principle of ideology critique, and they Legitimate this principle in turn by entrenching it in some form of overarching metanarrative. This is to reinstate the impossible bond between ethics and epistemology (between critique and Critique) in the very attempt to leave the modern metanarrative of epistemological Legitimation behind.

To be sure, the problem of relativism appears to be averted; however, an insurmountable difficulty ensues. It is that when the critique *is* epistemologically grounded on a "totalizing vision" (McLaren), a "theoretical framework for critique" (Giroux), a teleological account of "our ontological vocation" (Roberts), a developmental capacity for "social intelligence" (Carr), a "justificatory framework" based on 'our' form of life (Smeyers), or "a theory of the historical genesis of rationality" (Wardekker and

Miedema), some particular characteristic of the subject (such as self-determination, bodily experience, intelligence, rationality, humanization, responsibility or autonomy) will have been transcendentally essentialized. For the mobilization of the subjective capacity for self-legislation as a logical principle of ethico-political critique always already names "Man" as such *into* being (it transcendentalizes the subject), even if the subject is described in a radically contingent, open-ended or indeterminate way.

Neomodernists thus unwittingly perpetuate the Enlightenment's own mystifying tendency: whenever logic is posited as capable of mastering rhetoric or, that is to say, whenever reason (*qua* autonomy) is posited as the logical ground (as the a priori principle) of ethico-political critique, the normative aim of critical, educational thought will have been violently restricted with reference to some particular cultural, historical, racial, sexual and/or class-based interest(s). And this means that some *other* capacity, characteristic or developmental possibility will have been unjustifiably ("mystically") foreclosed. The fundamental problem, in short, is that the determination of a rational standard of critique depends upon the centring of a transcendental subject whose very centrality and coherence is denied.

To circumvent this difficulty, some theorists of pedagogy propose rejecting the entire apparatus of Critique. Specifically, this view is that a *political* educational theory and practice should take the place of the *philosophical* discourse of modernity. An emancipatory educational project, it is argued, would be better off if it ceased aiming at moral legitimacy and, concomitantly, at a *rational* standard of critique, altogether. For such an aim inevitably entails the imposition of a particular 'good' that cannot be universally compelled, and that may be oppressive in its effects. Thus, instead of either unproblematically linking together (modernism) or trying to separate the categories of ethics and epistemology *within* a Legitimating metanarrative (neomodernism), a number of critical educational theorists appeal to what is ostensibly *outside* philosophical discourse altogether. They appeal, in a word, to politics. Since, for reasons I have already indicated, this straightforward reversal of terms should not be confused with "postmodernism," I use the term "anti-modernist" to designate this distinct theoretical approach.

Elizabeth Ellsworth offers a particularly compelling version of anti-modernism so understood. She argues, persuasively, that there is something that "perpetuate[s] relations of domination" in such key values as "'empowerment', 'student voice', 'dialogue', and even the term 'critical'" (1992, 91). She contends that the assumption of rationalism underlying critical pedagogical theory is exclusionary in its effects, that even a "critical" understanding of the notion of "voice" cannot address structural differences of power among students themselves as well as between them and the professor (whose own "voice" tends not to be problematized at all), and that "dialogue" among unequals is not enabled simply by one's wish for it (see also Gore 1993, esp. 105–11 and Orner 1992).

Ellsworth reached these conclusions after attempting to put "neomodernist" educational theory to work in the classroom. Indeed, in her course on anti-racism she tried to apply just the sorts of emancipatory educational theories discussed in the last chapter. She observed that,

> when participants in our class attempted to put into practice prescriptions offered in the literature concerning empowerment, student voice, and dialogue, we produced results that were not only unhelpful, but actually exacerbated the very conditions we were trying to work against, including Eurocentrism, racism, sexism, classism, and "banking education." To the extent that our efforts to put discourses of critical pedagogy into practice led us to reproduce relations of domination in our classroom, these discourses were "working through" us in repressive ways, and had themselves become vehicles of repression. (1992, 91)

In contrast to critical theorists such as McLaren, Giroux, Carr and other "neomodernists," therefore, Ellsworth came to believe that because knowledge is partial and subjects are multifaceted, reason simply cannot serve as an emancipatory force. She writes,

> Literary criticism, cultural studies, post-structuralism, feminist studies, comparative studies, and media studies have by now amassed overwhelming evidence of the extent to which the myths of the ideal rational person and the "universality" of propositions have been oppressive to those who are not European, White, male, middle-class, Christian, able-bodied, thin, and heterosexual … In contrast, post-structural thought is not bound to reason, but "to discourse, literally *narratives* about the world that are admittedly *partial*." (Ellsworth 1992, 96; internal reference omitted)[1]

The term "anti-modernism" names this strategic, theoretical shift: from universality to partiality, from logic to narrative, and from philosophy to politics (Burbules and Rice 1991, 398). Similarly, Ellsworth seems to be suggesting that hope for emancipation rests with a rejection of the ethos of Enlightenment reason in the name of emancipatory politics. Nicholas Burbules and Suzanne Rice attribute this conviction to anti-modernists: that "there are no sustainable norms of rationality and value" and that, consequently, "educational discourse … exists … only for the purpose of enfranchising certain group interests over others" (Burbules and Rice 1991, 395). Indeed, this is how Ellsworth's course was concluded: "Media and Anti-Racist Pedagogies" eventually evolved into a number of affinity groups, each of which possessed "only partial narratives of its oppressions" (1992, 110). Together, these groups engaged in direct political actions (1992, 110–12).

"Anti-modernism" thus differs from neomodernism in at least one important respect: anti-modernists take contemporary challenges to Enlightenment universalism directly to heart. Because they believe that the modern philosophical tradition is constitutively exclusionary, anti-modernists do not grapple directly with the impossible bond between ethics and epistemology in the name of "postmodernism." They advocate, rather, negating modern values altogether. On this view, critical pedagogy should be understood as an explicitly political discourse *instead of* as a discourse of Enlightenment reason, and it should be so understood because "postmodern" social theory is said to support the ethico-political celebration of difference over sameness, of partiality instead of totality, and/or of rhetoric and the "literary" in the place of logic and scientific truth.

Ellsworth expresses the tendency to reverse the priority of logic and rhetoric when she rejects the ideal of "rationalized, individualized subjects capable of agreeing on universalizable 'fundamental moral principles,'" which underlies the conventional pedagogical goal of "dialogue" (Ellsworth 1992, 108), and calls instead for "a pedagogy of the unknowing" (1992, 110). Ellsworth writes,

> The terms in which I can and will assert and unsettle "difference" and unlearn my positions of privilege in future classroom practices are wholly dependent on the Others/others whose presence – with their concrete experiences of privileges and oppressions, and subjugated or oppressive knowledges – I am responding to and acting with in any given classroom. My moving about between the positions of privileged speaking subject and Inappropriate/d Other cannot be predicted, prescribed, or understood beforehand by any theoretical framework or methodological practice. It is in this sense that *a practice grounded on the unknowable* is profoundly contextual (historical) and interdependent (social). (1992, 115; emphasis added)

This understanding of the normative (and practical) implications of "postmodernism," which gives rise to the proposal to replace a critical theory of education grounded on rational principles with contextually-contingent political action grounded on the unknowable, is shared by other critical political and educational theorists as well. Suzanne de Castell, for example, claims that "[w]e have … a good deal to learn from postmodernism," *reversing as it does* the traditional values of text, of linearity, of coherence, and of argument, and replacing these with image, with simultaneity, with rupture, and with story (de Castell 1995, 242–3). On de Castell's view, this purported reversal can teach us that traditional practices of philosophy are "not merely inadequate but indeed corrupt" (1995, 255), for philosophy as it has been practised entails generalizing abstractly in the face of the concrete differences that structure people's various relations to power and to privilege. Moreover, de Castell argues, philosophers of education are necessarily complicit in evil, because their most valued artefacts and practices "have been produced and continue ... to be produced in and through the oppression and exploitation of others" (1995, 248). These texts and practices should be relegated to the history of a bygone era, she says, so that philosophers of education who are "seriously concerned with the appalling conditions of people's lives in the present" (1995, 255) can begin to address such concerns.

Like Ellsworth, therefore, de Castell seems to support the "anti-modernist" perspective that Burbules and Rice describe. For de Castell, the task of the philosopher in the wake of "postmodernism" is to right wrongs based on social difference *rather* than to pursue abstract universality or totalizing knowledge. Patti Lather, similarly, suggests that "postmodernism" displaces the Enlightenment project altogether. From a feminist pedagogical perspective, Lather insists that "[useful theories of social change] *celebrate* the dispersion and fragmentation that has *displaced* the ideal of a global, totalizing project of emancipation which attempted to unify and solidify what is contradictory, diverse and changing" (Lather 1991, 164; emphases added).

Or consider the argument of René Vincente Arcilla, which evidences this epistemological shift from universality to partiality, from logic to narrative, or from philosophy to politics, as well. "Jacques Derrida and allied thinkers," he writes, "invite us to balance the 'scientific' tendency in philosophy to value the features of language that promote ideal clarity, verified communication, and committed consensus, with a 'literary' appreciation of those features that disclose material opacity (particularly of the signifier), unconscious signification, and undecided possibilities of interpretation" (1995, 168). Arcilla goes on to underline the importance of recognizing the "indefinite and self-estranging" nature of cultural identity in the name of advancing "multiculturalist education," (1995, 169). An educational discourse based on this recognition, he proposes, would be one in which,

> a politics sensitive to cultural differences would meet a politics that finds in these differences the natural limit of our intelligible identities; an incongruous mix of cultures would thus yield a common sense of strangeness. And so is born hope for a new politics of commonality, *one grounded in nature conceived* not as an intelligible (to some privileged cultural language) cosmos but *as the withdrawing source of language and linguistic beings, the mysterious X*. Such a politics would be guided by a discourse of universal rights for a multicultural society. (1995, 170; emphasis added)

It is difficult to know just what Arcilla is saying, given his insistent appeal to the discourse of universal human rights just when he contends that no natural human, and no "recognizable" identity can be determined (1995,

167). Nonetheless, the normative implications are clear: what is "unknowable" or unintelligible is, according to Arcilla, just what we ought to embrace:

> Thus *philosophia* could be transformed from a project to eliminate or reduce indefiniteness, from an epistemological project, into a giving thanks for how the return of indefiniteness reminds us of *our awful and awesome, sublime communion with indefinite Being* (ontologically different, as Heidegger shows, from culturally defined beings). (1995, 171; note omitted, emphasis added)

This group of theorists understands "postmodernism" differently than neomodernists do. Neomodernists believe that traditional ethico-political values can be reclaimed for "postmodernity" once they are extricated from the original epistemological metanarrative in which they were lodged. Anti-modernists, in contrast, reject those traditional values and propose to replace them with their negative, arational or even irrational counterparts. Critical values proposed by anti-modernists include, for instance, partiality and the "unknowable" (Ellsworth 1992), disruption (de Castell 1995), fragmentation (Lather 1991, 1992), "indefiniteness" (Arcilla 1995), "multivocality" (McCarthy 1993) and radical pluralism (McGee 1993).

Ironically, this tendency to reverse the traditional categories aligns anti-modernists much more closely with anti-postmodernists – those who dismiss contemporary critiques of the Enlightenment out of hand – than it does with neomodernists, even though the latter (who acknowledge the validity of contemporary critiques of modernity) seem more likely theoretical companions. But neomodernists accept "postmodern" criticism insofar as it is seen to *continue* the emancipatory modernist project, not insofar as it negates it. Anti-modernists, in contrast, see "postmodernism" as modernity's outright replacement. They thus share with anti-postmodernists the erroneous belief that philosophers such as Derrida stand "the primacy of logic over rhetoric, canonized since Aristotle, on its head" (Habermas 1987, 187). It remains, therefore, that even though anti-modernists and anti-postmodernists draw diametrically opposed conclusions about the normative implications of "postmodernism," they go astray on the same basis. For, while the "postmodern" theory I have been discussing is not simply a continuation of the modernist project of Enlightenment (as neomodernists would have it), it is not its negation, either.

In fact, I have shown, the understanding of "postmodernism" as a straightforward negation of the modern ethos of Enlightenment leaves intact one of the two crucial premises that de Man, Lyotard, Derrida and other continental theorists have challenged. Specifically, I have argued that – whether they take it for good or for ill – those who believe that deconstruction "aestheticizes" political philosophy beg the question of logic's purity with regard to language's tropological effects. In other words, while anti-modernists reverse the *priority* of the categories (the first assumption), they still take the *autonomy* of the categories (the second assumption) for granted, just as anti-postmodernists do. Yet it is just this distinction *between* logic and "rhetoric" (that feature of language de Man calls its "literariness" or its tropological dimension), between the aesthetic and the sublime, or between philosophical and apocalyptic discourse, that (a certain) "postmodernism" attends.

Anti-modernists (no less than modernists) overlook this point, insofar as they uphold the status of the "literary" as (mere) aesthetic ornament *in opposition to* the philosophical. They thereby obscure what de Man calls the "epistemological thrust" of rhetoric itself, which is the provocative capacity of a "rhetorical reading" to disarticulate the theoretical system as a whole. Consequently, "postmodern" revelations concerning the rhetorical dimensions *of* logic, the apocalyptic opening *of* philosophy or, indeed, the "sublime" cause *of* "critique," are denied. The anti-modernist thus loses sight of the very critical resource – the "post-modern" in Lyotard's sense of the future anterior, whereby the "post"-modern is what *will have been* modernity's undoing – that they call upon to *counter* the exclusionary effects of Enlightenment.

It is important to underline once again, therefore, that once these terms are understood, their reversal is out of the question. Terms such as "rhetoric," the "sublime," the "apocalyptic" or the "mystagogical" do not signify possible objects of consciousness, because they are not concepts or categories at all. Although these terms appear to signify something determinate that is, on first glance, analogous to logic and its correlates, they refer to what is constitutively absent or indeterminable. What is mystagogical, sublime or rhetorically ambiguous is precisely what we *cannot* determine, objectify or know. This is why logic had to be prioritized over (so-called) "rhetoric" in the formulation of the link between the *trivium* and the *quadrivium*: knowledge cannot be founded on an outright incapacity to know. The primacy of logic over rhetoric (which obscures linguistic undecidability) was (and remains) indispensable for "scientific" (systematic) knowledge or *theõria*. The cost of *theõria*, in other words, is the erasure of a rhetorical "undecidability" that not only cannot be got rid of, but that is actually a necessary condition for the very knowledge, the very theory, that denies it.

Now, if a literary theory "that foregrounds the rhetorical over the grammatical and the logical function" (de Man 1982, 14) brings an undecidability at the root of the classical theory of language into view, what kind of "theory" could this be? Clearly, what I called (literary) theory$_2$ is not itself simply an(other) *theory* of the aesthetic function of language. Rather, it is the inevitable disruption or deconstruction *of* systematic knowledge *qua theõria* (or theory$_1$) and, as such, not a "theory" at all. On the other hand, insofar as "theory$_2$" is a *systematic* disruption of systematicity, it partakes of the very "resistance" *to* "literariness" that characterizes theory (theory$_1$) itself. To this extent, even so-called "rhetorical" readings do not actually negate the place of "logic," for they never *are* strictly "rhetorical." On the contrary, they partake of theory$_1$ as well. Ambivalently, then – insofar as they both are and are not 'theory' – rhetorical readings cannot but help upholding, even while they deny, the supremacy of logic over rhetoric entrenched in the classical *trivium*.

When this argument was mapped onto the relationship between ethics and epistemology – which underlies the political project of education as emancipation, and which apparently authorizes the outright dismissal of "postmodernism" – we saw that logic's impossible primacy was essential to the discourse of Enlightenment. In particular, Kant revitalized this classical relationship when he established for the first time a critical or normative *doctrine* of reason in its totality. In Kant's philosophy, the illegitimate (yet necessary) prioritizing of logic occurs when the potentially disruptive tension between the beautiful and the sublime is contained in the third *Critique* – that is, when it is *impossibly* contained, by virtue of a bracketing of what is, as "sublime," beyond the reach of aesthetic or logical meaning. Kant thus established as "science" (i.e., as *theõria*) a universal *system* of knowledge within which moral knowledge could be enclosed and thereby Legitimated as a distinct epistemological object. Precisely because his system *was* conceived in strictly epistemological terms, moreover, Kant had to distinguish what is distinctly *moral* about reason as compared to its merely theoretical status. To this end, Kant argued that the principle of practical reason in particular (i.e., the unconditioned condition or ground of a legitimate standard of critique) is rooted in the subject's excessive, sublime essence – that is, in its response-ability to the law of universalization. By virtue of this logical objectification of (undecidable) sublimity as autonomy (as the subject's essential "freedom"), Kant was able to ground the critical system as a whole (the *theõria*) on a normative or moral basis. Thus, by illegitimately restricting the sublime quality of response-ability to a logical concept of "freedom," Kant not only established a moral standard of critique; he simultaneously lent to merely theoretical reason a critical, emphatic force – a force that continues to be upheld in the name of the emancipatory promise of Enlightenment.

As in the case of a "literary" theory($_2$) of the relationship between logic and rhetoric within the *trivium*, however, the priority of the terms cannot be reversed. To be sure, a deconstructive reading reveals the way in which a bracketing of the sublime founds (it founds impossibly) the Critical doctrine as a whole, and it shows that the relationship between the Critical doctrine and the ethical critique is grounded on the subject's sublime essence. Nonetheless, the "sublime" nature of "Being" can no more usurp the place of a restricted conception of rational "autonomy" (as per Arcilla) than can the aesthetic sublime usurp the place of the beautiful within the Kantian architectonic as a whole – or, for that matter, than can a pedagogy of the "unknowing" usurp the prescription made possible in advance by a "theoretical framework or methodological practice" (Ellsworth 1992, 115). On the contrary, the possibility of a logic that is pure *must* be upheld, and logic *must* be prioritized over rhetoric, since these assumptions are the conditions of possibility for any meaningful, translatable, communicable, *sense*. They are necessary, therefore, even for the distinctly moral sense that Ellsworth, de Castell, Lather and Arcilla want to make of the so-called "unknowable." Similarly, I argued above, any theory which aims to understand with logic the rhetorical challenge to logic will *also* "resist" its own rhetorical undoing; consequently, the possibility that rhetorical reading (literariness) could take the place of theory (of logic) is ruled out from the start.

The necessity at issue is strictly logical: once the "sublime" is understood as, simply, what is unrecoverable by discourse – namely, discursivity, or the gesture of speech, as such – it becomes clear that any political project based on the priority of the sublime would be utterly unintelligible. In other words, what (by definition) is *truly* "unknowable" or "sublime" is what exceeds the possibility of cognitive or imaginative re-presentation (it is what is mysterious, unrepresentable and unimaginable) – for Kant and for contemporary theorists alike. The "sublime" in any of its various guises (such as multivocality, strangeness, "indefiniteness," border-crossing, "unknowing" or fragmentation) is not and cannot be a(nother) type of phenomenal sense, a(nother) kind of ethico-political principle or a(nother) representable object that is available to consciousness, nor can the indeterminacy that de Man calls "literariness" and Derrida calls "*différance*" ever take the place of determinate knowledge or aesthetic meaning as such. Insofar as the sublime really does inhere *in* the logical principle of practical reason, therefore, it undoes every determination, every objectification and every (re)cognizable value, including those values determined as "*the* unknowable" (Ellsworth), "*the* disruptive" (de Castell) or "*the* mysterious X" (Arcilla).

Furthermore, just as the "sublime" deconstructs every value on which it is brought to bear, so the reverse will follow as well. The moment the "unknowable," the "disruptive" or the "indefinite" are determined as identifiable 'goods', the moment these terms are imbued with moral meaning, they uphold (even while they deny) the possibility of knowing in advance what we ought, morally, to do. As soon as it is discursively positioned as *a* value, in other words, the sublime loses its deconstructive force, its capacity to undo determination, precisely because it no longer *is* what we understand as "sublime." This is the moment at which *différance* is reduced to "difference," and stripped of its radical import.

To suggest that one ought to celebrate the "literary" (*qua* the sublime, the mystagogical, the rhetorical or, indeed, the political) instead of upholding "science" (*qua* systematicity, philosophy, logic or reason), therefore, is to misconstrue the meaning of these terms. Indeed, it is just because this reversal does issue in unintelligibility, one imagines, that anti-modernists are ambivalent about how the ineffable idea of "unknowing" or "indefiniteness" can actually "ground" a political educational project aimed at social justice. On one hand, for instance, Ellsworth says that she "refuses to know and resist oppression from any a priori line of attack, such as race, class, or gender solidarity" – that, in effect, she rejects outright the strategies of an ahistorical or decontextualized identity politics – because "fundamental moral and political principles are not absolute and universalizable, waiting to be discovered by the disinterested researcher/teacher" (1992, 113, 108). On the other hand, her explicit goal in the course was to combat social oppression by "winning semiotic space for the marginalized discourses of students against racism" (1992, 94, 111), and the key moral term of that undertaking *was* that of "self-definition" (1992, 97, 101, 110 and 114). In this sense, a conception of social justice was clearly already in place. This ambivalence is captured economically towards the end of the article. After describing the three anti-racist actions undertaken by "Coalition 607" (the class), Ellsworth writes, "Thus students engaged in the political work of changing material conditions within a public space, allowing them to make visible and assert *the legitimacy of their own definitions, in their own terms*, of racism and anti-racism on the UW [the University of Wisconsin-Madison] campus" (1992, 111; emphasis mine).

This claim is important for Ellsworth's argument, since it is intended to distinguish her pedagogical programme to *disrupt* "the ways social technologies of gender, race, ability, and so on define Otherness and use it as a vehicle for subordination" (1992, 113) – that is, her programme to undertake a certain "critique" – from that of neomodern theorists, who impose an a priori principle (i.e., a critical standard) in advance. Neomodernists, she implies, appeal to the fixed identity of the rational subject, and thereby occlude relations of privilege and power that are already in play. However, Ellsworth's reference to the value of self-definition does more to align her approach with that of various anti-postmodernists than to distinguish it as a viable alternative.

To be sure, Ellsworth's appeal to self-definition allows her to ground the "pedagogy of unknowing" on a conception of justice that allows us to judge. The introduction of a principle of self-definition thus solves the problem that each group's narrative of oppression could only ever be partial – both in the sense that each group in class projected a one-sided interest (1992, 97) and thus necessarily excluded "the voices of others" (1992, 110), and also in the sense that each one of the narratives was "unfinished, imperfect, limited" (1992, 97). Consequently, the political strategies that the class undertook on the basis of those narratives could never be guaranteed to safeguard the struggles of *other* groups, or even the struggles of various affinity groups within the class itself. Indeed, it is particularly interesting that each of the political proposals were appraised by the class according to a "final arbiter" (or critical standard) of moral acceptability that had been intersubjectively determined. Before they were implemented, proposals first had to be judged as to whether or not they would "succeed in alleviating campus racism, while at the same time managing *not to undercut* the efforts of the other social groups to win self-definition" (1992, 110; original emphasis). But since on Ellsworth's own account this is *in principle* an unanswerable question, the judgements students made clearly did not and could not function as an arbitrating standard of critique. On the contrary, as Ellsworth insists, "accounts of one group's suffering and struggle [are not] immune from reproducing narratives oppressive to another's," and "there are no social positions exempt from becoming oppressive to others ... any group – any position – can move into the oppressor role" (1992, 99, 114; internal reference omitted). The principle of self-definition served, therefore, to enable the evaluation of *which* disruptions of the social status quo would be emancipatory, and which would not.

The principle makes it possible, in effect, to gauge whether the action proposed will be emancipatory or oppressive in its effects. Thus, while a pedagogy of the unknowing suggests that no *culturally or historically-determined* identity can be specified as unoppressive in advance, we can nonetheless appeal to our *human* capacity for and right to self-definition as the gauge for assessing the relative merit of given cultural determinations and socially-embedded narratives. By virtue of this standard, we *can* know what is bad when we see it.

Significantly, however, this entails that "legitimacy" *derives from* the groups' assertions of "their own definitions, in their own terms." What makes the definitions of "racism" and "anti-racism" legitimate, in other words, is that they are the students' *own*, self-determined ones. And, if this is what Ellsworth intends, then she is tacitly endorsing the classic, Enlightenment value of self-determination as the (epistemological) ground of (moral) action. On this view, in other words, it appears that Ellsworth is positing the subject as such, the subject to whom rights accrue, *as* that being distinguished by its essential (human) capacity for self-determination – as capable of constituting (or 'causing') itself, notwithstanding contingent social determinants, and so *transcending* contingency – even though she is directly critical of that Enlightenment perspective. And, if Ellsworth is read in this way, her position is as vulnerable as that of any other neomodernist: she fails to explain how or why the logical idea of self-determination (self-causality, as it were) should be taken as an ethico-political 'good' once the modernist metanarrative, with its illegitimate, transcendental justification of moral autonomy, is explicitly eschewed.

But the claim is ambiguous, and thus open to another interpretation. Specifically, Ellsworth may merely be reporting that her class provided a context in which counter-hegemonic terms and definitions could be asserted as (equally) legitimate bases for contesting racism on campus. If the term "legitimacy" is taken in this more colloquial sense, it would appear to lend rhetorical support to the political assertion of an opposing, yet arguably equally "legitimate," point of view. (To say that my view is *as legitimate as yours*, for example, is to say that no view is any more legitimate than any other.) On this latter reading, significantly, it follows that the educative project of inculcating critical reason – the capacity to distinguish rationally between legitimate and illegitimate views – should give way to a strictly political project of providing students with opportunities to identify and *assert* a variety of claims, whatever these may be. Taken this way, all claims apparently are relative, since none of them bear a Legitimate bearing on social justice at all. This second interpretation rescues Ellsworth's proposal from the Scylla of transcendentalism, but it does so by succumbing to the Charybdis of relativism instead.

As it should by now be clear, what is of special interest here is not which interpretation we choose. In fact, such a decision would be misplaced, since neither the grammar nor the logic of the argument can help us out. What is interesting, rather, is that Ellsworth's simultaneous claim to and denial of ethico-political legitimacy reveals the problem with installing the ineffable ("unknowing") as an ethico-political standard of critique. For the anti-modernist argument logically demands that one introduce an alternative standard that can be mobilized towards the vision of social justice that one upholds, even while it announces, correctly, that what makes indeterminacy a normative force at all is that it undermines, disrupts and challenges the ways in which any such standard, and any such vision, will be oppressive in its turn. Since these claims are mutually exclusive, anti-modernist attempts to combine them will undoubtedly give rise to the kind of ambivalence that was witnessed above.

This is perhaps why, according to Ellsworth, Patti Lather asks how "postmodernism" can,

> begin to clear the ground and challenge the plethora of concepts that appear as givens in our debates about the possibilities and limits of emancipatory education? How can such self-reflexivity both render our basic assumptions problematic and provisional and yet still propel us to take a stand? (1991, 44)

One might redirect these questions back to Lather herself. What could it mean to "[display] under the sign of (post)critical" a pedagogical practice in which "emancipatory space is problematized via *deconstruction* of the Enlightenment equation of knowing, naming and emancipation" (1992, 131; 1991, 118), if the very designation "(post)critical" *means* the "continued centrality of *critical reason*" in its sense of "the driving force behind modernism" (Lather 1992, 131, 121; my emphasis)? As I argued earlier, the "driving force behind modernism" *is* the equation of knowing, naming and emancipation. "Postmodernism" cannot both clear this ground or challenge its equation, and also instantiate it, at the same time.

This impossibility leads one to question just how deep Lather's wish to deconstruct Enlightenment precepts, particularly those concerning the centrality of the subject, actually goes. To be sure, we are told that "deconstruction can serve to problematize critical pedagogy in ways that *resituate* our emancipatory work" such that it can interrogate and reflect upon *itself* (1991, 47, 154) – and this, precisely, because the "goal" of deconstruction is "to keep things in process, to disrupt, to keep the system in play, to set up procedures to continuously demystify the realities we create, [and] to fight the tendency for our categories to congeal" (1992, 13). In this sense, according to Lather, the "postmodern" "break[s] with totalizing, universalizing 'metanarratives' and the humanist view of the subject that undergirds them" (1991, 5).

But the progressive potential of this "postmodernism" is never spelled out. On the contrary, Lather maintains that "relativistic assumptions of a free play of meaning that denies power relations are of little use for those struggling to free themselves from normalizing boundaries and categories" (1991, 116), and that

> the debunking of foundational grounding ... the insistence upon a fragmented, de-centred self, and the retreat from teleology via historical progress and human agency ... may be useful strategies 'for the inheritor of the voice of the transcendental ego', but they pose dangers for any appropriation of postmodernism on the part of the marginalized. (1991, 37–8; internal reference omitted)

This leads Lather to characterize "postmodernism" as 'irredeemably politically ambivalent' (1991, 31) and as requiring the correction of a *political* feminist practice. What is most notable here is that feminist practice (in all its variety), according to Lather, characteristically appeals "to the powers of agency and subjectivity as necessary components of socially transformative struggle." Feminist discourse, she avers, has "raised the most questions about the fractured, fragmented subject postulated by post-structural discourse" (1991, 28).

Notwithstanding these concerns about the political implications of a fragmented subject, Lather contends that "Ellsworth ... *begins to give a feel for* the political possibilities of the multiply-sited subject of post-structuralist theory, a subject characterized by heterogeneity, irreducible particularities, and incalculable differences." Ellsworth's work is thus said to demonstrate that "postmodernism has much to offer those of us who do our work in the name of emancipatory education" (1991, 48; emphasis mine). This claim seems somewhat misplaced. For the most forceful conclusion that Lather draws is that "there is nothing in postmodernism that makes it intrinsically reactionary" (1991, 49); thus, she has not countered her own worries by demonstrating that there *is* something in "post-modernism" that makes it intrinsically progressive instead.

It is understandable, of course, if the standoff between feminism and poststructuralism inspires in Lather an "ambivalence" about "the politics of postmodern thought and practice" (1991, 1, 38). For the conflict between the logical need *for* a standard of critique that feminist theory and practice provides (however problematically), and the "postmodern" interrogation *of* that possibility that Lather promotes, is arguably insoluble. But insofar as her ambivalence is *itself* ultimately offered as a category of critique, Lather is misconstruing the meaning of that term exactly as I outlined before. Specifically, she writes with respect to her own position that,

> I see this ambivalence as a way to interrupt the contestatory discourses of the various feminisms, neo-Marxisms, minoritarianisms, and poststructuralisms in order to begin to move outside of both the logic of binary oppositions and the principle of non-contradiction. Situated in our multiple sites for movements of social justice, we can begin to "reinscribe otherwise" while avoiding the fall into an infinite regress of demystification. (1991, 163)

In fact, however, we cannot avoid falling into the "infinite regress of demystification" that Lather fears. Not, that is to say, if it is recalled that the ultimate irrecuperability *by* discourse of the apocalyptic opening *of* discourse means that the task of 'denouncing false discourses' is, as Derrida says, constitutively interminable. Or, to put this more simply, insofar as we can never finish enlightening the Enlightenment about itself, there is no "outside" – no non-mystagogical space – to which to escape.

Certainly "ambivalence" itself cannot figure such a space, since ambivalence – like rhetorical undecidability within the *trivium*, sublime response-ability to the law of universalization or literary resistance to *theõria* – signifies an indeterminacy that we cannot (re)cognize, objectify or know. Ambivalence as such, so to speak, cannot lead us out of the domain of non-contradiction or logical determination any more readily than the uncommon can 'be' what is "common" to us all (Arcilla). To suggest that it can is to reinscribe ambivalence *not* "otherwise," but rather *as* the Other of the Same. To just this extent, ambivalence itself is rendered *as* a determinate position – it is turned into a(nother) contestatory discourse that is "deliberate" – and its critical capacity to "interrupt" various discourses of intelligibility is forgone.

But the fact that terms such as "unknowing," "indefiniteness" or undecidability are not discursively recoverable as determinations that can ground an alternative stance is not the only argument against the attempt to reverse the positions of logic and rhetoric. There is a second argument as well. It is that insofar as the "apocalyptic tone" *of* philosophy conditions the possibility of distinguishing *between* philosophy and mystagogy, or insofar as the sublime is what first *opens* the aesthetic (i.e., as the "beautiful") or the theoretical (philosophy proper) to its own possibility – apocalyptic polyvocality and the sublime do not stand outside philosophy as its symmetrical negation or as, themselves, analogous *kinds of* discourses. Rather, we have seen, our indeterminable, sublime response *to* the moral law is what first makes both critique – a knowledge of the difference between moral and immoral acts – and Critique (a knowledge of the principle of moral knowledge) possible. So understood, polyvocality, rhetorical undecidability or *différance* open the determinate difference *between* the categories of ethics (or politics) and epistemology (or reason); they do not serve as epistemology's complement or its alternative.

Rather, I argued in Part One, the category of the sublime is that *without which* Kant could not have determined what *is* "beautiful," what *is* true or, indeed, what one "ought" to do at all. I also argued that, contrary to those who read Lyotard as rejecting modernist philosophical tenets in the name of "postmodernity," he does not describe an external position that the subject can intentionally adopt (or not) at will with regard to modernity. As I showed, Lyotard diagnoses modernity's *own* erosion or deconstruction *from within*. It is in this sense that "literariness" (de Man), the "apocalyptic opening of philosophy" (Derrida), modernity's "internal erosion" (Lyotard) and the "sublime" causality of practical reason (Kant) all stand, as it were, 'inside' philosophy as its (internal) *constitutive* 'outside.' These terms *are figured by* and *figure for* philosophy's own "supplemental" lack. As such, they *signify what cannot be signified* but what nonetheless first enables – what "possibilizes" (Gasché 1995) – philosophical completeness as such. The sublime is simply not, on this account, the Other of the Same.

What is most important here, then, is that the apocalyptic, the mysterious, the "sublime" or the undecidable are philosophical reason's *own* impossible necessity – not its rejection, not its absolute other and not its logical equivalent. For this reason as well, what Ellsworth calls the "unknowable," de Castell calls "disruption," Lather calls "dispersion" and Arcilla calls "indefiniteness" cannot take the place of the ethico-political values that underpin the philosophical discourse of modernity. To say that rhetoric possibilizes logic, that the sublime possibilizes the aesthetic, or that something we might call 'arche-critique' possibilizes the Critical architectonic as a whole is to say that the very determination *of* value – the very appeal to any ethico-political term that is (literally) meaningful – simultaneously presupposes *and* erases just that unknowability, just that disruption, just that sublimity and just that indefiniteness these theorists want to evoke. Or, to put this differently, *normative* (ethico-political) claims *for* the unknowable are themselves always already inside, and always already structured by, the very discourse of definition, restriction and exclusion *of* the unknowable that Ellsworth, de Castell, Lather and Arcilla wish to avoid.

Contrary to Burbules and Rice, then, the fundamental problem with the anti-modernist approach to educational theory is not primarily that it generates educative practices that "seem largely dependent upon the preferences of those who advance them" (1991, 399). In a certain sense this is true, but the problem is not only this. It is that, with their normative appeal to what escapes logic, determination and reason's exclusionary effects, anti-modernists presuppose a hard and fast distinction *between* (for example) universality and partiality, logic and rhetoric, or philosophical reason and ethico-political 'goods.' This distinction is always already indebted to the irrecoverable, apocalyptic opening *of* philosophy – and, indeed, of discourse in general – that is thereby obscured from view. In short, the anti-modernist determination of *différance* as *a* value reinstates the impossible difference between the epistemological and the ethico-political, and so covers over the *différantial* structure of the very divide that "postmodernism" brought into view. In effect, then, if an anti-modernist approach to education generates practices that cannot be universally Legitimated, this is not because the approach is "postmodern." It is because, on the contrary, the belief in a *pure* contest of wills (a *pure* ethical or political stance) against which there can be no rational appeal depends on a classically modern erasure of the undecidable difference between "philosophy" and "politics." In anti-modernist theory, this impossible root of legitimate ethico-political critique is restricted as, itself, a(nother) distinct normative end, and so the ideological effects of emancipatory discourse are once more upheld.

This misreading of *différance* (structural undecidability) as "difference" (politics instead of philosophy) is ubiquitous, of course, but it is particularly unfortunate in the context of anti-modernist theories of critique. For the error does not only produce fundamental confusion. It also obscures the normative potential of deconstruction itself; namely, the possibility that the 'ungrounded ground' of the philosophy–politics difference, once brought into view, will undo the purity of both categories, and so will provoke precisely the kind of *critical* challenge (a certain "critique") that anti-modernists actually support. This possibility suggests in turn, however, that if we are to sustain the idea of reason as critique, the ethico-political ends of education will have to be reformulated.

For, despite their misunderstandings, anti-modernist theorists Ellsworth, de Castell, Lather and Arcilla, together with neomodernist theorists McLaren, Carr, Giroux and others, are also right. Critical political philosophers of education *are* necessarily complicit in a kind of "evil" (de Castell), and they *do* inevitably exacerbate the conditions they are trying to work against, including "Eurocentrism, racism, sexism, classism, and 'banking education'" (Ellsworth 1992, 91). Theorists will continue to be complicit in these ills, however, as long as they believe that the task of a progressive political or educational theory is to formulate a particular, ethico-political agenda that is morally legitimate. For, in order for a particular political 'good' to serve as a legitimate educational aim, it must be tied to a critical standard that is rationally grounded. Such a standard grounds that "critical consciousness" through which one can distinguish the genuinely just from the genuinely unjust. Yet, as we have seen, the ethico-political standard of critique needed to inform this decision can only be determined and Legitimated – it can only be epistemologically-grounded in what is unconditionally true, and so can only embody reason in its normative sense – by tacitly appealing to the subject's inherent, transcendental essence (its moral end), and every such reference is exclusionary in its effects. Thus, a critical theory of education aimed at social justice *does* entail generalizing abstractly in the face of concrete differences, as de Castell, among others, suggests.

Critics of Enlightenment are thus not wrong to underline the oppressive effects of reason in philosophical discourses of emancipation. Where anti-modernists and neomodernists err, rather, is in the belief that one can understand political norms in different terms – for example, as strictly political, without any bearing on legitimate (philosophical) grounds at all. On this basis, anti-modernists argue, the emancipatory aim of the educational project can still be upheld *despite* the contemporary challenge to its traditional philosophical justification.

For the reasons given above, this proposal is untenable. Most importantly, we have seen that every political claim implicates a determinate standard of critique since, in the absence of a logical (and, hence, necessarily restrictive) principle of ethico-political judgement, one cannot speak to the difference between justice and injustice, and so one can neither contest nor support any particular state of affairs. To say that one's claim supports *justice*, in short, is just to say that one has taken a stand. And, once this distinction between the just and the unjust has been made, the question of legitimacy will ineluctably arise. On what basis, we must ask, is this not simply a version of "might makes right"? This Kantian question is not bypassed just because the standard in question is determined *as* the rhetorical, the literary or the sublime – as, for example, anti-modernists suggest. For the very naming of these categories as critically perspicacious values ensures that they will remain *inside* the speculative game. For anti-modernists and neomodernists alike, therefore, the emancipatory intent of Enlightenment is salvaged from the contemporary, deconstructive critique only insofar as the political theory that upholds it is still founded on a philosophy of the subject in its essence – on, for example, our (unconditional) capacity for self-determination, or on the (true) "existence" of *an* "indefinite, mysterious *self*" (Arcilla 1995, 169; my emphasis).[2] Something, in each case, is still said to be (truly) "common" to "us all."

The transcendentalizing move is not, I have argued, the consequence of our reasoning about or our inquiry into the rational grounds of our claims. On the contrary, a Critical inquiry into grounds reveals that it is only ever by virtue of an illegitimate closure of Critique, only by virtue of a mystagogical move, that the logical principle of moral determination is established. Transcendentalism, rather, attends those ethico-political claims that can be meaningfully expressed, shared or taught, themselves. It is just because metaphysics *is* the *sine qua non* of ethico-political norms themselves – at least insofar as they are not purely relative – that neither neo-modernists nor anti-modernists can escape the Kantian problematic, no matter how creatively, or how strenuously, they try.

What is of special interest in the anti-modernist case, however, is that the failure to escape the Kantian impasse is consequent upon the particular manner in which they attempt to do so. Specifically, anti-modernists insist on a radical distinction between politics and philosophy, and so unwittingly determine as *difference* the indeterminacy of *différance*. It was for this reason that I claimed that anti-modernists and anti-postmodernists are secretly allied: both beg the question of the autonomy of the logical and the rhetorical dimensions of language. The crucial difference between them, then, is not that one is modern and the other is its "post." Rather, it is that unlike anti-postmodernists, anti-modernists have nowhere intelligible to go. In other words, the anti-modernist strategy entails the determination of the indeterminable *as such*, and this is logically meaningless. This is why anti-postmodernists necessarily have the upper argumentative hand. In the next chapter, I therefore examine Jürgen Habermas's vigorous attempt to counter the contemporary delegitimation of modern legitimacy. In response to the "postmodern" challenge, he offers a reformulation of reason's normative force in non (or only quasi-) transcendental terms. In so doing, Habermas appears to offer to educational theorists a solution to the transcendentalism–relativism problematic that was first instantiated by Kant.

Notes

1 The internal reference is to Stanley Aronowitz. He would likely take issue with Ellsworth's willingness to sacrifice a "vision" of democratic ends in the name of partial truths (see Aronowitz 1997, 194).

2 Arcilla denies that this "self" can be judged to be authentically truer than other "fictive identities" we assume (1995, 169). If we take Arcilla at his word, however, then we must dismiss as nonsensical the "existence" of an "it" or a "self" that assumes various practical roles and identities. Second, we must also ask why the fiction of a "self" that "has no positive qualities" and that 'exists' purely as "aporia" should be celebrated before or above any other fiction (1995, 169, 170). Presumably, it is precisely because this "self" *is* to be taken in an ontological or quasi-ontological sense that it deserves the pedagogical attention that Arcilla recommends.

8 The Habermasian Gambit

A Critique of Discourse Ethics

> The fallibilism built into the theory of discourse is merely the converse side of the postulate that every sufficiently precise question admits of just one right answer … [I]nsofar as what is at issue is in fact a moral matter in the strict sense, we must proceed from the assumption that in the long run it could be decided one way or the other on the basis of good reasons.
>
> (Habermas 1993, 59)

> If we analysed the concepts of decision and responsibility in a cool manner, we would find that undecidability is irreducible within them. If one does not take rigorous account of undecidability, it will not only be the case that one cannot act, decide or assume responsibility, but one will not even be able to *think* the concepts of decision and responsibility.
>
> (Derrida 1996, 86)

The previous examinations of neomodernist and anti-modernist educational theory reveal that the tension between 'all' and 'nothing' is evident across the theoretical board – from adaptations of Gramsci, Freire, Dewey, Wittgenstein and Vygotsky for critical educational theory through to anti-racist, feminist and multicultural critical theories of education – and, thus, just how pertinent the Kantian formulation of the relationship between ethics and epistemology still is. Since this relationship is still very much at play in the meaning of "criticality," one must contest the Kantian formulation directly if one is to uphold the distinction between knowledge and ideology that the conception of education as emancipation demands. Otherwise, the critical standard of demystification being espoused will entail the very mystification – the occlusion of C/critique and the transcendentalizing of the subject – which Kant himself inscribed in the meaning of "critique."

To the extent that it alone addresses this necessity, a third strategic response to "postmodernism" – one which embodies a much more direct engagement with the Kantian legacy – is arguably the strongest position of the three. This "anti-postmodernist" approach to critical theory is based on a clear recognition of the problematic status of critique once it has been decoupled, either ambivalently (as in neomodernism) or definitively (as in anti-modernism), from the Enlightenment metanarrative of Critique. Specifically, what I call "anti-postmodernism" is the attempt to retain reason's emancipatory promise by contesting rather than embracing "postmodern" insights. To this end, anti-postmodernists offer a reformulation of reason's own normative ground, but this time in fallible and phenomenal, rather than in (Hegel's) ideal or (Kant's) noumenal, terms. Thus, it is argued, it is possible to formulate a post-metaphysical, detranscendentalized version of the Kantian standard for critique. In various forms, this rebuttal to the 'totalizing' "postmodernist" critique of the Enlightenment ethos can be identified in the work of such theorists as (among others) Nigel Blake, Helmet Peukert, Wendy Kohli, Les Burwood and Harvey Siegel.

These philosophers of education are among many who routinely appeal to Jürgen Habermas's theory of discourse ethics in order to make an anti-postmodernist, ethico-political case. As I have indicated, for example, Blake is expressly critical of Carr's (Deweyan) neomodernist approach to educational theory, insofar as Carr endorses democracy as a social norm, but fails to make a compelling case for "the superiority of a modern democratic form of social organization" (Blake 1996, 218, 217). "[W]e need stronger reasons than Dewey's to back our appeal to democracy," Blake says, and Habermas has provided them (Blake 1996, 234, 225).

Helmet Peukert mobilizes the Habermasian argument as well. He says,

> The basic task for a theory of education as well as for a theory of democracy remains to develop a critical concept of communication which would be able to describe the structure and goal of transformatory educational processes and, at the same time, to establish *the regulative ideals for communication in non-ideological decision-making*. The most promising candidates for this task seem to be theories of communication which include a discursive ethics of self-reflective communication. (1993, 167, emphasis mine)

Habermas's theory of discourse ethics is said to establish the needed ideals because it includes a normative core that defines the basis of ethics. Indeed, the argument that the principle of autonomy can be "apprehended *a priori*" as inherent in the structure of language (Habermas, qtd. in Peukert 1993, 163) – rather than as an essential fact about the subject – and, consequently, that any communicative act entails a set of *universal* normative presuppositions, is deemed by Peukert to be "fundamentally correct in its central intuition" (1993, 164, 163).

Another two theorists for whom Habermas's work plays a crucial role are Les Burwood and Wendy Kohli. For Burwood, for example, Habermas's analysis of the "*a priori* presuppositions of discourse" provides a "relatively uncontaminated point of reference beyond and independent of any particular culture" (1996, 426). Specific principles, Burwood says –

including "truthfulness, consistency, meaningfulness, weighing evidence and sincerity" (1996, 426) – can be mobilized in collective judgements about what is educationally and socially valuable in a multicultural society, thus lending to those judgements a "rational" quality that rebuts relativism. And for Kohli, similarly, Habermas provides a key starting point for critical reflection on the possibility of a "truly 'rational' society" (1995, 109). Unlike Burwood, she recognizes and shares many of the concerns that have been raised (particularly from a feminist perspective) about the "dominant Western view of reason, even *critical* reason" that Habermas's work provokes (1995, 107).[1] But Kohli also believes that, historically, reason has served "as a liberating force for women and other subordinated groups" (1995, 107). Hence, she contends, it is both possible and worthwhile to reconstruct reason's "liberatory potential" in a way that builds on such key Habermasian criteria as "the dialogical and the historical" as these are explicated in the theory of communicative ethics, but that also takes important criticisms into account (1995, 107–8). Such a "reconstruction" of discourse ethics will allow philosophers of education to continue to appeal to the "normative and the universal" in the wake of "postmodern discourse" (1995, 108, 103).

Perhaps the most strongly argued "anti-postmodernist" position, however, is that of Harvey Siegel. Siegel has written extensively on "rationality as an educational ideal" (1988, 1997), and he has paid particular attention to what he calls the broad "'anti-Enlightenment' currents in philosophy of education and in general philosophy" (1997, 1). In particular, he rightly points out that theorists who adopt what I call the "anti-modernism" position are engaged in a performative contradiction, because they are mobilizing the very epistemic and argumentative resources they are trying to escape. This is why, Siegel maintains, the "substantive, epistemic sense of rationality" he defends should continue to stand (1997, 188).

If Siegel's defence of "that old-time Enlightenment metanarrative" (1997, 2) is largely persuasive in the context of this all-or-nothing debate, however, it has considerably less force against a position that is not reducible to a "simple antirationalism or relativism" (Burbules 1996, 41). Specifically, I argued earlier that the classical ideal of critical reason is not undercut by (certain) "postmodernists" in the simple sense that they reject it; rather, "critical reason" is undercut by – or, more precisely, it undercuts – *itself*. De-legitimation, thus, is what modernity *will have been* about. Siegel must therefore do more than defeat the straw "postmodernists" with whom he engages. He must justify his own commitment to the Kantian version of "critical reason" that he favours (e.g., 1997, 145–6) in a way that resolves (rather than simply reiterates) the Kantian problem.

Interestingly, Siegel acknowledges that it is not only legitimate but indeed necessary to justify the normative prescription of criticality itself. "The demand for reasons which warrant a commitment to rationality," he writes, "is as legitimate … as … the demand for reasons which warrant any other claim, position, or commitment" (1997, 76–7). Indeed, he agrees, such a demand is not only legitimate but in fact "*basic* to regarding critical thinking as a fundamental educational ideal" (1997, 198, nt.1, and 191, nt.13; emphasis mine) and, in this respect, he agrees fully with Derrida: "whenever reason can be rendered, it *must*" (Derrida 1983b, 8; my emphasis).

It is significant that for a text that purports to "redeem rationality" against authors who have challenged the Enlightenment project, therefore, Siegel's justification is actually quite thin. He offers two distinct lines of support for rationality (or "criticality") as an educational ideal. His primary defence is the argument that rationality can be defended in a non-circular and non-question-begging way. Specifically, Siegel insists that reason is "self-justifying" because

> the very raising of the question ['why be rational'?] … commits one to a recognition of the epistemic force of reasons. To recognize that force is to recognize the answer to the question: we should be rational because (for the reason that) reasons, as the rationalist holds, have force. (1997, 82, 83)

Siegel's support for rationality thus amounts to the defeat of a straightforward scepticism: those who question "seriously" the reason for rationality already grant the overpowering force of reasons, and thereby support the rationalist position by implication.

There are many objections one might make about this claim, but the most important issue is that in order to ensure the rationality of the response to the demand for reason, reasons that are illegitimate must first be ruled out. In other words, the persuasiveness of Siegel's position hinges on a series of assumptions. First, the question "why be rational?" must be reduced to a demand for "justification," and then the demand for justification must be further reduced to a demand for "rational justification" (1997, 85). In short, the proposed justification of rationality that the question "why be rational?" ostensibly performs implicitly requires that one has requested a formal (philosophically sound) "justification" of rationality. For, according to Siegel, rationality is evinced not simply by the disposition to be compelled by any reasons at all, but only by the disposition to be compelled by *good* reasons. The demand for a reason is thus, in effect, the demand for a "serious" response. And, once the self-justification of rationality is seen to hinge on this requirement, the way in which Siegel begs the question becomes clear: he supposes that someone who does not accept the rationalist's position to begin with is nonetheless, in asking for *a* reason, demanding a "rational justification" in the formal, philosophical sense.

Yet someone who does not share Siegel's view might well be satisfied by a completely different response, such as, "I try always to be rational because it really bothers me when I contradict myself"; or, "If we do not behave rationally, there can be no hope for the human race"; or, "Behaving rationally/thinking critically is what we do here." Indeed, the possibility that emotional, political or cultural reasons may be taken as good ones is presumably exactly why Siegel thinks critical thinking must be taught. We are *not* all already critical thinkers (in Siegel's sense) to begin with, and so we must learn which reasons qualify as good ones, and by virtue of what criteria to tell the difference. Additionally, we must also (on Siegel's view) be taught to *care*. Thus, it is by no means clear that the mere demand for *a* reason for rationality necessarily and inevitably entails the demand for a "rational justification" in the formal, philosophical sense.

These considerations suggest that Siegel's demonstration is more modest that it appears. What follows from his argument is this: those who seek "justified grounds" for a commitment to rationality do instantiate that normative desire *for* reason that Kant first characterized as our "sublime interest" in moral legitimacy. In other words, when someone presupposes (however unwittingly) the legitimacy and epistemic force of reasons by asking for the (good) grounds of rationality, they do perform the commitment to rationality that Siegel upholds. The question Siegel must address, however, is not whether that commitment already obtains some of the time, but why it ought to obtain all of the time – why, in short, "critical thinking" ought to be taught. For his argumentative purposes, the demonstration that rationality *sometimes* obtains does not suffice, since, on Siegel's view, the desire for reason(s) characterizes the critical subject as such, and the production of "critical" subjects is the proper end of education. Thus, what is required is more than the demonstration that such a commitment obtains if (and only if) one is already answering *to* the principle of reason by seeking out a rational justification of rationality to begin with. What is required is that, to paraphrase Derrida (1983b), one answers *for* the principle of reason as well.

Kant, of course, attempted to undertake this task. As we saw, he argues that the commitment to rationality is by definition morally legitimate, because the demand for reason (for grounds) imposes itself affectively *on* the subject *as* that subject's noumenal essence. Specifically, reason (in the form of the law of universalization) was said to "humiliate" and so to "[humble] every man when he compares the sensuous propensity of his nature with the law." In so doing, reason's own law of universalization thus "awakens respect for itself insofar as it is a positive motive" (Kant 1993a, 78), and this feeling of "respect" for the moral law, when in force, is what defines an act as distinctly moral. Thus, unless Siegel is merely adopting – with all its attendant problems – Kant's own explanation of why one 'ought' (morally) to be rational, the burden is on him to provide an alternative explanation to Kant's.

This is where Siegel's secondary defence of rationality as a morally legitimate educational ideal becomes relevant. On Siegel's view, a particular judgement – in this case, the judgement that the ideal of rationality ought to be embraced – not only *can* have universal application and legitimacy, but indeed *must* have universal application and legitimacy if it is to be considered justified. Siegel admits that while he has not "systematically defended" that thesis himself, it *is* defended "by Habermas and Apel" (1997, 216, nt.31). It appears, therefore, that Siegel's anti-postmodernist defence of the Enlightenment metanarrative – along with the arguments offered by Blake, Peukert, Burwood and Kohli – also stands or falls on the basis of discourse ethics.

To be sure, this wide reliance on Habermas seems to be well placed; he offers compelling support for the thesis that reason can be "redeemed" in post-metaphysical terms and that, on this basis, it can still be said to enlighten the path to social and political betterment. Against this anti-postmodernist view, however, I have argued that the ground *of* "critique" is constitutively undecidable – that it is not possible to determine a logical principle of moral judgement without illegitimately restricting the subject to some particular essence such as its "sublimely" indeterminable response-ability, and so illegitimately closing the responsibility *to* reason that the very term "criticality" is intended to convey. If this is so, then Habermas's theory will be no less vulnerable than Kant's, and the consequence will be that "anti-postmodernists" do not resolve the difficulties that a wide variety of critics of the Enlightenment have identified either.

This case has not yet been made. On the contrary, notwithstanding the fact that discourse ethics has, over the years, provoked extensive critiques and reformulations (Benhabib 1987; Wellmer 1991; Rehg 1994; Heath 1995; Payrow Shabani 2003), the Habermasian approach to moral theory has largely remained intact. Unlike generally supportive criticisms of the programme, therefore, the present contestation of Habermasian discourse ethics goes further: it is intended to show that the theory is bolstered by a set of metaphysical assumptions that it cannot sustain; consequently, Habermas does not provide an adequate rebuttal to the challenge posed by a certain "postmodernism." In particular, I argue that Habermas's reconstruction of "*the* moral point of view" – the perspective of impartiality and universality that is ostensibly tied to communicative action as such (Habermas 1990, 198; 1993, 118)[2] – cannot *but* privilege the (Kantian) subject characterized by a "sublime" capacity for moral reason. This metaphysical legacy, I submit, is structurally indispensable; it is embedded, ironically, in the very strategies through which Habermas distinguishes his position from that of Kant.

Among these strategies, most importantly, is Habermas's proposal to shift from solitary reflection to intersubjective agreement on moral norms. This allows him to explicate the moral dignity of our ability to universalize (i.e., to reason impartially) *not* in terms of a noumenal Kingdom, but rather in the phenomenal terms of the intersubjective, hence *materially* or *socially*-constituted nature of psychic integrity. In contrast to Kantian morality, then, discourse ethics attempts to treat the reality of pluralism in a post-traditional world, and it does so by way of a move from monologic to dialogic modes of normative legitimation.

Yet, once the material reality of pluralism is acknowledged, and once it is agreed that normative claims therefore may be contingent upon one's social, historical or cultural context, it becomes apparent that the possibility of universal moral validity depends directly on the difference between particular and universal norms. In other words, if he is to detranscendentalize Kantian "Man" by discarding the doctrine of the two realms without, at the same time, sacrificing the possibility of moral universalism, Habermas must draw a sharp distinction, here and now in everyday practice, so to speak; he must distinguish between norms that are amenable to rational argumentation and that are therefore universally justifiable – norms that constitute the so-called "moral" sphere – and norms that follow from particular conceptions of the 'good life' and, as such, resist rational, consensual resolution (i.e., so-called "ethical" norms). The weakness of discourse ethics as a critical theory of society stem from this distinction – a distinction between 'justice' and the 'good life' which, as Seyla Benhabib remarks, has not been sufficiently attended (1997, 104). In particular, the questions at issue are why this sharp distinction is necessary and what, given its necessity, are its consequences.

With regard to the first question, let us note that Habermas must maintain the rationality of the moral sphere against incursions from the contingencies of ethical life, because this is the only way that discourse ethics can lay claim to a universal perspective and, thereby, to avoid metaphysics or ethnocentrism. In other words, in light of the reality of moral pluralism in the post-metaphysical (post-traditional) world, the theory of discourse ethics must be conceived in purely procedural and formal terms, lest it be argued that, in being permeated by contingent, "ethical" goods, the moral sphere as explicated by Habermas reflects and imposes only the particular form of life which Habermas, among others, prefers. Benhabib, significantly, takes issue with this claim; she argues that there can be universal as well as culturally-specific 'goods,' and she offers human rights as an example of the former. Yet Benhabib herself is very clear that, when conceived as a 'good' rather than exclusively in terms of what is just, the value of human rights is to some extent culturally-constituted; as such, it is not strictly rational and is, therefore, *ethically* contestable relative to other goods. Indeed, based on the argument that a universalist morality of human rights and of liberal tolerance follows from the perspective of the third person legislator, and that this perspective, in turn, entails culturally-specific, albeit thin, notions of the good, Benhabib accuses Rainer Forst of coming closer in some respects "to an ethnocentric communitarian position" than she herself does, insofar as Forst would limit himself to that standpoint alone (Benhabib 1997, esp. 105–8; Forst 1997). Since it is the charge of ethnocentricism that the autonomy of the moral sphere is intended to refute, however, such a softening of the line between morality and ethical life as Benhabib proposes will not serve Habermas's theoretical purposes.[3] On the contrary, the distinction is essential to the discourse ethicist's position. The problem, however, is that the maintenance of the distinction entails the transcendentalization of the subject, and it does so for Habermas no less than for Kant.

In order to see why Habermas is vulnerable to the same charge notwithstanding his concerted efforts to move beyond Kant, let us begin by underlining that Habermas is fully aware of the problem. For him, as for Max Weber, modernity is characterized by the fragmentation of reason into its different applications in the spheres of science, morality and art (see Habermas 1982, 240; 1987, 339). As a result, Habermas claims, pre-Kantian concepts of substantive reason are simply not plausible; we no longer have recourse to "collectively binding religious or metaphysical worldviews" (1993, 70). This, quite simply, is what it means to Habermas to "take modern pluralism seriously" (1993, 123). Indeed, Habermas asserts,

> Only at the cost of Occidental rationalism itself could we rescind the differentiation of reason into those rationality complexes to which Kant's three critiques of reason refer. Nothing is further from my intention than to make myself an advocate of such a regression, to conjure up the substantial unity of reason. (1982, 235; see also 1990, 206)

This is why Habermas insists upon a narrow, purely procedural role for moral reason; given a plurality of world views, the theory of communicative ethics is intended to explicate only the *process* of *normative legitimation* and is to be held entirely separate from evaluative questions of the good. "Moral theory is competent to clarify the moral point of view and justify its universality," he says, "but it can contribute nothing to answering the question 'Why be Moral?'" (1993, 76).[4] Indeed, even more pointedly, Habermas says,

> What moral theory can do and should be trusted to do is to clarify the universal core of our moral intuitions and thereby to refute value scepticism. What it cannot do is make any kind of substantive contribution. By singling out a procedure of decision making, it seeks to make room for those involved, who must find answers on their own to the moral–practical issues that come at them, or are imposed on them, with objective historical force. (1990, 211)

Yet notwithstanding its evaluative neutrality, the formal delineation of communicative reason is intended to serve a crucial moral role. Indeed, one could characterize the driving motivation of the discourse–ethical project as a whole in terms of Habermas's desire to establish an incontrovertible moment of normative unconditionality for the theorization of social life. For Habermas, this moment is the *sine qua non* of a justified critique of society. Without the unconditional, he says, "we must be prepared to renounce the emancipatory potential of moral universalism and deny so much as the possibility of subjecting the structural violence inherent in social conditions characterized by latent exploitation and repression to an unstinting moral critique" (1993, 125).

Significantly, this means that the distinction between "morality" and "ethical life" is crucial for Habermas's argument. In other words, if it is only by virtue of "the *moral* point of view" that one can arrive at agreements which are universal – that is to say, unconditional and therefore "rational" – in nature, then what Habermas calls "moral–practical discourses" do indeed "require a break with all of the unquestioned truths of an established, concrete ethical life"; they require, in fact, the "distancing [of] oneself from the contexts of life with which one's identity is inextricably woven" (1993, 12). Most importantly, to fail to determine a sphere composed of universalizable norms would be to "[succumb] to a relativism that robs moral commands of their meaning and moral obligations of their peculiar force" (1993, 76). This is why the morality–ethics divide is structurally indispensable: it concerns nothing less than the very basis, in Habermas's eyes, for a legitimate critical political response to social and political forms of injustice.

It is therefore significant that Habermas fails to make the case for the autonomy of the moral sphere – that is, that he fails to distinguish clearly between "justice" and "the good" – except at the cost of burying a metaphysical premise in the theory of communicative ethics. For this means that one is caught between the equally undesirable choices of either having to derive the legitimacy of "the" moral point of view from an unthematized reference to transcendence, or of falling prey to the charge of relativism Habermas has consistently sought to refute. To avoid relativism, discourse ethics must privilege a subject that is removed, in essence and by definition, from the contingencies of everyday life.

This claim may seem strong, given that Habermas is fully aware that the insistence on universality carries a particular danger for contemporary deontologists. He knows, in particular, that Kant could appeal to the ideal of universalizability (in the form of the categorical imperative) as the very 'form' of reason only because the Enlightenment philosopher saw reason itself as the constitutive feature of the noumenal subject. Habermas, of course, no longer depends on such a strategy of argumentation; a post-conventional, post-metaphysical perspective cannot rely on the subject's noumenal 'essence' – what Kant called "the fact of reason" – to support the relation between reason and normative validity. At the same time, however, for Habermas the moral sphere only qualifies *as such* insofar as it comprises norms that are amenable to rational justification through a procedure of universalization.

In order to solve this problem, Habermas proposes a reformulated principle of universalization (U). Specifically, for Habermas normative validity is conferred not merely by virtue of the fact that a moral actor employs the rational *ideal* of universalizability in a process of solitary reflection ("Act only according to that maxim whereby you can at the same time will that it should become a universal law" [Kant 1993b, 30]), but rather by virtue of the *concrete enactment* of universalization in the form of an uncoerced consensus among a genuine plurality of communicative subjects (1993, 51). Habermas formulates the principle (U), therefore, as follows: "a contested norm cannot meet with the consent of all of the participants in a practical discourse unless (U) holds," which is to say, as he continues,

> Unless all affected can *freely* accept the consequences and the side effects that the *general* observance of a controversial norm can be expected to have for the satisfaction of the interests of *each individual.* (1990, 93; emphases his)

Thus, as Albrecht Wellmer has carefully argued, in order to qualify as valid, a norm must not only be considered through a process in which all interests are fairly and fully (reciprocally and symmetrically) represented – that is, a process in which all the reasons of all concerned are weighed equally and impartially so as to determine which reasons are the most 'forceful.' Additionally, the norm must also be one to which all have *actually agreed* – that is, the interests of all concerned must also, in fact, have been served (Wellmer 1991, 113–231).

This requirement becomes apparent once we notice, with Wellmer, that the justificatory process itself can only be redeemed (i.e., determined as a valid one) *retroactively.* In other words, Wellmer argues, when taken as a principle of justice, Habermas's (U) is "quasi-circular": we can only say that all interests have been impartially represented in the first instance (i.e., that all reasons and interests have been brought forward and equally weighted in the argument) in light of a consensus (i.e., the determination of a norm which actually serves all interests) in the second instance (1991, 149). Thus, Habermas's explication of a "common" will escapes the charge that it is a metaphysical postulation precisely because it is a factual achievement; unless an actual agreement results from the discussion, there is no "common" will to speak of at all. As Habermas writes,

> as long as the isolated subject, in his role as custodian of the transcendental, arrogates to himself the authority to examine norms on behalf of all others, the difference between his supposition concerning a *general* will and an intersubjective agreement concerning a *common* will never comes to light … [O]nce we abandon the metaphysical doctrine of two separate spheres of reality, subjects encounter each

other as individuals who can no longer rely on [an] antecedent transcendental agreement. (1993, 51; emphasis his; compare 1990, 203)

It cannot be argued, therefore, that (U) provides only a formal presupposition of, or a regulative idea for, argument – that, insofar as "communicative reason, unlike practical reason, is not itself a source of norms of right action" (1993, 81), (U) is merely a rule of argument the *goal* of which is consensus. While this claim is fair as far as it goes, it obscures the fact that we cannot establish that a norm *is* legitimate unless we can establish that the principle of (U) has been applied, and – most crucially – *(U) cannot be said to have been applied unless an actual consensual agreement among impartial discussants has been reached.* [5] Significantly, therefore, while the conditions of the procedure itself are a necessary feature of its rationality, the conditions are insufficient as criteria of normative validity. Equally important is the achievement of an agreement as to what the common (universal) interest really *is*, since only a consensus qualifies the strictly valid norm, and only the identification of such a norm, in turn, can retroactively establish the moral sphere. It is in this sense that Habermas speaks of the "discursive redemption" of validity claims (1993, 29, 51).[6]

Once this is acknowledged, another significant difference between Kantian and Habermasian morality becomes apparent. In discourse ethics the meaning of 'universalizability' shifts from what I (or we) can generalize *without contradiction* to what we have all (universally) *actually agreed* we *should* generalize. Most importantly, this means that rationality can no longer be said to follow from the mere achievement of universality (i.e., consensus) – as it did in the Kantian paradigm from the mere fact of being able to will without contradiction – since agreement might be reached on a variety of bases, such as the fear of reprisals, for example. Thus the "rational potential inherent in everyday practice" (Habermas 1987, 341) resides not in the criterion of universalizability alone but, additionally, in the *discursive process* whereby a universal agreement is achieved.[7] More specifically, an agreement is deemed fully rational only when it is based solely on the force of the better argument; namely, when the conditions *for* the agreement are (or at least adequately approximate) the ideal conditions of mutual recognition and reciprocity.[8]

This demand for an impartially-determined norm achieved through actual consensus is where Habermas runs into trouble. For it is here that the definitive distinction between the categorically moral and the contingently evaluative must be established; here that an unconditional moral 'ought' must be shown to be identifiable under real and not merely ideal discursive conditions, and here that the theory of discursive ethics must be identified as a moral theory in its own right rather than as a specific application of a consensus theory of truth to the realm of justice (Wellmer 1991, 149). Yet it is at this crucial moment that Habermas's theory of discourse ethics relies tacitly upon the possibility of transparent, ahistorical and culturally-unencumbered rationality.

This conclusion can be demonstrated with reference to Seyla Benhabib's work, notwithstanding her obvious sympathy with the Habermasian approach in general. Benhabib has argued that the justice–ethical split that characterizes the onset of modernity translates into a split between the public and the domestic or private, with the consequence that the latter is simply left behind as part and parcel of an atemporal state of nature that is prior to history (1987, 86). To be sure, Benhabib is treating Lawrence Kohlberg's theory in particular, but it is one which Habermas follows closely. He too characterizes the achievement of postconventional morality with its justice orientation – both socially and ontogenically – in terms of a catastrophic but 'natural' break from a state of nature (Habermas 1990, 126). This means that in Habermas's theory too, the public, male figure of moral and political, justice-oriented theory is split "into the public person and the private individual" – a dualism that Benhabib characterizes in terms of what she calls a "generalized" and a "concrete" other. Specifically, the "generalized other" signifies the abstract, public persona of modern moral and political thought; it is based on the male head of the bourgeois household, and it suggests the standpoint of "formal equality and reciprocity." The standpoint of the "concrete other," in contrast, is based on the private world of personal and domestic life; this standpoint "requires us to view each and every rational being as an individual with a concrete history, identity, and affective-emotional constitution" (1987, 87).

On Benhabib's view, moral theories such as Kohlberg's and Rawls's, which entrench this dualism by focusing exclusively on the standpoint of the "generalized other," are epistemologically incoherent (1987, 88–9), because human identity cannot be reduced to the "capacity for agency alone" (1987, 88, 89). Rather, Benhabib insists, identity refers to

> the actuality of my choices, namely to how I as a finite, concrete, embodied individual, shape and fashion the circumstances of my birth and family, linguistic, cultural and gender identity into a coherent narrative that stands as my life story. (1987, 89)

If the idea of a "self" prior to its concretization is incoherent as Benhabib suggests, and if, therefore,

> there is no human *plurality* behind the veil of ignorance but only *definitional identity*, then this has consequences for the criteria of reversibility and universalizability said to be constituents of the moral point of view. Definitional identity leads to *incomplete reversibility*. (1987, 90; emphases hers)

In other words, the distinction between justice and the good life which characterizes modern Western societies institutes a "generalized" concept of the self which, in turn, renders universalistic moral theories constitutively incapable of accounting for concrete differences among actual moral discussants.

This contention is directly relevant here, since Habermas, like Rawls, calls for complete reversibility in the specific sense that "in communicative action speaker and hearer assume that their perspectives are interchangeable" (Habermas 1993, 131). Indeed, we have already established that the discourse ethical claim to rationality stands or falls with the impartiality of the process whereby consensual agreement is achieved. To this end, Habermas contends, at the level of argumentative praxis

> perspectives, relations of recognition, and normative expectations built into communicative action become completely reversible in all relevant respects, for participants in argumentation are credited with the ability to distance themselves temporarily from the normative spectrum of all existing forms of life. (1993, 131)

But there is a curious equivocation at work; unlike Rawls, Habermas also insists that the role of such idealizations – for example, 'crediting interlocutors with the ability to distance themselves from values of an evaluative, substantive kind' – does not entail the problem of empty formalism. On the contrary, he claims, "First, (U) regulates only argumentation among a plurality of participants; second, *it suggests the perspective of real-life argumentation*, in which all affected are admitted as participants. In this respect my universalization principle differs from the one John Rawls proposes" (1990, 66; emphasis mine). Thus, Habermas maintains that the idealization entailed by moral–practical discourse, the supposition that the conditions of the "ideal speech situation" sufficiently obtain,

> does not bear on the objects treated in argumentation; it leaves the identity of the participants and sources of conflict originating in the lifeworld untouched. The moral point of view calls for the extension and reversibility of interpretive perspectives so that alternative viewpoints and interest structures and differences in individual self-understandings and worldviews are not effaced but are given full play in discourse. (1993, 58; see also 1982, 255)

This equivocation signals a crucial problem. If Habermas can be said to escape Benhabib's critique of Rawls by virtue of the fact that in his theory individual self-understandings and identities are not suspended but are, on the contrary, given "full play in discourse," then the procedure of moral discourse cannot be said to establish rationality by virtue of its impartiality. For in this case the strict criterion of impartiality will not have been met. On the other hand, if the individual participants in a moral discourse *are* fully to 'distance' themselves from the contingent, "normative spectrum of all existing forms of life," the result for discourse ethics will be a transcendentalizing of the subject and the consequent "epistemic incoherence" that Benhabib finds in moral theories that focus exclusively upon that standpoint. Either way, therefore, rationality cannot be said to be established solely by virtue of the discourse ethical procedure.

In response to Benhabib's analysis, Rainer Forst has argued that Rawls's description of an "original position" is intended only to establish the legitimacy of the principles of equality and reciprocity in discourse; "any further 'concrete' moral, political or legal questions," he says, "have to be dealt with in different ways," and "these ways obviously include others as concrete persons." To this extent, Forst argues, Kantian theories (such as Rawls's) do not entail the sharp opposition between the "general" and the "concrete" that Benhabib describes (Forst 1997, 93, 94). Such a critique, however (even if plausible) cannot be mobilized here. For there is a significant difference between Habermas's theory of justice and that of John Rawls, and to this extent Forst too quickly dismisses Benhabib's analysis as it bears on Habermas's work. Whereas Rawls merely *posits* 'primary goods' and an 'original position' in order to arrive at principles of justice, Habermas seeks to *derive* those same principles from the structural features of communicative action as it might actually take place (i.e., in "real life argumentation"). Importantly, this means that fully embodied, concretely-situated persons are necessary not only for the resolution of "further questions," but for the legitimation of the principles themselves. For this reason, Habermasians cannot appeal to "an unavoidable 'ideal' moment in the sphere of morality," whereby the "criteria of moral validity necessarily transcend[s] moral agreements … that have been reached" (Forst 1997, 92). For it is that very ideal, *qua* normative criterion, that Habermas is trying to establish in actual (pragmatic) rather than in transcendental terms (see Habermas 1990, esp. 75–6).

Habermas in fact forgoes Rawls's strong version of "generalizing the other" for precisely this reason; he insists that the legitimacy of norms *follows* from having given specific viewpoints and interests full play in a moral discourse. As Romand Coles notes, "In the idealizing supposition of a consensus open to criticism, the possibility of diverse voices on a given issue is not repressed, but rather the very condition of possibility for the legitimacy of the agreement" (1995, 25; compare Habermas 1990, 203). Therefore, the discourse ethicist cannot do without the kind of concretization that Benhabib is calling for, since only "concrete" selves can engage in the full reversal of interpretive structures that Habermas demands. Consequently, however, Habermas must give up the discourse ethical claim to impartiality too. For concretely-situated "others," in contrast to general or abstract ones, are decidedly partial, precisely to the extent that they *cannot* be said to be removed from the normative spectrum of their everyday lives. The implication of Benhabib's argument for Habermasian discourse ethics is thus that the impartiality of the moral point of view is bought at the cost of transcendentalizing the subject. Indeed, Benhabib notices that it was the very shift to a "justice" or "moral" orientation within modern political thought that gave rise to the general–concrete difference in the first place. On the other hand, insofar as Habermas intends a genuine and not merely a nominal pluralization of moral interlocutors, his distinction between morality and ethical life – the very distinction upon which the rationality of discourse ethics depends – is untenable.

Habermas must therefore reject Benhabib's own version of discourse ethics, which involves replacing a strictly "moral" theory with a "communicative ethic of need interpretation," whereby "the object domain of moral theory is so enlarged that not only rights but needs, not only justice but possible modes of the good life, are moved into an anticipatory-utopian perspective" (1987, 93; see also Benhabib 1990, 349, 350).[9] For his refutation of the charge of relativism rests directly on the contention that the universal core of 'our' normative intuitions can be distinguished absolutely from the contingencies of ethical life on the basis of the application of the principle of universalization (U).[10] Now in Habermas's reconstruction of (U), it will be recalled, the rationality of moral action shifts from its basis in the Kantian injunction to universalize without contradiction to that of a procedure aimed at a universal consensus guided by impartial reasoning and ideal role-taking. Yet we have also seen that the impartial reasoning and ideal role-taking Habermas has in mind are the characteristics of a 'generalized' other that is (by definition) incapable of undertaking the full reversibility upon which Habermas insists. Indeed, the principle (U) may be said to have been applied only when concretely situated individuals (each of whom necessarily brings his or her substantive, ethical concerns and perspectives into the discussion) have actually participated in a debate. Consequently, no purely 'rational', non-relative, unconditioned sphere of morality can be said to emerge *from* the procedure itself.

Without recourse to an unthematized transcendentalism, then, (U) cannot be relied upon to mark *retroactively* the distinction between questions of justice and questions of the good life and, thereby, to confer moral validity (in the form of unconditionality) on the process of normative legitimation. Such unconditionality would require a *prior* distinction between morality and ethical life; without a distinction between justice and the good *already* in place, there is no basis for the postulation of a generalized (transcendental) other capable of the pure impartiality moral legitimacy requires. Without the prior availability of this distinction, in other words, we must face the reality of concrete discussants who are not impartial, transcendental subjects, but are situated, partial individuals whose moral arguments are inextricably layered with contingent evaluations. Consequently, the theory of discourse ethics must either fall prey to the charge of relativism, or it must continue to rely on an abstract notion of the human subject, whose transcendence of the historical, gender, racial, class and cultural (*inter alia*) contingencies of everyday life is not merely a temporary achievement but a constitutive attribute.

Habermas's attempts to address Benhabib's and Carol Gilligan's critiques of Kohlberg's developmental theory do not resolve this difficulty; they merely shift the terms of the debate:

> Practical reason is not fully realized in discourses of justification. Whereas in justifying norms practical reason finds expression in the principle of universalization, in the application of norms, it takes the form of a principle of appropriateness. Once we grasp the complementarity of justification and application, it becomes clear how discourse ethics can address the misgivings you [Torben Hviid Nielsen] share with Seyla Benhabib and Carol Gilligan. (Habermas 1993, 154)

Not only does this response leave the problem of transcendentalizing the subject intact with regard to justification, but it brings to light a further issue: the determination of "appropriateness" (A) in the context of application no more reflects a contextual mode of thought than does the determination of universalizability (U) in the context of justification. Rather, just as (U) entails abstracting from normative worldviews, so (A) requires that

> [a]n *impartial judge* must assess which of the competing norms of action – whose validity has been established in advance – is most appropriate to a given concrete case once all of the relevant features of the given constellation of circumstances have been accorded due weight in the situational description. (1993, 128f., esp. 129–30; emphasis mine)[11]

Leaving aside the arguable assertion that "the" relevant features of a moral question can definitively be determined, we need only note that the original charge may be redirected to the issue of application as well: if the judge of 'appropriateness' is *also* to be impartial (by 'distancing' him or herself from contingent notions of the 'good'), it is not clear either how that achievement is to be determined, or in what way, precisely, the necessity of concretizing moral discussants in their socio-historical contexts has actually been addressed.

It would certainly seem, then, that the programme of discourse ethics is caught at an inescapable impasse regarding the demand to distinguish between questions of justice and questions of the ethically good life. Habermas must either concede the relativism of discourse ethics, or he must support the autonomy of the moral sphere on the basis of a metaphysically determined concept of transcendental reason.[12] In either event, the demonstration of a *post*-metaphysical break between questions of the good and questions of justice has not been provided; rather, the neutrality of the discourse ethics programme relies upon an unacknowledged metaphysical premise, whereby the subject is once again illegitimately restricted to some particular essence.

Thus, while the problem of transcendentalism attending Kantian (and Hegelian) philosophy is indeed addressed directly by Habermas and his proponents in the field of critical political theory – much more directly, in fact, than these problems are generally treated by educational theorists who seek either to replace Enlightenment idealism with the philosophy of Dewey, Freire, Wittgenstein or Vygotsky (for instance), or alternatively, by those who try to escape the modern discourses of Enlightenment altogether – the metaphysical dimensions of the modernist conception of "critique" are not eliminated here either. On the contrary, Habermas extricates discourse ethics from the charge of relativism by pluralizing an abstract subject that is only ever illegitimately universalized. Against those such as Blake, Peukert, Burwood, Kohli and Siegel who would mobilize the discourse ethics of Jürgen Habermas for a critical political philosophy of education, therefore, I contend that Habermas's 'post-metaphysical' deontological ethics does not serve this end.

Taken together, therefore, it remains that none of the three strategic responses to "postmodernism" – neomodernism, anti-modernism or anti-postmodernism – ultimately dodges the dilemma at hand: the *political* purchase of critical educational theory is gained at the expense of a certain critique. In effect, I have argued, it is simply not possible to bypass the double bind in which the pedagogical goal of ethico-political knowledge is caught. Consequently, a *critical* theory of emancipation must account for, rather than escape or deny, critique's (own) "mystagogical" effects. To be sure, such a theory will sacrifice the possibility of a Legitimate (epistemologically-grounded) purchase on the question of what is 'good.' In so doing, however, it arguably exemplifies a "certain critique." In fact, as I now want to show, it is precisely in this way that deconstruction's own "quasi-responsibility" can come into view as an indispensable resource for theorists of progressive, emancipatory change.

Notes

1 Kohli (1995) references Seyla Benhabib's criticisms in particular (106–7).
2 For the sake of clarity, I retain Habermas's phrase ("the moral point of view") throughout.
3 Peter Dews's solution to the problem of distinguishing sharply between justice and the good coincides with Benhabib's (Dews 1995, 207).
4 In "Remarks on Discourse Ethics" Habermas attempts to clarify and correct his theory in light of critical objections from a variety of perspectives. It is

therefore fair to say that this essay, along with, for example, "Discourse Ethics: Notes on a Program of Philosophical Justification" and "Morality and Ethical Life: Does Hegel's Critique of Kant Apply to Discourse Ethics?" (Habermas 1990), represents Habermas's considered word on his position.

5 For Wellmer, the fact that discourse ethics requires an actual and not merely an ideal consensus means that Habermas is open to the charge that discourse ethics is nothing other than "the application of a general consensus theory of truth to the specific case of the concept of justice" (1991, 149).

6 For this reason above all it is clear that Wellmer's proposal that Habermas discard the requirement of consensus (1991, 153f.) is simply implausible.

7 "Universal" here is to be taken to mean, 'among all concerned with or affected by the norm in question'; that is, the rightful participants in the moral discourse.

8 Habermas qualifies the "redemption" of a validity claim in terms of "the framework of a discourse which is sufficiently close to the conditions of an ideal speech situation for the consensus aimed at by participants to be brought about solely through the force of the better argument, and in this sense to be 'rationally motivated'" (qtd. in Wellmer 1991, 166). I leave aside the obvious objection that the "better" argument in moral disputes is rarely transparently evident.

9 Forst notes that this move seems to reflect an Hegelian-influenced vision of reconciled life which is not supported by the theory (1997, esp. 79–81). See also Benhabib's response (1997). For further criticism of Benhabib's suggestion, see Herta Nagl-Docekal (1997, 70–71).

10 This argument poses a decisive challenge to any attempt to render discourse ethics more responsive to social and cultural difference by softening the morality/ethics divide, such as those of Kohli (1995) and Strike (1995).

11 This seems to be Wellmer's view as well. In his essay "Ethics and Dialogue," for example, Wellmer presupposes there can be only one "correct" interpretation of a given situation. The question of appropriateness raised by the application of norms in concrete situations thus lends itself to the moral point of view as well (1991, 202, 203). Compare Habermas: "Interpreted from the perspective of discourse ethics, practical reason does indeed require practical prudence in the application of rules. But use of this capacity does not restrict practical reason to the parameters of a specific culture or historical period. *Learning processes governed by the universalistic substance of the norm being applied* are possible even in the dimension of application" (1990, 181–2; emphasis mine). If I understand him correctly, Habermas is saying that the prudential question of "appropriateness" can be answered impartially, eventually, as well. This interpretation is also supported elsewhere (Habermas 1993, 172).

12 Significantly, this is only one half of the problem. As I have argued elsewhere, even if (U) *could* be said to act "like a knife that makes razor sharp cuts between evaluative statements and strictly normative ones" (Habermas 1990, 104), Habermas would still face an additional and perhaps impossible task. He would have to substantiate his contention "that the *procedural* explanation discourse ethics gives of the moral point of view – in other words, of the impartiality of moral judgments – constitutes an adequate account of moral intuitions which are after all *substantive* in kind" (1990, 199; his emphasis). Since Habermas cannot appeal to the self-respect that accrues to subjects by virtue of their noumenal essence, he must look elsewhere; his solution hinges on an appeal to Lawrence Kohlberg's developmental theory. However, Kohlberg's theory implicates teleology in a way that is also fatal to the discourse ethical programme. For a full elaboration of this point, see Gaon (1998).

Part III

On Deconstruction and Justice

9 Responsibility as Messianic Injunction

> All the same, and in spite of appearances, deconstruction is neither an *analysis* nor a *critique* and its translation would have to take that into consideration. It is not an analysis in particular because the dismantling of a structure is not a regression toward a *simple element*, toward an *indissoluble origin*. These values, like that of analysis, are themselves philosophemes subject to deconstruction. No more is it a critique, in a general or in a Kantian sense. The instance of *krinein* or of *krisis* (decision, choice, judgment, discernment) is itself, as is all the apparatus of transcendental critique, one of the essential "themes" or "objects" of deconstruction.
>
> (Derrida 1988a, 3)

The extended survey of critical educational theory undertaken in Part Two was not intended to demonstrate simply that this critical theorist or that philosopher of education has read "postmodernism" (or, indeed, modernism) wrong and that, from this point of view, deconstruction is "most valuably an exposure of error, certainly not other people's error, other people's essentialism" (Spivak 1993, 4). It has been intended to demonstrate, rather, that the political demand for legitimacy, the demand that we render the reason *for* our ethico-political commitments and so cover over the undecidability at their root, imposes itself inexorably on both sides of the modernism–postmodernism divide. The "error" of Enlightenment thought, as Spivak says, is "extremely useful"; it is one without which political theory cannot "live on" (1993, 4). In other words, what a deconstructive reading *of* "critique" (of "criticality," or of "legitimacy") reveals is that the bond between ethics and epistemology that the term "critique" embodies is inescapable for political thought, notwithstanding the fact that it is ideological as well.

In particular, I have argued, political and educational theorists cannot speak to the *difference* between justice and injustice in a way that is not simply culturally, historically, socially or otherwise contingently based without a determinate and rationally-grounded *standard* of critique. Without such a standard in place, the theory cannot issue in the legitimate ethico-political *decision* (the "critique") that it requires. Without reference to a standard of critique, in effect, no assessment of responsibility is possible at all. This is (so to speak) a logical rather than a political necessity. For this reason, the Kantian problematic – which concerns the difficulty of finding the logical ground for the criteria of the ethico-political decision itself – emerges in progressive pedagogical theory despite many theorists' explicit rejection of Kant's own emphasis on the "scientific" (and transcendental) status of moral judgement. The problem reappears, in other words, even when the theorist has ostensibly ceased aiming at moral legitimacy, or at rational grounding, altogether.

To support this claim, I have demonstrated on one hand that, notwithstanding the fact that various theorists of education – particularly those who adopt what I have called an anti-modernist theoretical strategy – mobilize substantially different philosophical resources than those provided by Kant, they nonetheless appeal to an ethico-political standard that can be determinately established. To the extent that such values as "openness," "unknowing" or "indefiniteness" serve as criteria for ethico-political judgement, the theory profits all the same from the ungrounded link between ethics and epistemology that Kant first *ideologically* established, and that has yet to be non-transcendentally justified. For, as I argued in Chapter Five, what is peculiarly Kantian is not the specific procedure for or standard of moral judgement that Kant himself upheld. Rather, it is the assumption that we can know (and hence teach) what *is* properly ethical, that there can be such a thing as moral legitimacy (a principled or grounded good) at all. And, as soon as any value is posited as the ground or principle of a critical theory of society, the spectre of moral legitimacy will already have been roused. Once it has, the only remaining question concerns the theoretical solidity or soundness *of* the value named. In particular, I have explained why anti-modernist arguments that prioritize rhetoric (in the form indefiniteness, unknowing or openness, for example) over logic do not bear up well in this regard.

On the other hand, I have also shown that neomodernist attempts to produce alternative theoretical justifications of why such principles as "autonomy," "voice" or "self-determination" ought to figure as the universal, ethico-political aim of education – and, consequently, as the ground of a "critical consciousness" – have failed as well. Theorists who undertake this justificatory project do understand that a "responsible" critique is one that is by definition based on a standard of justice that can be clearly identified; however, their various theoretical efforts to bypass Kantian metaphysics cover over the undecidable grounds (the apocalyptic opening) of their ethico-political claims nonetheless.

Specifically, from McLaren and Giroux through to Siegel and Habermas, the charge of relativism is countered only insofar as *a* (markedly Kantian) subject is ultimately (re)instituted as *the* universal, normative ground of the critique. In the three strategic approaches to emancipatory educational thought, therefore, some form of the link between ethics and epistemology that Kant first illegitimately established must still stand as the ungrounded ground (the apocalyptic opening) of the critical–theoretical enterprise, or else the enterprise will founder. And this means that political and critical theorists of every sort will necessarily implicate the very ideology they intend to challenge in the name of justice. This necessity prompts my claim that ideology is just what a political theory aimed at emancipation through the inculcation of reason – at the end of ideology and at the horizon of Enlightenment – needs.

Moreover, once a deconstructive interrogation of Enlightenment reason reveals the inescapability of an ideological moment at the heart of modernist and so-called "postmodernist" critical political theories alike, it becomes clear that the normative relevance of deconstruction does not relate to its putative "reversal" of classical, philosophical hierarchies. As I have argued, those who understand deconstruction in this way collapse *différance* – that "non-full, non-simple, structured and differentiating origin" *of* difference (Derrida 1982, 11) – into, simply, another *kind* of "difference." *Différance*-cum-"difference" is then *itself* celebrated as a critical standard in the place of universality (or not). Or, to put this another way, those who understand deconstruction in this way turn theory's own rhetorical undoing (theory_2) into, simply, another kind of theory (theory_1) – only this time so that rhetoric, rather than logic, becomes the operative, logical term. In both the modernist and the anti-modernist case, therefore, the (rhetorically undecidable) co-implication of ethics and epistemology is missed. Thus, whether claims concerning deconstruction's ethico-political pertinence stem from either position (pro or con modernity), critical theorists who presuppose that deconstruction "aestheticizes" philosophy take for granted the very possibility of moral legitimacy (or, alternatively, of *theory* as such) that "postmodernism" puts into question – or, to be more precise, the erosion of which itself results in "postmodernism."

From this point of view, the "ethics" of deconstruction (such as it is) can be seen to lie solely in the revelation of a certain ideology at the root of any ethico-political critique that claims to be legitimate, whether that critique is undertaken in the express name of universality, totality and autonomy, or not. In other words, deconstruction can be qualified as a certain "critique" insofar as it exposes an ideological moment at the root *of* "critique" whenever and wherever moral legitimacy is said to obtain. For the investigation of the principle, root or grounds of moral knowledge – even, paradoxically, an investigation that culminates in knowledge's own undoing – is just what has characterized reason in its "critical" mode (in its "responsibility") all along. To say that deconstruction's ethico-political pertinence should be understood in this way, therefore, is to say that the (self-) deconstruction of critique – that is, the way in which the postulation of moral legitimacy itself brings about the exposure of "legitimacy's" own mystagogical or apocalyptic grounding on the abyssal structure of arche-critique (C/critique) – can be formulated in the opposite way as well. If we grant that "critique" (is) what *will have been* its own deconstruction, we must equally grant that deconstruction (is) what *will have been* critical to begin with. In this sense, deconstruction might be said to be "post" critical (in the Lyotardian sense).

The definition of the term "post-critical" that I suggest here, however, must be rigorously distinguished from the definition proposed by Patti Lather, which I discussed above. For Lather, it will be recalled, "post-criticality" refers to a position on the part of the critic that can be characterized as a kind of neomodernist ambivalence or equivocation; the term is said to refer to *both* the continued *centrality* of critical reason in its modernist sense (whereby "criticality" is understood as the equation of knowing, naming and emancipation), *and* to the interrogation of that equation at the same time. The definition of the term I offer here, in contrast, has nothing to do with the attitude or the activity of the critic, least of all with an attitude of incredulity or doubt. Rather, "post-criticality" refers to the inevitable *decentring* and *delegitimation* of critical reason (in its modernist sense) that occurs when the concept of "critique" (*as* that equation) is brought, self-reflexively so to speak, to bear upon itself. Deconstruction is thus "post-critical" in the precise sense that it issues in a legitimate (or quasi-legitimate) delegitimation of legitimacy. This postulation entails the assumption that the deconstruction of moral legitimacy is "always already" a response to the demand for reason (or *for* Legitimate grounds) that Kant established as the meaning of "critique" to begin with. Or, to phrase this differently, the postulation that deconstruction (is) what will already have been critical suggests that *the normative or ethico-political responsibility at work in deconstruction rests, paradoxically, on its interrogation of responsibility as such.*

Now, if such an interrogation results in the deconstruction of critique in its very possibility, this would seem to suggest that in terms of both politics and pedagogy, the "postmodern" decentring of the subject leaves us with nothing – with no basis whatsoever on which to challenge the injustice and oppression to which critical political thought addresses itself. For, on this "postmodern" view, it is clear that deconstruction is not simply another political theory with another standard of critique; rather, it is a *Critical* interrogation *of* the possibility of "responsible" critique as such. Is this to say, then, that deconstruction *is*, simply, the critique of a critique – only one which replaces the standard we have used to gauge injustice with, instead, nothing but the poor recognition that critique no longer has (will no longer have had) any force?

Not simply. For once it is understood as "post-critical" in the sense I propose, it becomes clear that deconstruction can be neither, simply, a form of (responsible) "critique," nor said to rest outside the sphere of responsibility, outside the jurisdiction of ethico-political legitimacy. Thus, deconstruction does have a "certain" normative force. But just what its claim to responsibility is, and just what its implications for political and educational thought are, remain to be seen. Indeed, as Derrida has rightly remarked, it is important that,

> it not be said too precipitately that these questions or these propositions ["What is the ethicity of ethics?, the morality of morality? What is responsibility? What is the 'What is'? in this case? etc."] are *already* inspired by a concern that could by right be called ethical, moral, responsible, etc. I know that, in saying that ("And let it not be said too precipitately…" etc.), one gives ammunition to the officials of anti-deconstruction, but all in all I prefer that to the constitution of a consensual euphoria or, worse, a community of complacent deconstructionists, reassured and reconciled with the world in ethical certainty, good conscience, satisfaction of service rendered, and the consciousness of duty accomplished (or, more heroically still, yet to be accomplished). (Derrida, 1992b, 14–15)

Most importantly, the reason that the deconstructive interrogation of "morality," "ethicity" or responsibility cannot be said to be "*already* inspired" by an ethical, moral or responsible concern is because this characterization would have to draw on the very form of legitimacy whose "complacent" self-certainty deconstruction challenges. Such a challenge, then, is issued in the name of what?

Interestingly, Derrida has posed this question himself. He asks, "is answering *to* the principle of reason the same act as answering *for* the principle of reason? Is the scene the same? Is the landscape the same?" (1983b, 8). Peggy Kamuf offers a particularly lucid depiction of the paradox that Derrida's question entails, and it is therefore worth citing her at length. She writes,

> [I]t is here, within this circle [of the legitimated figure of legitimacy, or auto-destination], that the question of a destination *not already comprised* by the space of legitimated knowledge arises. But how can that question arise *within* the circle? Unless an opening has been left, a space wherein the auto- or the self- of destination *dis-closes* itself? Unless the dis-closure of the circle opens up a space that is neither within the legitimated domain nor simply outside it, but along the edge where the two divide? … [T]o the extent that this dis-closure of the circle along its unfigurable edge lets one challenge the legitimacy that is conferred by circular destination, it can be seen to arise as an illegitimate question, as falling outside the realm of legitimate reason. And this despite the fact that, as already suggested, the question can only be posed because the realm itself in effect produces the question of its limit at its limit … The legitimacy that concerns us most – the legitimacy of the very figure of legitimacy – is open to question and to challenge only in a space opened *within* the circle, but which is

> therefore not a part of that figure. It is within without being a part of the circle and as such it is the very possibility of the figure's reconfiguration. (Kamuf 1995, 102–3; original emphases)

Similarly, Derrida asserts, if analysts end up working "on the structures of the simulacrum or of literary fiction, on a poetic rather than an informative value of language, on the effects of undecidability, and so on, by that very token they are interested in possibilities that arise at the outer limits of the authority and the power of the principle of reason" (1983b, 14). This must not be confused with a mere nihilism or obscurantism on their part, for these categories are still dependent on the principle of reason as its symmetrical opposite (Derrida 1983b, 14–15, 9).

By the same token, I submit, the deconstructive intervention in philosophy must be understood neither as the reinstatement of responsibility *qua* subjective mastery elsewhere, nor as an outright destruction of the Enlightenment ethos. To be sure, a deconstructive reading can and does reveal indeterminacy at the root of any of ethical, political or educational norms insofar as these are said to be rationally grounded; it thus can open them to the possibility of an ethico-political critique. Insofar as it can do so, however, a deconstructive reading is paradoxically both within and without the very circle of legitimation (the auto-legitimation of the principle of reason) that it questions, and thus is neither strictly "critical" nor strictly "ideological." In fact, I will demonstrate here, deconstruction enacts "critique" otherwise. It can be qualified, therefore, as what I have been referring to as a certain "critique."

Specifically, my purpose now is to explain in what sense deconstruction can be said to entail a politically affirmative gesture and why, in turn, it therefore can be qualified as "quasi-responsible." As I will show, deconstruction is a response to the very "law" that Derrida invokes; namely, that we cannot "forgo the *Aufklärung*, in other words, what imposes itself as the enigmatic desire for vigilance, for the lucid vigil [*veille*], for elucidation, for critique and truth" (Derrida, 1983a, 22, cited above). This claim concerning deconstruction's peculiar enactment of critical responsibility, I submit, opens the door to a radical reformulation of the very character of political critique, and thus has direct implications for emancipatory political thought more generally.

The discussion begins in the present chapter with Drucilla Cornell's argument in *The Philosophy of the Limit* (1992a). For she argues there with respect to critical legal studies, just as I have argued here with respect to political theory, that deconstruction challenges the law in its very legitimacy (in its putative "justice"). However, she goes further than this; she contends that it does so *responsibly*. On Cornell's view, deconstruction responds to an infinite, messianic notion of justice against which positive laws can be gauged, and so can itself be "translated" as a version of critique insofar as it exemplifies "an attitude that permits us to choose (*krinein*), and so to decide and to cut decisively in history and on the subject of history" (Derrida 1992a, 54). Thus, despite her acknowledgement that deconstruction cannot be translated directly into a positive political or legal programme, Cornell argues that the law's own inescapable openness (its justice) "can be 'translated' as a standard" by which to judge different legal systems and even "the justices themselves" with regard to the exercise of judicial responsibility (Cornell 1992a, 181, 166).

Cornell's reading of deconstruction as the exposure of a messianic injunction to honour justice and, thus, as the *basis* for a justified critical decision in the field of (American) jurisprudence, leads her to formulate deconstruction itself as a radical standard of critique. To be sure, such a formulation is not entirely misplaced. Derrida has often referred to deconstruction as a kind of "radical critique" – in, for example, his 1984 interview with Richard Kearney (in Kearney 1984, 118) and again in *Specters of Marx* (1994) – and he has even proposed that its motivating affirmation takes the form of a response to the call of an alterity that necessarily summons it (in Kearney 1984, 118). Moreover, when Derrida specifies that legal theorists such as Cornell and Samuel Weber in particular are furthering a deconstructive programme that would aspire "to *change* things" – to intervene politically, as it were, in the world (Derrida 1992a, 7, 8) – he implicitly aligns deconstruction with a classical version of Marxist critique.

Yet notwithstanding his apparent endorsement of Cornell's theoretical trajectory, Derrida has also consistently maintained that deconstruction – a practice of reading which disseminates, which multiplies meaning, which 'writes the trace of a decision as the margin of its own impossibility' (Derrida 1981a, 5) – is neither critique nor the critique of a critique (as the epigraph to the present chapter indicates). Rather, he insists, it is a strategic practice of reading that tries to think the possibility *of* critique "from another point, that of the genealogy of judgement, will, conscience, or activity" (1995a, 286, see also 1992b, 17). Thus, Cornell's equation of deconstruction with ideology critique and Derrida's own approval of her theoretical agenda deserve a closer look.

To this end, I elucidate Derrida's distinction between "law" and "justice" in order to show precisely what Cornell has in mind when she invokes the possibility of an ethico-political critique of law derived from deconstruction. Specifically, it emerges that Cornell does *not* understand deconstruction as a quintessential form of responsible critique in the sense that she sees it as grounded on a more secure principle of reason than is the Kantian notion of ethico-political "critique." Rather, Cornell's view is that the deconstructive "critique" of law is normatively demanded by an infinite otherness that both precedes and exceeds the laws and principles of judgement themselves.

There is, according to Cornell, in this sense a messianic injunction to deconstruct. Significantly, however, the concept of "responsibility" Cornell is mobilizing here, whereby the deconstructive reading is characterized as a response to the injunction of an otherness that inheres *in* the law, is not derived solely from Derrida's own work. It is derived, rather, from Emmanuel Levinas's formulation of "responsibility" as a *response to* a messianic injunction that imposes itself in the primary, phenomenological experience of radical alterity. The infinity of the Other makes an ethical demand on me, Levinas argues, at the moment I encounter an other (person). Moreover, as I go on to argue, Levinas presents the concept of "responsibility" as a religious relation, and he conceives it as an *external* site from which to launch a critique of philosophy. This is the argument that Cornell mobilizes to justify her contention that deconstruction enacts a "critical" intervention in the law. In fact, we will see, the reason deconstruction is *not* said by Cornell to be "already inspired by a concern that could by right be called ethical, moral, responsible, etc." in a Kantian sense, is that she sees deconstruction as "already inspired" by a messianic ethicity instead.

In Chapter Ten I will take issue with this view. Specifically, I argue that in proposing that deconstruction mobilizes a Levinasian, rather than a Kantian, standard of critique, Cornell has in fact neglected Derrida's own reading of Levinas. For Derrida's reading suggests that the messianic dimension of experience on which Levinas's (and Cornell's) external critique of philosophy is based 'takes place,' so to speak, neither 'outside' nor 'inside' philosophy but rather, *as* philosophy's *own* apocalyptic opening. Indeed, Derrida's reading of Levinas results in an understanding of deconstruction itself as the exposure of the impossibility of the very 'outside' on which Levinasian responsibility (no less than Kantian autonomy), *qua* critique, depends. Consequently, it emerges, deconstructive strategies of reading have the paradoxical effect of putting the meaning of critical responsibility – including the putative responsibility of the deconstructive intervention itself – into profound question. They do so, I suggest, by virtue of their very adherence to the (Kantian) protocols of critique.

Derrida's own work thus points ultimately to the need to rethink the concept of critical "responsibility" itself in terms of the way in which it fails, constitutively, to account for its own desire. In other words, although it is possible to say that deconstruction bears a "certain" critical or normative force (a quasi-responsibility) and is, therefore, of consequence for the fields of education, politics and the law, it remains that it is finally deconstruction's (or, more precisely, the *deconstructionist's*) own desire *for* reason that must be addressed.

In Chapters 11 and 12 I therefore undertake to explain the normative status of the deconstructive intervention itself in terms of a psychological, not a strictly moral, imperative. This reformulation of the desire for reason (for C/critique) in a psychoanalytic register does not leave us with nothing, I argue. For the psychoanalytic explication of the desire for reason that I propose suggests there is a commitment to ethico-political responsibility that we "heirs" of the Enlightenment cannot *not* share, even if we cannot adequately Legitimate it, either. What is more than nothing, then, is the conditional sense in which the imperative of unconditionality, the imperative *to determine* a self-grounding ground, inexorably imposes itself on those of us grappling with "justice," notwithstanding the constitutive impossibility of satisfying this demand. So understood, deconstruction cannot be said to provide us with some *thing*, another ontological ground, either. On the contrary, because the "reason" – the normative demand *for* grounds – to which critical theory responds is itself contingent in nature, any theory that purports to be "critical" cannot at the same time advocate the perpetuation of reason *as* an emancipatory, educational ideal. The imperative to question the ethical dimensions of political and educational thought, therefore, is all that a critical educational or political theory can impel.

*

Given the character of Cornell's approach to deconstruction as it already has been sketched, it is clear that her understanding of deconstruction's ethico-political purchase is not the common one. Cornell's formulation can be contrasted, for example, with Habermas's belief that deconstruction levels the distinction between literature and philosophy and thereby aestheticizes the fields of ethics and politics (Habermas 1987, esp. 205). It can also be contrasted with the neo and anti-modernist belief that, in undermining the possibility of any textual authority whatsoever, deconstruction renders meaning in terms of an undecidable "free play" whereby all readings are as valid as any others. Finally and most crucially for the field of critical legal studies, Cornell's outlook can be contrasted with the standard anti-postmodernist charge: if deconstruction is an exposure of the law's imbrication in socio-political power[1] – if, that is, it shows that legal interpretation is ultimately unjustifiable in unconditional terms – then the result is that legal critique will be informed by whatever interpretive scheme happens to strike the preference of the critic.

In comparison with these views, Cornell's understanding is radical. She contends not only that deconstruction is not the levelling of moral differences between different legal systems or alternative judicial interpretations – not only is it *not*, therefore, the abdication of critical theoretical responsibility – but that it is on the contrary the essential condition of any justified critique of the law whatsoever. A "justified" critique. That is to say, a critique of law that is undertaken in the service of, and aimed at, justice, and one which is so on legitimate grounds.

Significantly, two different claims appear to be embedded in Cornell's explication of the normative status of deconstruction. While they are fundamentally entwined, it is important to distinguish between them. The first claim is that deconstruction has a critical function, and that this functions rests in its unique ability to expose what Derrida calls the "mystique" or the 'mystagogical foundation' of law, 'there' where justice is said to have taken place. This first thesis, which corresponds to the way in which deconstruction qualifies on my own view as a certain "critique," is based on Derrida's discussion of "justice" and the "law" (1992a). Derrida shows that, for essential and structural reasons, justice as such (that is, in its essence or pure form) is never literally present or 'there' to be found in the law. Any enforcement of the law in the name of justice, therefore, will necessarily miss its mark. Succinctly phrased, the crucial paradox or "aporia" at issue in the question of the relationship between justice and the law is that *the 'general form of the rule, norm or value' that constitutes the law "prescribes a singular application in each case"* (Derrida 1992a, 17; emphasis mine). Most importantly, this means the law must suppose the "generality of a rule, a norm, or a universal imperative" in order to sustain its legitimacy (the law cannot be legitimate if it is for me or you alone), just as ethico-political legitimacy must presuppose epistemological Legitimation. At the same time, however, if it is to be "just," the law must also be specifiable in the singular; it must be susceptible of being addressed to each (and any) idiomatic case.

What is most important in this analysis of the law *as* justice, then, is that it leads to the conclusion that, rigorously speaking, "justice" is impossible. On one side: the general, determinate and calculable rule. On the other, an infinite idea of justice as the singular, the idiomatic and the incalculable. Between these poles, no rule exists or could exist to guide a passage. There is, quite literally, no way forward. In aiming *at* justice, in promising to address itself *to* the other, law must in effect calculate the incalculable. Now if a law *truly* specifies, if a law *is* 'just' in the sense that it is adequately idiomatic, this means that it is not yet a universal *law*. If, on the other hand, the law entails a repeatable calculation that can be universally applied then, strictly speaking, the law is no longer *just*. For no 'idiom' can be translated into a universalist discourse without a loss. In this sense, the law is either too early or too late for justice. So the inescapable aporia *of* law – its impossible passage, its deepest secret and its profound 'mystique' – is that, as the *realization* of justice, the law in its very meaning cannot 'be' (here now). Its very possibility and promise of 'justice' (is) this impossibility.

More significantly still, this impossibility cannot appear, for it cannot be recovered by the universalist discourse (the repeatable formulations and codes) it sets in motion. Moreover, if the relation between the calculable rule (a given law) and the incalculably idiomatic (the singular case) is as unavoidable as it is impossible, this means that any 'preservation' of the law (as justice) by virtue of its enforcement is at once its 'invention' and so, strictly speaking, not simply a (re)enactment of the (same) law. In other words, any *application* of a law – if it is to be 'just' with respect to any singular case – will mark its 'first' instantiation and, hence, its (non) original legitimation. Consequently, legitimations of the law (precedents) are on Derrida's view always *coups de force* (1992a, 13) – which is to say, violent 'blows,' but also 'cuts,' or decisions. Applications of the law *retroactively* legitimate that which they ostensibly preserve. For this reason, Derrida contends, an aporia, a 'not-is-ness' of law *as* justice, so to speak, remains at the heart of law; the law, therefore, is interminably open to deconstruction. And justice, as this undecidable promise *in* the law, 'is' the deconstruction, which is to say, the de-sedimentation or "internal erosion" *of* the law.

This understanding of the nature of justice gives rise to Cornell's first assertion concerning the normative nature of the deconstructive impulse. In light of the non-coincidence between justice and the law that Derrida describes, Cornell maintains, there is always an opportunity for a (certain) *critical* engagement. There, in its very claim *to* legitimacy, the law (any law) will necessarily (it will always) have covered over the non-legitimate foundation of its own force. Similarly, I have shown, this kind of occlusion occurs with respect to the moral legitimacy defended by Kant as well: as soon as it is announced, the moral law (whichever one) covers over the non-legitimate ground (the "mystical origin") of its own determination. And this means that if we begin by accepting (as political and educational theorists, I have shown, inescapably *do*) that Legitimacy is what a moral claim *must* bear, or that justice is what the law *must* effect, then we can always take issue with a given law or a given ethical standard by looking for the traces of its founding violence.

Cornell demonstrates how one might undertake such a deconstructive "critique" with reference to the 1986 legal case of *Bowers v. Hardwick*. This is a case in which two gay men were criminally convicted on the basis of the ruling that "the state of Georgia has the right to make homosexual sodomy a criminal offense" (Cornell 1992a 159). In his judgement, Justice White essentially concluded that the defendants' fundamental rights to privacy and to 'life, liberty and property' (the 9th and the 14th Amendment to the US Constitution) were not violated, since neither the constitution nor the legal precedents cited in their defence specifically enumerated 'the right of privacy to homosexual activity' (see Cornell 1992a, 159, 160–61 and 207n. 25).[2]

With regard to this case, Cornell argues that Justice White used a predominant justificatory myth: the myth Stanley Fish calls "the plain meaning of the words" (Cornell 1992a, 158). Formulated differently, Cornell says, this is "the myth of full readability" (1992a, 159). It is the fiction that the law can be evoked as an ideally transparent origin of legitimacy, because its meaning is always completely translatable and clear. This myth allowed the Justice to overlook the unavoidable, interpretive and evaluative moment of his own reading of the Constitution. He did not acknowledge, in particular, his crucial claim that "family, marriage, and procreation" have *on his view* nothing to do with homosexual practices (1992a, 160–61).

A moment of (re)interpretation such as this, Cornell suggests – the inevitable calculation of the incalculable – is an ineradicable feature of any legal decision. Hence, it can be seen that in upholding the prejudices prevalent at the time of the Constitution's writing, Justice White in fact *re-legitimated and re-founded* those very prejudices in the name of a just decision. By appealing to a seeming origin – the 'real' meaning 'there' to be simply read in the law – the judge effectively re-founded the legitimacy of the oppression of gay men in the very gesture of his ostensible "conservation" of that law.[3] For Cornell, therefore, deconstruction contributes a strategy for criticizing oppression enacted by the law. As she says,

> The exposure of the mystical foundation of authority … [shows] that the establishment of law is violence in the sense of an *imposition* without *present* justification … The point, then, of questioning the origin of authority is precisely to undermine the conflation of justification with an appeal to the origin, a conflation made possible because of the erasure of the mystical foundation of authority. (1992a, 164)[4]

Now, Cornell's contention, that a deconstructive practice of reading can illuminate the violent, ungrounded force with which laws themselves are repeatedly (re-)legitimized, is arguably apt. What I want to contest is not this critical function of deconstruction, whereby it can expose an 'originary' non-foundation at the base of legal legitimacy *if* such legitimacy is assumed to be given, but Cornell's further claim. For it is not merely that, for Cornell, deconstruction exposes a certain 'violence' and that, in so doing, it enacts a certain critical responsibility. To be sure, this claim is already contentious, and will require further elaboration. But there is a second, more emphatic claim embedded in Cornell's argument. It is that a deconstructive practice of reading is itself *the* justified – possibly even the most justified because the most responsible – form of critique. For Cornell, deconstruction is not just a mode of critical responsibility; it is also the most responsible critique. It is necessary to engage, then, with what Cornell sees as deconstruction's exemplary critical status.

As Cornell notes, deconstruction inspires a particular anxiety for critical legal theorists. It is that, as Dominick LaCapra has argued, if the origin of all legitimate authority is 'mystical' insofar as it is ultimately based on a groundless violence, then the ethico-political significance of deconstruction might be seen to rest in its "dangerous equalizing force" (Cornell 1992a, 163). In particular, LaCapra's uneasiness has to do with the possibility of "an *irresponsible* turn to violence, because," in the absence of a legitimate origin of legal authority, "there can be no projected standards by which to judge in advance the acceptability of violent acts" (Cornell 1992a, 167; emphasis added). This, of course, is the danger of rhetoric described above, but expressed in a different register. The peril, again, is that no judgement or legal system can be deemed more 'just' than any other once the originary violence on which they are founded have been (deconstructively) revealed. Fred Dallmayr describes the anxiety attending this purported radical perspectivism as well. He asks: does not the rule of law

> become a captive or instrument of arbitrary caprice, of the whim of particular interpreters? Are we not witnessing here the triumph of power over law, of [a radical or "deconstructive"] *voluntas* over *ratio* (which the hermeneutic circle had hoped to obviate)?[5]

Cornell's explanation of why deconstruction is not simply irresponsible can be addressed not only to LaCapra, but to Stanley Rosen (the critic Dallmayr is paraphrasing) as well. She insists,

> [I]t is not that the question of the ultimate ground or foundation is pointless for Derrida [as it is for LaCapra]; instead, it is the question of the ultimate ground, or correctly stated, lack of such, that *must* be asked, if we are to heed the call of Justice. That no justificatory discourse *can* or *should* insure the role of a metalanguage in relation to its dominant interpretation, *means* that the conserving promise of the law can never be fully actualized in a hermeneutic circle that successfully turns back in on itself and therefore grounds itself. (1992a, 163; emphases hers. Compare Derrida 1992a, 13)

Even more directly, she adds, "Thus we can respond to LaCapra's concern that all legal systems not be conceived as equally 'rotten.' All judges are not equal in the exercise of their *responsibility to Justice*, even if justice can not be determined once and for all as a set of established norms" (1992a 166; emphasis added).

Cornell's response suggests that she thinks deconstructive reading itself provides a critical standard (a legitimate "must") by virtue of which we can determine or decide the *relative* justice of the judges. This standard is formulated in terms of a "responsibility to Justice." Indeed, the weight of Cornell's rebuttal hinges on the performative strength of that "must." For without recourse to such an imperative, Cornell's response to LaCapra and to Rosen is no response at all. In other words, it is only by virtue of an unassailable appeal to the ideal or horizon of an *absolute* responsibility (signalled by the capitalization of "Justice") that we can make sense of Cornell's claim that legal systems and judgements can be judged as *relatively* (rather than as merely equally) rotten. On this basis, Cornell claims to have answered the charge against deconstruction. Not only is it not the case that deconstruction forecloses the possibility of responsibility or, worse, that it authorizes irresponsible violence, but deconstruction actually demands that one be critically responsible with regard to the justice of legal decisions and systems. Against LaCapra, Cornell suggests that we have a legal response-ability to the singularity of every case, and that this responsibility can serve as the 'standard' by which to judge, decide or choose between 'competing' legal systems (Cornell 1992a, 166). To this extent, deconstruction may itself function as *critique* (as the "philosophy of the limit," as Cornell says). It follows that deconstruction's "must" has been decided.

But this means a crucial shift has occurred. The Derridean view I have presented throughout this study leads, arguably, to the conclusion that deconstruction 'is' (or that deconstruction takes place 'as,' so to speak) the exposure of an essential impossibility of the "just" law (or the "legitimate" moral decision) as such. The exposure of this aporia and, consequently, the revelation of the inescapable failure of legal (or moral) legitimacy, is what deconstruction does, here from 'inside' (at the internal–external limit of) the law. On this basis it is clear that, if it is "of obligation that we must speak" whenever we speak of justice (to paraphrase Derrida), it is the law's own obligation as *droit* to aim *at* justice, to address itself *to* justice (and, consequently, to encounter the aporia of the undecidable relation within it) that Derrida actually evokes. It does not seem to be *our* obligation to expose the law's constitutive failure (its failure to address the singular fully, adequately or without a loss) that Derrida has in mind. Justice as deconstruction – or, rather, justice as the (non)site *of* deconstruction – was merely Derrida's formula for "the *self*-authorization of law (droit) *as* the possibility of the exercise of deconstruction" (1992a, 15; emphasis added).

With regard to our responsibility *to deconstruct* – our charge *to* pose the 'question of the lack of ground'[6] – Derrida is much more oblique. The practice of deconstructive reading, it is true, is said to find its motivation in, and to be "mad about the desire for," the possibility of a certain justice (1992a, 20–21, 25). This 'madness' – Derrida's name for the idea of an "infinite" justice characterized by the "demand of gift without exchange, without circulation, without recognition or gratitude, without economic circularity, without calculation and without rules, without reason and without rationality" – this madness, then, is said to be the "basis" of deconstruction's "operation" (1992a, 25, 26). But is this madness, this infinite justice, itself the deconstructionist's own ethico-political charge? Or is it, rather, that "deconstruction," "justice" and "madness," all name a structural impossibility that we "experience" 'there,' where justice is said to 'take place'?

On this latter view, one might say, justice as undecidability is no more and no less than a structural feature of law in (or 'as') its address to an infinite idea of justice (*qua* the singular or the radically heterogeneous). "This kind of justice, which isn't law, is the very movement of deconstruction at work in law," 'here' where the impossible takes place (Derrida 1992a, 25). This is precisely why justice for Derrida cannot function as a horizon or a limit, as he cautions repeatedly, and as Cornell acknowledges too (Derrida 1992a, esp. 25–7; Cornell 1992a, 134–5). For justice as aporia is never *there* (anywhere), but only ever 'here': it is the impossible (not 'present,' not 'as such') experience (meaning) of an absolute alterity (the infinite opening at the origin of what 'is') (1992a 27). It is in this sense that Derrida contends that "the interest of deconstruction, of such force and desire as it may have, is a certain experience of the impossible" (1992a, 30). It is in this sense too that deconstruction has the motivation of an "always unsatisfied appeal" (1992a, 21).

But it is not at all clear how one might move from Derrida's *description of* deconstruction to Cornell's *prescription to* deconstruct. To say that deconstruction exposes (or, rather, that it "is" the exposure of) the impossibility of an ultimate ground that is promised is not synonymous with saying that deconstruction can be determined *as the responsibility to expose.* It is not to say that it must. Thus, without recourse to an argument that goes beyond Derrida's own, we are no closer to understanding why, for Derrida at least, the question of the ground "must" be asked.

To say – although it is by no means all he says – that deconstruction is motivated by an unsatisfied appeal, that it corresponds to the *structure* of an incalculable promise, or that it 'is' an interest in the experience of the impossible is, to be sure, to tie the force of deconstruction to the inherently "affirmative" meanings of motivation, of promise and of interest. Yet it must be noted, too, that when in "Force of Law" (1992a) Derrida explicitly evokes the "must" of an ethical–political imperative, he does not do so in the name of deconstruction or incalculable justice *per se.* He does so, rather, in the explicit name of a "classic emancipatory ideal" – an ideal, in fact, for which we must risk the worst. Specifically, he admonishes, the fact that justice exceeds the law and that "the unpresentable exceeds the determinable" is no excuse for political quietism. For,

> Left to itself the incalculable and giving (*donatrice*) idea of justice is always very close to the bad, even to the worst for it can always be reappropriated by the most perverse calculation. It's always possible. And so incalculable justice *requires* us to calculate ... Not only *must* we calculate, negotiate the relation between the calculable and the incalculable, and negotiate without the sort of rule that wouldn't have to be reinvented there where we are cast, there where we find ourselves; but we *must* take it as far as possible, beyond the place we find ourselves and beyond the already identifiable zones of morality or politics or law, beyond the distinction between national and international, public and private, and so on. This requirement does not properly belong either to justice or to law. It only belongs to either of these two domains by exceeding each one in the direction of the other. (1992a, 28; emphases his)

What is most significant about this passage, in my view, is its indication that the aporetic relation between justice and the law (and, hence the deconstructibility of the law) does not name an imperative 'to deconstruct.' It is, rather, the condition *of* an emancipatory ideal that Derrida himself wishes to uphold, and that he wishes to uphold despite the fact that it cannot be grounded, legitimately calculated or guaranteed. What is required, Derrida says, is *that* we judge, that we decide, or that we choose – that we choose *a* good – in order that we may avoid the "worst" which the incalculability of "justice" (Cornell's infinite ideal) itself *necessarily* risks.[7] Thus it is, finally, in the name of emancipation, in the name of "a new Enlightenment for the century to come" (Derrida 1994, 90), and in the name of a critical responsibility – a "responsibility for responsibility" (1992a, 20) – that the incalculability of justice *must* (impossibly) be calculated and not, precisely, "left to itself" (cited above).

I treat the relation between justice and this emancipatory ideal directly in the next chapter, as it is central to this discussion. What is important now, however, is that the Derridean "must" is not (at least not simply) a moral imperative that arises strictly from the aporia at the heart of law. The imperative is not to ask after the origin if we are to heed the call of "Justice." The imperative, rather, is that we must heed the call of justice as the absolutely singular – as what exceeds the law infinitely – *if* we are to serve the particular emancipatory ideal that the law *as* justice already embodies.

This reformulation is crucial, I shall argue. To understand its nature is to distinguish between the Derridean notion of deconstruction as an affirmative and perhaps even an indispensable *questioning* of ethicity, of morality or of the law, and Cornell's notion of deconstruction as a determinate *ideal* (as justice with a capital "J") – that is, as the basis for a critical practice that aims to determine responsibly the *relative* justice of a given case. Insofar as Cornell sustains the latter view, her argument hinges on the possibility that deconstruction itself can give rise to the ethico-political decision (to *krinein*, or to critique), and that it can do so legitimately, in excess of pre-existing ethical, social or legal codes.[8] On her understanding, it is precisely this deconstructive 'must' that is at stake. The need to substantiate this prescriptive claim when it is not supported by Derrida himself, I submit, prompts Cornell to mobilize the thought of Emmanuel Levinas. It is therefore to Levinas's own ethical thought that it is necessary to turn.

Notes

1 Although the implication of knowledge in socio-political power is often attributed to deconstruction, and although this thought is certainly not foreign to it, the theoretical insight and its development belong more directly to Michel Foucault (1980).

2 This decision was finally overturned by the US Supreme Court on June 26, 2003, although only by a five–four majority, along with a six–three ruling against the Texas anti-sodomy law that had been upheld in 1998 in Lawrence et al. v. Texas. Justice Anthony Kennedy, who wrote for the majority, said among other things, "the state cannot demean their [gay people's] existence by making their private sexual conduct a crime" (see Houpt 2003, A1).

3 The reference is to Walter Benjamin's distinction in "The Critique of Violence" between "law-making or founding violence" and "law-preserving or conserving *force*" (Cornell 1992a, 156).

4 The phrase "the mystical foundation of authority" is the subtitle of Derrida's keynote address, "Force of Law," which I have been citing (Derrida 1992a). The phrase refers to the "performative power itself" insofar as that power retroactively instantiates what *will have been* ('mystically') legitimate (1992a, 14). This 'will-have-been,' it will be recalled, is the grammatical category that for Lyotard characterizes the "postmodern condition."

5 Dallmayr's question, it should be noted, is in that context a rhetorical one. He goes on to position his own understanding of hermeneutics against precisely this kind of (in his view) "farfetched and excessive" concern as it is expressed, for example, by Rosen (see Dallmayr 1992, 298f).

6 Derrida elsewhere calls this "the injunction of *différance*" (cited in Critchley 1995, 10, 11).

7 In the *Politics of Deconstruction: A New Introduction to Jacques Derrida*, Susanne Lüdemann makes the same move: she elides the difference between the ethical imperative *of* deconstruction (deconstruction *as* justice), and an injunction *to* deconstruct, whereby deconstruction is said to be undertaken 'in the name of' justice (2014, 65).

8 Notwithstanding her explicit rejection of Critchley's Levinasian understanding of the ethics of deconstruction (Critchley 1992), Nicole Anderson may be making the same assumption (2012, esp. 128–30).

10 Derrida Contra Levinas

In Chapter Nine I suggested that it is necessary to distinguish between Levinas's "messianic conception of justice" and "the notion of justice as aporia that Derrida emphasizes" (Cornell 1992b, 87). This is not because Derrida rejects the Levinasian conception outright. On the contrary, he tacitly approves it. However, an examination of Derrida's "Violence and Metaphysics" (1978, 79–153) reveals that, nonetheless, his conception of justice is not "exactly" the same as Levinas's (Cornell 1992b, 87). Levinas asserts the absolute priority of ethics over, above and before knowing and being (epistemology and ontology). While Derrida acknowledges the "irreducible heterogeneity" between the ethical and the epistemologico-ontological orders as well, he also insists, paradoxically, on the "original and irreducible complexity" that links "practical conscience and theoretical consciousness" together (1995b, 25). Insofar as Derrida challenges the absolute otherness on which Levinasian responsibility depends, he puts Cornell's (and arguably also his own) understanding of deconstruction's normative status into doubt.

In order to formulate the way in which deconstruction constitutes a mode of critique, therefore, it is first necessary to clarify what Levinasian "responsibility" entails in distinction. Most importantly, Levinas breaks decisively with Kant's notion of moral action whereby, in responding to "duty," one takes direction from an epistemologically-grounded principle. On Levinas's view, responsibility derives instead from one's willingness "to depose or dethrone [oneself] – to abdicate [one's] position of centrality – in favour of the vulnerable other" (Levinas, in Kearney ed. 1984, 63). The Other[1], for Levinas, thus not only precedes my existence; "his"[2] ethical demand on me *produces* my capacity for knowledge, for an ontological relation to the world, to begin with.

This thesis embodies the reformulation of at least three major Heideggerian ideas. The first concerns the difference between the "ontic" and the "ontological," or what Heidegger calls the "ontico-ontological" difference. Generally put, this can be understood as a distinction between beings as entities or *Seinde*, the ontic, and Being (the 'Being' *of* beings, or *Sein*), the ontological (Beardsworth 1996, 104). For Heidegger, Being is not simply another *kind* of being, but rather the meaning of what it is to 'be' in general. Because it has forgotten this difference, however, the metaphysical tradition has been unable fully to think the ontological question (what *is* the meaning of being?) that inaugurates philosophy. Rather, traditional metaphysics poses the question 'what is' in terms of the very categories of Being that *already* presuppose its meaning. Thus, the metaphysical as such, for Heidegger, is characterized by a certain occlusion of the question of Being. In this sense, ontology in the metaphysical tradition is actually "onto-theology"; it asks the question of Being (*ontos*) in terms of the possibility of a highest being (*theos*), because it presupposes that Being *is* being in its exemplarity (see Gasché 1994, esp. 154; Colebrook 1997, 85). Heidegger thus attempts to think Being more fundamentally, by directly questioning the essence or 'presence' of the entity as such.

The second Heideggerian idea that Levinas reformulates has to do with how Heidegger redresses Western metaphysics through a meditation on the question of time (see Derrida 1982, 31 nt.3, 33 nt.6). Heidegger argues that the thought of Being as a self-coincident, present entity (as *a* being that *is* here-now, so to speak) depends on the "vulgar notion of time," whereby the present (now) is conceived *as* present (see Derrida 1982, esp. 35). Against this notion, Heidegger contends that time is not reducible to momentary 'nows', any more than Being is reducible to *the* being of beings. In fact, "now" never arrives; the present no more coincides with itself than law coincides with justice, because "now" is never (not yet, or no longer) *now*. Properly speaking, "now" is always coming. This is the mode of its temporalization, according to Heidegger; "now" becomes what we understand and, indeed, what we experience as "now" by virtue of its imminent arrival, its 'to come.' And yet, since experience itself is only possible insofar as one experiences "now" as *present* to consciousness, it follows that experience is enabled (or "possibilized") by the *becoming*, the temporalization, of time. Heidegger calls this understanding of time "primordial time."

The third important idea follows from this. For Heidegger, the fact that time only becomes present through its temporalization (its 'to come') means that 'authentic dwelling in being' entails the recognition of primordial time. "Primordial time" 'awakens' the present. It calls me as a being to the inmost of Being, from or as futurity. My response to this call, in turn, requires that I know myself as a being-towards-death, that I "possibilize" my (own) future, because my death marks for me the "limit experience" (Beardsworth 1996, 130), the becoming-now of my own being, as such. In other words, death marks my temporal horizon; consequently, my knowledge of myself as a being-towards-death is how I live my own being (as *Dasein*) authentically. This is why, for Heidegger, "authenticity" names my response to the call of Being (Beardsworth 1996, 104–14); it is my response to the "call of conscience," by virtue of which I experience (my own) Being, fundamentally. As Richard Beardsworth writes,

> To open up the "as" of entities from under metaphysical concealment (ontological "or" technical) means reflecting upon the "as" according to primordial temporality. Such reflection (the questioning of being) develops the ecstatic unity of past, present and future … For the early Heidegger this articulation is the *ecstatic structure of Dasein itself.* Heidegger's presentation of the existential "being-towards-death" confirms that the above "unity" of time is nothing else than the self-projection of Dasein from the future. For Heidegger, in other words, being-towards-death confirms that the unified ecstasis of authentic time is structured from the future as Dasein's self-affection. (1996, 108–9; emphasis his)

Levinas builds on, but significantly reformulates, Heidegger's analysis of being and time. For Levinas, too, time entails radical alterity or excess insofar as it is irreducible to presence ("now"). However, Levinas rejects the proposition that we can think (cognize) the infinite character of time, least of all through a gesture in which we appropriate our own death as the possibility of our own future. Thus, whereas for Heidegger the call of Being (conscience) is a call from myself to myself, so to speak, Levinas insists that although death signifies futurity, it is never mine. Rather, it is always that of an other. On Levinas's view, I cannot experience the possibility of my own death (Beardsworth 1996, 130). This difference is crucial; the irreducibility of time to presence can only be encountered in and through an *ethical* experience of the relation to another person in their alterity (*qua Autrui*), rather than in terms of an ontico-ontological conceptualization of Being.

Indeed, the relation to the other (*as* Other, as the trace of infinity) is for Levinas *the* ethical relation. Ethics (not metaphysics, as Aristotle maintained) is for Levinas "first philosophy," because it precedes and conditions ontological or philosophical speech (the "said" of 'what is,' here-now). Thus, Levinas finds in Heidegger's thought the same appropriative, calculative and ultimately violent gesture that he finds in all Western philosophy, beginning with the Greeks. He says,

> Perhaps the most essential distinguishing feature of the language of Greek philosophy [before the incursion of the Jewish and Christian cultures] was its equation of truth with an *intelligibility of presence.* By this I mean an intelligibility which considers truth to be that which is present or co-present, that which can be gathered or synchronized into a totality which we would call the world or *cosmos.* According to the Greek model, intelligibility is what can be rendered present, what can be represented in some eternal here-and-now, exposed and disclosed in pure light … The Greek notion of Being is essentially this presence. (Levinas, in Kearney ed. 1984, 55)

Levinas takes specific issue, then, with the Heideggerian proposition that one can (re)cognize or re-present Being in terms of a calculable relation to (primordial) time. For Levinas the radical impossibility of a self-coincident "now" means that my relation to the other, to time *as* the other, is "absolutely incalculable" (Perpich 2008, 154) and, in this sense, radically asymmetrical. The Other commands me *before* I am determined as (my)self.

Specifically, the "face" of the Other invokes the excess of ontological existence, which cannot be rendered present; it provokes my first response – in Levinasian terms, the "said" of the 'yes' or the 'no' (Derrida 1978, 96) – that necessarily follows the ethical "Saying" of the Other. For Levinas, importantly,

> the face is the other who asks me not to let him die alone, as if to do so were to become an accomplice in his death. Thus the face says to me: you shall not kill … To expose myself to the vulnerability of the face is to put my ontological right to existence into question. In ethics, the other's right to exist has primacy over my own, a primacy epitomized in the ethical edict: you shall not kill. (In Kearney ed. 1984, 59–60)

This primacy of the Other thus opens, apocalyptically, the possibility of my own speech, my own question of the meaning of Being. If Heidegger understood the call of conscience as my appropriation of primordial time in terms of living as a being-towards-death, then, Levinas here inscribes my response to the other – whose face bears the "trace"[3] of time's excess as infinitely Other and thus who presents me with the possibility of "*his*" death – as my responsibility *for* "him." I am responsible not to myself, but to the other *qua* Other.

Importantly, then, the face is significant for Levinas because it figures as the trace of what is *beyond* being, unrepresentable and un(re)cognizable in or through an onto-logical grasp of conceptuality. Moreover, my encounter with the face of another in and through the interhuman relation implicates what Levinas calls an "ethical or biblical" encounter with the Absolutely Other. As he specifies, the interhuman realm is both "part of the disclosure of the world as presence," *and*

> part of the disclosure of the world from … the ethical or biblical perspective which transcends the Greek language of intelligibility – as a theme of justice and concern for the other as other, as a theme of love and desire which carries us beyond the finite Being of the world as presence. The interhuman is thus an interface; a double axis where what is "of the world" qua *phenomenological intelligibility* is juxtaposed with what is "not of the world" qua *ethical responsibility*. It is in this ethical perspective that God must be thought and not in the ontological perspective of our being-there or of some Supreme Being and Creator correlative to the world, as traditional metaphysics often

> held. God, as the God of alterity and transcendence, can only be understood in terms of that interhuman dimension which … cuts through and perforates the totality of presence and points towards the absolutely Other. (In Kearney ed. 1984, 56–7; original emphasis)

In this respect, Levinas concedes, "biblical thought has, *to some extent*, influenced my ethical reading of the interhuman" (in Kearney ed. 1984, 57; emphasis added). Yet this seems not to go far enough. For it is not clear that the ethical relation can stand unless one understands it in explicitly religious terms, that is, in relation to a sacred, otherworldly reality.

For Levinas, to be sure, the encounter with absolute alterity is ostensibly experiential; it is explained in phenomenological rather than onto-theological terms. Levinas argues that it is *in* my experience of the other's face as 'trace' that I encounter time's irreducibility to presence and am, thereby, directed toward what is strictly unrepresentable as God. Yet in the absence of religious conviction, the proposal seems to beg a crucial question, namely, that the other's mortality (even granting that this experience obtains), is my *responsibility*. Notably, this is not simply the sceptical challenge with which Diane Perpich contends: "What is the other to *me*?" (2008, 130; emphasis added). This question is performatively contradictory, Perpich argues, because in asking for proof of the other's value, the sceptic has already conceded the very imperative of critical reflection that only the *prior* exposure to the other made possible (2008, 133–44). This rebuttal is fine as far as it goes, but it begs the same question. The demand for critical reflection may well presuppose the injunction to account for oneself, but it does not explain why that injunction has normative force (and, hence why the sceptic asks for proof). The real challenge to Levinas is not "Why am *I* responsible?" but "Why am I *responsible*?" What is there in or of the other's face that, as Other, *compels* my non-indifference, my incapacity for indifference and thus, the necessity of my ethical response?

Levinas's answer appears to be that the religiously-imbued, ethical imperative renders individuation possible in the first place. He argues that the radical obligation that the Other demands of me, namely, that I do not kill "him," is the origin of my freedom as a willing (self-determining) subject. The Other's accusation is thus prior to my autonomy; it calls responsibility out *from* me (it calls *me*), before I am a subject, subjecting me, as it were, *to* my own subjectivity. In Perpich's formulation, "the subject is constituted in a manner that makes it unable to be totally deaf to the other's demands, whether those be demands for reason, a cry for compassion, an expression of pain, or the pangs of hunger" (2008, 145). Similarly, Levinas says,

> The Other becomes my neighbour precisely through the way the face summons me, calls for me, begs for me, and in so doing recalls my responsibility, and calls me into question. (1989, 83)

> What one sees in this questioning is being as *mauvaise conscience*; to be open to question, but also to questioning, to have to respond. Language is born in responsibility. One has to speak, to say I, to be in the first person, precisely to be me (*moi*). But, from that point, in affirming this me being, one has to respond to one's right to be. (1989, 82)

The experience of responsibility, then, is the experience of encountering a human "face" *as* a messianic, religious or biblical call. What is thereby impressed *is* an inescapable, ethico-political injunction to respect "his" life, and so not to kill, which in turn requires that one answers for oneself. Moreover, Perpich writes, Levinas 'does not believe it is possible' *not* to feel "this call of the other" (2008, 130); for him "the moment of normativity … is incontestable" (2008, 147–8; original emphasis omitted). This is why, for Levinas, the "ethical call of conscience" is a "religious vocation" (in Kearney ed. 1984, 61; see also Derrida 1978, 96). It cuts through phenomenological intelligibility, perforating the world of beings, with divinely-imbued, *ethical* force, such that I am hostage to the Other.

This ethical injunction comes from one knows not where; it is the apocalyptic, messianic opening *of* philosophy, of principled morality and of ontology. Levinas says,

> It is in a *responsibility that is justified by no prior commitment*, in the responsibility for another – in an ethical situation – that the me-ontological and metalogical structure of this anarchy takes form, undoing the logos in which the apology by which consciousness always regains its self-control, and commands, is inserted. This passion is absolute in that it takes hold without any a priori. The consciousness is affected, then, before forming an image of what is coming to it, affected in spite of itself. (1989, 92; emphasis his)

Thus, we can say that ethicity as first philosophy "remains hidden," that ethicity is *beyond* discourse and *beyond* the "what is"; it comes from one knows not where. This is why, in turn, Levinasian ethics escapes the cognitive reach of theology to which even Heidegger, on Levinas's view, returns Being. As Jill Robbins explains,

> [W]hen Levinas writes that the face commands me, "thou shalt not kill," he seems to suggest that the law is revealed not by God, as in the biblical claim, but in the face of the other (man), and that this relationship is prior to any relationship between man and God. This is indeed the case, but it need be the case only if that relationship between man and God is conceived as a theology, a discourse on God's attributes, or a thematization. As Levinas implies [elsewhere], the relationship to God is, however, not a *credo*, nor is it any kind of ontological assertion. It is the primacy of doing for the other. That is

> the sole relationship between man and God. In many ways, this "Judaism" is closer to atheism. (1991, 146–7)

The ethical relation to the Other is prophetic or ethico-eschatological rather than theological, in other words, because Levinas's notion of the face-to-face evokes "a discourse *with* God rather than discourse *on* God and his attributes as *theology*" (Derrida 1978, 108; last emphasis his). Ethics thus precedes and in fact enables or opens onto-theo-logical discourse, but it does not precede the religious relation.

My recollection here of the "apocalyptic tone of philosophy" is thus deliberate. There is a decisive difference between Derrida's elucidation of the "apocalyptic opening" without which philosophical discourse cannot begin, and Levinas's postulation of an ethico-messianic *origin* of philosophy that precedes ontology, and is "otherwise than being," absolutely (Levinas 1981). Derrida, we saw, revealed the apocalyptic as inscribed in philosophy itself. As I explained, the apocalyptic tone names into being the "we" that comes to say the truth (the truth of the end of mystagogy and the beginning of philosophy). In this sense, the "messianic" is (for Derrida) a certain apocalyptic tone that is structurally necessary for discourse, including – perhaps especially – for the discourses of we "*Aufklärer* of modern times" (Derrida 1983a, 29).

But this peculiar messianism is not strictly external, or strictly an origin, any more than *différance* is, simply, the *origin* of difference, or than the sublime feeling of moral respect is, simply, the *origin* of the logical principle of autonomy posited by Kant. The *impossible* necessity of "C/critique," one might say – the *mystical* foundation of authority or the *différantial* structure of difference – are not prior forces. Rather, they signal or figure what is undecidable *as*, the "playing movement" *of*, the determinate categories of cognition themselves. What is strictly "undecidable," we have seen, is "a proposition which, *given a system of axioms governing a multiplicity*, is neither an analytical nor deductive consequence of those axioms, nor in contradiction with them, neither true nor false with respect to those axioms" (Derrida, qtd. in Gasché 1987, 9; emphasis added). Undecidability thus *both produces and is produced by* the system or doctrine it undoes. To "give" as possible the legitimate authority of the law, the philosophical grounds of a moral critique, the logical determination of difference, or the self-evident axioms of geometry, is at once to "give" as possible their internal erosion, their deconstruction, as well. The messianic or apocalyptic indeterminacy that 'founds' philosophy comes, on Derrida's view, from nowhere else.

Levinas, in contrast, postulates an ethico-messianic *origin* of philosophical intelligibility that is absolutely Other, and that precedes – as prophetic or ethical "Saying" – the philosophical enunciation of the "said." Indeed, Ciaramelli notes, "Levinas continually underlines the ethical dimension of Revelation in Hebraism … Prophecy is the real modality of the manifestation – and universal significance – of the ethical" (1991, 103 nt.41). Levinasian messianism, thus, does not derive from *this* authority, *this* understanding of ethics, or *this* instantiation of law. It derives, rather, from an excessive ethical relation (with God) that *precedes* authority, ethics or the law.

Cornell's understanding of the (moral) imperative *to* deconstruct now becomes clear. For her, justice is impelled by a radical, incalculable *obligation* that is pre-philosophical in Levinas's sense, and that comes from one knows not where. Specifically, she suggests that we are infinitely obligated to a messianic form of "Justice," the "trace" of which we encounter *in* the positive law. Its (infinite) voice is our imperative command. In the first place, therefore, the normativity of deconstruction stems from a certain religiosity that qualifies the ethical encounter. Beyond this, however, the criticality of deconstruction – by virtue of which we can gauge the relative *degree* to which justice in the legal system has been served – hinges on the difference between the ethical experience of responsibility, and a philosophical (or onto-theological) discourse about it. Indeed, we have seen, Levinas rebuts the charge of theology not because he eschews religious belief, but because he offers an even *more* authoritative, more primary and more originary account of messianism than theology does, based on his phenomenological explanation of subjectivity. The claim that Levinasian "responsibility" can serve as the ground for a "justified" (indeed, for *the* justified), deconstructive critique thus depends upon the theoretical explanation of ethical responsibility in phenomenological *rather* than onto(theo)logical terms. On Derrida's reading of Levinas, however, this requirement is a problem for Cornell's argument as well.

The issue emerges in Derrida's examination of the relationship between phenomenology and onto(theo)logy. Specifically, Derrida argues that the Levinasian notion of absolute alterity – which ostensibly signifies a religious relation at the very heart of human experience – is a feature of conceptuality itself. Derrida's engagement with Levinas is extremely complex but, in effect, he returns Levinas's prophetic discourse ("Saying") – the discourse *with* God that Levinas poses over and against an onto-theological discourse *on* God – to the "said" of ontology. The difference between these two discourses, it will be recalled, is the difference between the infinite, incalculable, ethical relation to the radically Other, and the ontological, calculative reduction of the Other to the Same that Levinas finds in Heideggerian thought. What Derrida notices is that the condition of possibility for my ethical encounter with the Other *as* absolute exteriority – the condition whereby the other can appear as wholly Other, and as "he" to whom I am (always already) infinitely indebted – *is still the appearance of the other as an other ego.* "The Other is not myself," Derrida writes, "and who has ever maintained that it is? – but it is *an* Ego, as Levinas must suppose in order to maintain his own discourse" (1978, 110; his emphasis). In order to encounter the Other as "Him" to whom I am radically obliged for my very existence, in other words, I must have *already* (re)presented the Other to myself as a *general* other (as a universal subject or *I*) – which is to say, as an other *like* the 'self,' the ego, that I am in general.[4] This is what Husserl means by the term "analogical appresentation"; it means the act of the ego in its constitution of the world as a world, my presentation to myself of what 'is' there *as* I am here. Husserl maintains that an egoic *opening* of the world is the precondition of all experience, including that experience which Levinas would consider the most sublime of all: the encounter with Absolute Alterity that instantiates the ethical relation.

Now, if "egoic opening" is required for experience, the ethical relation that Levinas describes cannot be said to be absolutely outside, or finally to precede, the philosophical (epistemologico-ontological) domain. Therefore, it cannot serve as the external origin of, and the legitimate lever for, the interrogation of philosophy or law. On the contrary, there is already a form of ontological discourse at work *in* the ethical relation as such. What is at work there, Derrida argues, is what one might call an originary metaphoricity – the metaphor, in this case, in which the face of God is like the face of (a) man. This metaphor is that through which the possibility of the wholly Other, the Absolutely Other, must pass. Absolute alterity is *figured by* the face (Derrida 1978, esp. 143; see also Robbins 1991). Conceptuality, therefore, through which the other *appears* to me *as* another "I" *like* the ego that I am, is indispensable even in the ostensibly pure realm of phenomenology that Levinas characterizes as a transcendental discourse with God, and that he postulates as supposedly *preceding* any possible conceptual account of what ontologically 'is' there *in* (appears *as*) the world. The indeterminable excess of the ethical relation beyond conceptuality, Derrida shows, cannot be experienced as what it *is* without a (non)originary moment of language as metaphoricity – which is to say, without the rhetoricity that (pre)conditions logic.

This insight undermines Cornell's analysis. For Derrida's Husserlian argument concerning the necessity of an egoic opening of the world does not entail that the relation between the self and the other can simultaneously be seen (contra Levinas) as a fundamentally *symmetrical* relation. It does not imply that one can therefore posit a "moment of universality" (the possibility of generalizing the "I") against the potentially violent asymmetry of the ethical relation that Levinas describes, as Cornell proposes (1992a, 174–5). On the contrary, Derrida is very clear on this point. First, *against* Levinas he argues that there is no protection against the originary, "pre-ethical violence" of conceptual reduction, because ethicity can only be opened by virtue of what Derrida calls an "*economy* of violence" (1978, 128, 129). One might say that, just as "alterity had to circulate at the origin of meaning" (Derrida 1978, 153), so meaning (the theoretical determination of what *is*) had to circulate at the origin of alterity (the phenomenological experience of ethics). The experience of the other as absolutely Other, and the calculative reduction of the Other to the Same (to an-other ego) take place in one and the same move. They are 'complexly, originally and irreducibly' linked. Levinasian "responsibility" obtains by virtue of a reduction or calculation of the incalculable that cannot even be recognized as *a* form of violence, *yet*, but which nonetheless is not beyond violence either.

Second, Derrida insists *with* Levinas that the 'greater' violence *is* the universalizing and calculative gesture that produces the conceptual 'symmetry' Cornell wants to celebrate. Symmetry is not an antidote to violence, but rather its essential character. As Derrida writes,

> That I am also essentially the other's other, and that I know that I am, is the evidence of a strange symmetry whose trace appears nowhere in Levinas's descriptions. Without this evidence, I could not desire (or) respect the other in ethical dissymmetry. This transcendental violence, which does not spring from an ethical resolution or freedom, or from a *certain way* of encountering or exceeding the other, originally institutes the relationship between two finite ipseities. In effect, the necessity of gaining access to the meaning of the other (in its irreducible alterity) on the basis of its "face," that is, its nonphenomenal phenomenon, its nonthematic theme, in other words on the basis of an intentional modification of my ego (in general) … and the necessity of speaking of the other as other, or to the other as other, on the basis of its appearing-for-me-as-what-it-is: the other … *these necessities are violence itself, or rather the transcendental origin of an irreducible violence*, supposing, as we said above, that it is somehow meaningful to speak of preethical violence. (1978, 128, last emphasis added)

And third, Derrida argues *further to* Levinas that the asymmetrical nature of the non-phenomenal phenomenon of the ethical relation and the potential violence that it entails – that the Other accuses me first, before I even know that "I" am – is in no way levelled by the fact that it is *conditioned* by what can only be termed the 'pre-ethical violence' of conceptual reduction. Violence is ineradicable, because a "pure" ethicity would not know what it was. Or, as Derrida puts it, "War, therefore, is congenital to phenomenality, it is the very emergence of speech and appearing" (1978, 129).

Thus, the significance of Derrida's insight that a strange symmetry obtains – that there is an inescapable reference of the other to the economy of the Same 'prior' to and necessary for the ethical encounter as such – lies elsewhere. It is that the alterity that for both Derrida and Levinas provokes ethical responsibility is encountered inside – or, rather, at the limits of – the philosophico-conceptual domain. Ethicity in Levinas's sense is provoked in and *as* the very move of egoic constitution *against* which Levinasian (and Cornell's version of legal) "responsibility" is supposedly opposed. And this means that there is no way to experience what 'is' beyond being, no way to experience that which exceeds the onto-theology of Being/being as its originary, ethical sense, except by mobilizing the very apparatus of onto(theo)logical conceptualization that both Husserl and Heidegger describe, and that Levinas sets out to displace.

For these reasons, the messianic, ethical injunction with which Levinas interrogates philosophy cannot be distinguished absolutely from theology on the grounds he suggests. On the contrary, onto(theo)logy is the inescapable risk of *any* investigation into the conditions or limits of thinking or experience themselves. As Gasché explains,

> If the positive infinite has to rely on a negative term (in-finite) through "the negation of (finite) spatial exteriority [Derrida 1978, 114]," this positivity is perhaps not positively infinite, but finite. If the "infinitely Other" can be what it is only if it is Other, that is, other *than* ... the Other "is no longer absolved of a relation to" another ego and, therefore, "no longer infinitely, absolutely other [Derrida 1978, 126–7]." Hence, "the other cannot be what it is, infinitely other, except in finitude and mortality (mine *and* his)," Derrida notes [1978, 114–15]. In short, since it is impossible to separate infinity and alterity from negativity, from death in the last resort, a positive infinity and absolute alterity called God *must compromise with such negativity*. (1994, 159–60; internal references his; last emphasis mine)

Without putting too fine a point on it, then, there is a moment of negative theology – a moment in which the discourse with God is considered in terms of a relation to what God (in his Being) 'is' not, and whereby "God" is the ineffable – in and as the ethical challenge to onto(theo)logical discourse. Levinas's move to interrogate philosophy *from* its ethico-messianic 'outside' is, in a certain sense, always already philosophy's own move. Thus, the notion of justice at work in "Force of Law," while indeed linked to responsibility, does not enable a judgement concerning the 'relative' justice of the judges. For the purely "ethical" appeal to the absolutely Other is always *already* in a certain way onto-theological, or negatively theological, too.

This is why Derrida's messianic concept of "justice" must be rigorously distinguished from Cornell's. Just as the ethical interrogation of philosophy is philosophy's own postulation of an 'outside' from inside it, so the promise of law *as* justice, and the impossibility it entails, was always already the condition of the law to begin with. The law's resource for critique is the trace of the promise *it* bears, not the revelation of its ethical (or non-violent) *origin*. This promise is the inscription (the "trace") *in* the law of an *infinite* idea of justice that appears 'beyond' it, but that issues from *within* ontological discourse itself. It is this impossible 'outside' – this apocalyptic responsibility whereby justice is *promised* as the origin and end of a law that can never 'be' its realization – *this* is "exactly" the conception of justice as aporia that Derrida emphasizes. Derrida thus sidesteps philosophy's "theological trap" (Gasché 1994, 161); he eschews the possibility of *the* (most) justified critique. He writes,

> Between original tragedy and messianic triumph there is *philosophy*, in which violence is returned against violence within knowledge, in which original finitude appears, and in which the other is respected within, and by, the same. This finitude makes its appearance in an irreducibly open question which is the *philosophical question in general: why* is the essential, irreducible, absolutely general and unconditioned form of experience as a venturing forth toward the other still egoity? *Why* is an experience which would not be lived as *my own* (for an ego in general, in the eidetic-transcendental sense of these words) impossible and unthinkable? This unthinkable and impossible are the limits of reason in general ... The philosophy which is the discourse of this reason as phenomenology cannot answer such a question by essence, for every answer can be made only in language, and language is opened by the question. Philosophy (in general) can only open itself to the question, within it and by it. It can only *let itself be questioned.* (1978, 131)

One might thus say that the "critical responsibility" of deconstruction, if such can be said, its nominal "justice," is conceived as the question of the radically impossible possibility *of* philosophy in its "apocalypticity" (or, alternatively, the messianicity of the law) itself. So understood, the "messianic" or apocalyptic dimension of philosophy or the law can be taken as that trace which is produced *in* the here-now *as* the structural futurity (and the elsewhere) of a justice "to come."

The messianic notion of justice as aporia that Derrida emphasizes is thus strictly "undecidable" in the technical sense. "Justice" as what "is" 'good' here-now (justice as present), is only ever (non-temporally) 'subsequent' to the "messianic notion of justice" (what we might call arche-justice) that Derrida describes, since justice as aporia never takes place *as such*. It is, rather, merely the name for a radical indeterminacy that opens the future to both good and ill, but without which "justice" (as "a" or "the" good) has no chance. And this means that to the extent that it is possible to derive a conception of responsibility from deconstruction, it will be a form of (quasi-) responsibility that is no longer strictly Kantian (theoretical), but that is not strictly Levinasian (ethical), either. This is why deconstruction cannot be said to be "*already* inspired by a concern that could by right be called ethical" (Derrida 1992b, 15) The decision – that this *is* good, or that this *is* evil – can only ever obtain by virtue of what Derrida calls a traversal of the "ordeal of the undecidable" (1994, 87). What he means by this is not that a decision does not happen; even less is it a matter of advocating indecisionism – as various critics have implied (see, e.g., Soper 1996). It is simply that, from the structural perspective of an event's *possibility*, the decision *is* not yet (has not yet come into being and, hence, is undecided, and undecidable).

Derrida characterizes this structural condition of determinate judgement as its "messianic" opening.[5] Thus the messianic dimension of the decision is said to 'tremble on the edge of an event'; indeed, it *is* this hesitation. However, he insists, "the messianic hesitation does not paralyze any decision, any affirmation, any responsibility. On the contrary, it grants them their elementary condition. It is their very experience" (1994, 169). In other words, it is precisely the traversal – the opening of and passage through a possible futurity – that enables or renders the presence of the present such that I can say (can decide) it '*is*.' Experience as such, is, in a sense, this determination.

Why call this a possible futurity? Because the point of Derrida's analysis is that the event, the coming to pass of what occurs – which is nothing less and nothing more than the saying, the decision, of what is – this coming to pass must not or cannot already have occurred if it is to be possible. *First* it must be possible and thus, not yet. That is its condition. A condition in the form of a promise. This will be. And yet it is only ever afterwards, only when the event has always already happened, that we may say 'it is.' We must have already decided, having inscribed the presence of the present, in order that the *is*, as well as the *is not*, take place. This is because Being is *for us* none other than the presence of the present, since we can only experience at all on this condition. That is why the future is also impossible. It is what must take place now, as *future*, but which we can know as "now" only when it has passed. In this sense, the future – one should say, 'futurity' – is (always already) no longer; it is a spectre, a trace, neither being nor non-being, but – to put it in a word – the movement of *différance*. *Différance* is this promise, the promise of what is to come.

This thought of *différance* as a trace or a possible futurity is precisely the site of Derrida's intervention into Heidegger's consideration of the "gift" – a notion that is central to the *spirit* of critique that Derrida elucidates in *Specters of Marx* (1994), just as it is central to the "giving" (*donatrice*) notion of "justice" that he describes in "Force of Law" (1992a). Specifically, it is important to note that, in his discussion of the classical Western notion of "justice," Heidegger links the disjoining of the present just outlined – the impossible future inscribed in the present as such – to a notion of excess and, more specifically, to a notion of excess as the incalculability that characterizes the gift. According to Heidegger, Derrida says, the disjunction of the present with itself, this inescapable out-of-jointedness of time, entails a debt. In particular, the necessary disjointure of the present entails the injunction or duty to *give back* jointure, to establish an accord. And it is to give back what one does not have. As Derrida summarizes, "giving rests only in presence, it does not signify simply to give away (*weggeben*) but, more originarily, to accord, that is here, *zugeben* which most often indicates addition, even excess, in any case that which is offered *in supplement, over and above the market, off trade, without exchange*" (1994, 26; my emphasis).

It follows, says Derrida, that for Heidegger "justice" in its classical, Greek sense means 'jointure'; justice is the *accord* that consists in giving to the other, over and above what one does not have and does not have to give, beyond what is owed, exchanged or reducible to a market economy, what is 'proper' to him or her. To leave the other this accord – that is the 'giving' of presence, and that 'gift,' in a word, is "justice" on Heidegger's reading of Western philosophy. Yet here Derrida intervenes with a question that bears quoting in full:

> Once one has recognized the force and the necessity of thinking justice on the basis of the gift, that is, beyond right, calculation, and commerce ... is there not a risk of inscribing this whole movement of justice under the sign of presence, be it of presence to meaning of the *Anwesen* [Heideggerian 'presencing'], of the event as coming into presence, of Being as presence joined to itself, of the proper of the other as presence? ... Beyond right, and still more beyond juridicism, beyond morality, and still more beyond moralism, does not justice as relation to the other suppose on the contrary the irreducible excess of a disjointure or an anachrony ... some "out of joint" dislocation in Being and in time itself, a disjointure that, in always risking the evil, expropriation, and injustice (*adikia*) against which there is no calculable insurance, would alone be able to *do justice* or to *render justice* to the other as other? (1994, 27–8)

A number of points bear underlining with regard to this intervention in Heidegger's analysis. The first is that the question of the gift that opens *Specters of Marx* and establishes its entire problematic is for Derrida an unflinchingly political one. What is at stake, here as always in Derrida's work, is the question of the just relation to the other, against the violence of a "totalizing" politics that would effect presence (or symmetry) at the expense of an irresponsible exorcizing or erasing of the condition of undecidability.

Second, Derrida mobilizes a distinctively Marxist analysis in his discussion of justice; the meaning of the gift is explicitly characterized as that which exceeds the market-based circuit of economic exchange. Indeed, Derrida's elaboration and development of Heidegger's analysis is intended as a corrective to Heidegger's own tendency to return justice to a "totalizing horizon" of "adequate restitution" – a tendency whereby juridical–moral rules risk being *re*instated as the possibility of an economic return (1994, 28). It is against an economic tendency in Heidegger himself then – whereby the singular and incalculable nature of justice risks being violently reduced to capitalism's ideological order of the 'Same' – that Derrida intervenes.

And third, this explication of justice in the Marxist corpus as incalculable 'gift' is directly implicated in – even if it is in a certain sense (non-originarily) 'prior' to – the decision of good or evil, of "socialism or barbarism." The issue for Derrida is that of a passage or an ordeal of undecidability that *must* have conditioned our experience in order that we may choose. The problematic of the gift is implicated as the very condition of this ethico-political choice. Concomitantly, however, there is no avoiding the risk of totalitarianism, no insurance to be had; on the contrary, the demand of justice is precisely that we chance it. As Derrida says,

> To be out of joint, whether it be present Being or present time, can do harm and do evil, it is no doubt the very possibility of evil. But without the opening of this possibility, there remains, perhaps, beyond good and evil, only the necessity of the worst. A necessity that would not (even) be a fated one. (1994, 29)

The risk of totalitarianism that Derrida identifies as an absolute evil (1994, 175) is here inextricably linked to a notion of justice that is a *structural* feature of experience. Derrida writes,

> [W]hat remains irreducible to any deconstruction, what remains as undeconstructible as the possibility itself of deconstruction is, perhaps, *a certain experience of the emancipatory promise; it is perhaps even the formality of a structural messianism*, a messianism without religion, even a messianic without messianism, an idea of justice – which we distinguish from law or right and even from human rights – and an idea of democracy – which we distinguish from its current concept and from its determined predicates today. (1994, 59; my emphasis)

If an understanding of justice in terms of the 'gift' – an inescapable moment of undecidability and disjointure that conditions the ethico-political decision *for* 'good' – is granted, then one cannot take issue with the indeterminacy of Derrida's political thought. For indeterminacy, the undecidable ordeal that constitutes experience, is justice's enabling feature. For the very justice that critical political thinkers advocate, one must take (one must have taken) a chance. As Ernesto Laclau submits, "The political and ethical significance [of deconstruction] is that by enlarging the area of structural undecidability, it enlarges also the area of responsibility – that is, of the decision" (1995, 93). Such a formulation may stand, provided we heed the proviso that it is the *conditions for*, not the *consequences of*, the ethico-political decision that are at stake in Derrida's analysis.[6] At stake, in other words, is a structural undecidability that must be *taken account of*, rather than exorcized, if political efforts are to be (quasi-) responsible.

Yet precisely because it is incumbent upon those who claim to be for "justice" to know whereof we speak, the question must be further pressed. For, given the nature of deconstruction, one cannot avoid addressing an issue that Laclau formulates as follows: if the "messianic" in question is merely "the structure of a promise which is inherent in all experience and whose lack of content … is the very possibility of justice and gives its only meaning to the democracy to come," then one must be very careful not to make an "illegitimate logical transition" to the particular ethical contents of a "classic emancipatory project" (1995, 91, 92). Indeed, Laclau continues, "from the fact that there is the impossibility of ultimate closure and presence, it does not follow that there is an ethical imperative to 'cultivate' that openness or even to be necessarily committed to a democratic society" (1995, 93). Whence, in short comes the imperative to deconstruct? To put the question again: why would the disjointure described above, even granting that undecidability takes place, be said to entail a debt that is *normative* or moral in nature? In the absence of recourse to Levinas's formulation of messianism, deconstruction's normative status no longer immediately obtains, since it is only authorized, if it is authorized at all, by the very concept of "criticality" whose authority it puts into question.

Ironically, then, it emerges that the problem with calling deconstruction "just" is its very formality; the problem does not concern its contingency, the indeterminacy of deconstruction's political *ends* (on which virtually all of Derrida's critics have remarked), but rather the almost inescapable, structural nature of its *conditions* – which is to say, the purely logical status of *différance*. For, most importantly, to say a "messianic" moment can be discerned in the structure of all experience – that undecidability is logically and constitutively an inescapable condition of the decision – is not to say how or why this feature of signification makes an *emphatic* demand on me. On what grounds, then, can deconstruction be "translated" as a form of normative ideology critique?

Derrida does not answer this question directly, nor does he provide resources with which to do so, because the religious explanation has already been displaced. In order to link the *structure* of a messianic promise to the *contents* of an ethico-political call, he merely refers to the spirit of "radical critique" he finds in Marx.

> To continue to take inspiration from a certain spirit of Marxism would be to keep faith with what has always made of Marxism in principle and first of all a *radical* critique, namely, a procedure ready to undertake its self-critique … Such a critical "wanting-itself" [to be open to its own transformation] necessarily takes root, it is involved in a ground that is not yet critical, even if it is not, not yet, pre-critical. This latter spirit is more than a style, even though it is also a style. It is heir to a spirit of the Enlightenment which must not be renounced. (1994, 88; emphasis his)

In the first place, notably, the "spirit of Enlightenment" Derrida most cherishes is one he identifies as a spirit of "radical critique." In the second place, Derrida defines 'radicalization' as follows:

> The point would be to do more or less than "radicalize", or something other, for the stakes are precisely those of the root and its proposed unity. The point would not be to progress still further into the depths of radicality, of the fundamental, or the originary … One would try instead to go there where the schema of the fundamental, of the originary, or of the radical, in its *ontological* unity and in the form in which it continues to govern the Marxist critique, calls for questions … that are *not* or *not sufficiently* put to work in what dominates the discourses that call themselves Marxist. (1994, 184, nt.9; emphases his)

On Derrida's reading, then, what is demanded *by* Marx (by his spirit) is a radicalization of the principle of reason *in* Marx, such as that principle was formulated by Leibniz in the seventeenth century. For on Leibniz's view, it should be recalled, the principle of reason comprises the law of non-contradiction and the principle that, for every true proposition, reason can be rendered. Taken together, these principles inform the classical Enlightenment conception of "critique" in its normative sense (i.e., *qua* "C/critique"). But if we are to "go there where the schema of the fundamental, of the originary, or of the radical" *itself* governs a critique, then we cannot but question the grounds of the injunction *itself*. "Radicalization" is thus formulated *as an injunction* to ask after the basis *of the injunction* to render reason (by going 'to the root'). The demand to interrogate the schema of the radical, in short, is the demand to bring the principle of reason to bear on its own *raison d'être*; it is the responsibility to return reason to itself. As Derrida says,

> Who is more faithful to reason's call, who hears it with a keener ear, who better sees the difference, the one who offers questions in return and tries to think through the possibility of that summons, or the one who does not want to hear any question about the reason of reason? (1983b, 9)

What emerges here, then, is that the Marxist spirit of radical "critique" entails the normative demand to *give* (reason) precisely what one does not *have* (reason). In this sense, it is not enough to say that a Marxist spirit of justice or of responsibility is rendered in terms of the gift. More specifically, the giving in question must be understood, in turn, as a response to the *critical* injunction to render, impossibly, the reason of reason itself. The ethico-political force of *différance*, therefore – its specifically normative bearing – is effectively tied to an Enlightenment notion of critique that Derrida finds in the spirit of Marx (Derrida 1994, esp. 91). Stated this way, it becomes apparent that the notion of "justice as aporia" as Derrida understands it is ultimately another name for reason in its critical, its normative and its emphatic sense. Justice as aporia, one might say, 'is' the impossible necessity of C/critique; it is the necessity, that philosophy cannot evade, to let itself be questioned. And it is in this sense too that the putative responsibility of deconstruction was always already "critical" to begin with.

Derrida's emphasis on criticality is not limited to *Specters of Marx*. On the contrary, the theme of an injunction to question the ground, to go to the root, to question the law of the law, and so forth – this spirit of Enlightenment critique that "must not be renounced" – can be found in virtually everything he has written. One recognizes here the move that opens the field of undecidability. Philosophy or reason in its normativity, I have argued, has no reason, no ground of its own, and yet it is impelled by an ideal of legitimacy that presupposes that grounds are there to be found. Indeed, I argued in Part One, this is exactly why the desire *for* reason is incapable of being lit or illuminated *by* reason. In terms of my argument here, however, what is most significant is this: once the messianic openness of constitutive undecidability has been linked to the radical spirit of critique governing critical political thought since the Enlightenment, the question at hand is why we are bound to such a spirit at all. *Why* do we feel, if we do, *why* do we experience ourselves, if we do, as impelled – in the emphatic or ethical sense of that word – to honour reason? The status of this desire has yet to be explained. An obligation to truth, to be sure, can always be heard as the voice of the oracle, as Derrida has remarked (1983a, 12). We have seen, moreover, that such a messianic–theological possibility is philosophy's foundational risk. But, if there is another way to think the desire for criticality from *inside* the philosophical–conceptual–metaphysical domain of language where we are, might it not be to think the desire for reason, historically, socially, politically?

This problematic of a socially-constituted *desire*, I suggest, this critical "wanting-itself" to provide grounds or to avoid contradiction – the inquiry, in short, into my or our *stakes* in the principle of reason – would lead towards an understanding of the peculiarly *ethical* nature of the messianic injunction to deconstruct. In this way, a certain deconstructive "critique" – which is to say, a Critique *of* "critique" that no longer lies either strictly within or wholly beyond the sphere of ethico-political responsibility – might be said to bear a limited, normative force. It is this possibility, and its implications for a critical political theory in general, that I address next.

Notes

1 Richard Beardsworth explains: "*Autrui* or *Autre* is the alterity of time *qua* the infinite responsibility of the ego to *autrui* [the other]. Phenomenal human beings

to whom the I is responsible *ad infinitum* are called *autrui* (lower case). *Autrui* (upper case) [Other] is the *face* of alterity 'in' phenomenal human beings, such that I am always responsible *to* others. In other terms, *Autrui* is the 'ad infinitum' of *autrui*; and *l'Autre* is the alterity particular to the face, the transcendent infinite in the finite (what Levinas also designates as *l'Autre* [the Other] as against *le Même* [the Same])" (1996, 133).

2 I retain the masculine pronouns throughout because Levinas's usage appears to be sexually specific rather than generic. Indeed, a number of commentators have remarked that Levinas's philosophy is essentially masculinist in that his references to "fraternity," the "son" and the "other man" appear to exclude even the possibility of a female subject. Luce Irigaray, for example, charges that Levinas subsumes sexual difference under ethical difference insofar as he "substitutes the son for the feminine" (1991, 111), while Catherine Chalier proposes that the feminine *is* the (non)site – the 'beyond being', so to speak – of absolute responsibility to the Other (1991, 123). Derrida (1991a) undertakes a form of "radical ingratitude" by 'returning' Levinasian discourse on the other not to Levinas, but to (a) "woman" as the "wholly other."

3 Diane Perpich provides an excellent explanation of the Levinasian concept of "trace" (2008, esp. 111–13, 127–8).

4 Thomas McCarthy makes a similar point from a Habermasian rather than Husserlian perspective (1988, 647).

5 Derrida is responding to Walter Benjamin in this regard, particularly to the "Theses on the Philosophy of History," as various readers have observed (Callinicos 1996, 40–41; Lüdemann 2014, 70).

6 For an interesting discussion of the difference between Derrida and Laclau with regard to the question of the decision, see Berns (1996).

11 Conscience and the Aporia of Subjectivity

> I have never said that the subject should be dispensed with. Only that it should be deconstructed. To deconstruct the subject does not mean to deny its existence. There are subjects, "operations" or "effects" (*effets*) of subjectivity. This is an incontrovertible fact. To acknowledge this does not mean, however, that the subject is what it *says* it is. The subject is not some metalinguistic substance or identity, some pure *cogito* of self-presence; it is always inscribed in language.
>
> (Derrida, in Kearney 1984, 125)

It is not by chance that Kant remarks that reason is "driven by its own need [*durch eigenes Bedürfnis getrieben*]" (1998, 147), that Habermas underlines the "exhortation" and "constraint" to which participants in communicative situations are subject (1990, 198, 203), or that Levinas insists that the face of the other immediately 'impassions' me, "without any a priori" (1989, 92). These formulations each explain why individuals are impelled to assume the moral responsibility that they do. Yet in all three cases the explanation rests on an unjustified assumption about the nature of the subject that purportedly responds. For Kant it hinges on what is "most sublime" in "man," namely, on the capacity to determine oneself freely; for Habermas a transcendental form of subjectivity ultimately grounds the communicative principles of morality; and for Levinas responsibility issues from the inescapable experience of the religious relation to the Other, by virtue of which the injunction to answer for oneself resonates. For Derrida, we have seen, the "*radical* critique" to which we must remain bound is one which "*wants itself* to be in principle and explicitly open to its own transformation, re-evaluation, self-reinterpretation" (1994, 88; emphases his). Yet in this case no explanation is given of what, in or of the subject, actually responds to that demand. On the contrary, Derrida puts that very subject into question.

Yet with respect to the question of the "who" that responds, Derrida's reference to "a donating affirmation that remains the ultimate unknown" (1998, 29) provokes more problems than it solves. It invites the interpretation that one ought to *replace* the possibility of a simple and original element with a non-simple, unrooted, ineffable (non)originarity that impels from without, rather than to *displace* the distinction between them. It risks forgetting that while an affirmative gesture "yes" (*oui*) or "come" (*viens*) opens the fields of language, meaning, inheritance or ethics (for example), it does so only from their own margins, and it suggests only that *différance* makes signification possible in general; it neither affirms nor rejects any *thing*. In other words, a "Yes, yes" does signify a certain force or affirmativity before or outside (marginal to) language (Wills 2006, 14), and it does thereby enable particular performative speech acts, such as promises or commitments to or against any determinable good. But as I have already argued, no particular end is thereby affirmed. This is why the originary affirmation does not itself constitute the one must (*il la faut*) of the logic (*la logique*) of ethical–political critique (Derrida 1988b, 122). It merely "situates" a hyperbolic responsibility, a responsibility that is neither identical with the "Come," nor reducible to the traditional category of the subject (Gaon 2018).

In order to demonstrate how deconstruction qualifies in a certain way as normative "critique," therefore, it is necessary to establish why a "vigil or beyond of the question" imposes itself (Derrida 1991b, 109). Why is one *necessarily* subject to a vigil that opens both the subject and its critical object to "processes of *différance*, trace, iterability, ex-appropriation, and so on" (1991b, 109)? [1] Or again: what, beyond reason and beyond even the authority of the question, *drives* the "enigmatic desire for vigilance" (1983a, 22)? The question is inescapable since, as we have seen, Derrida's reading of Levinas shows that an absolutely heteronomous, ethical force cannot obtain; the originary *economy* of violence, *within* knowledge, is ineliminable. This insight undermines Levinas's purportedly "ethical" rebuttal to the onto(theo)logical determinations of the subject found in Heidegger, Habermas and Kant. It means that the (quasi-) ethical response is not purely non-violent or extra-philosophical, but merely a *lesser* violence still rooted in reason; critical responsibility would thus be the "*vigilance*" that is "chosen as the least violence by a philosophy which takes history, that is, finitude, seriously" (Derrida 1978, 117; emphasis his).

Yet there are, seemingly, only two ways to characterize this vigilant subject, both of which are untenable. Specifically, if one determines the subject's attachment to reason *as* the logical principle of ethical–political judgement, one loses sight of the fact that "identities in general (of whatever kind, at whatever level), arise out of difference" and "nowhere ever is there anything simple" (Bennington 2016, para. 3, cited above). One would be grounding the normativity of deconstruction on a violent restriction of the subject to what it "is" (to an ontological essence that occludes *différance*), foreclosing the *critical* endeavour. Conversely, if one understands the subject as an irreducible surplus of meaning and being, so to speak, and thus as *not* present to or coincident with itself, one can no longer account for the subjective fidelity *to* reason that patently obtains in every demand for philosophical rigour. In this case one could not explain in *normative* terms what drives a radical critique to the very limit at which one realizes that reason cannot account for its own desire for light.

Neither characterization is tenable, it appears, yet both seem to be required. On one hand, as Derrida says in the epigraph above, the "who" is not some self-identical, "pure *cogito* of self-presence." As he elaborates elsewhere,

> It is not an atom. It is a singularity that dislocates or divides itself in gathering itself together to answer to the other, whose call somehow precedes its own identification with itself, for to this call I can *only* answer, have already answered, even if I think I am answering "no." (1991b, 100–101; emphasis his)

On the other hand, there *are* "subjects, 'operations' or 'effects' of subjectivity," as Derrida also avers (in Kearney 1984, 125), which is why a certain responsibility occurs nonetheless. More precisely, I contend, it is in the very 'self-gathering' that one undertakes *in response to* the call of reason that critical responsibility takes place. On the view that I support in what follows, responsibility does not issue from the subject's indebtedness to the other (contra Levinas), but rather from its *denial* of that indebtedness for the sake of its own primacy. In order to explain why this response is imperative, however, one would have to understand why that primacy is at stake. What is needed, in short, is a socially, politically and historically contextual explanation of why the divided singularities that we are *are* impelled to answer reason's call, at least insofar as the rendering of reason, the giving an account of oneself, so to speak, is what "responsibility" continues to mean.

The absence of this explanation (beyond Derrida's various references to an indeterminable "affirmation") is a lacuna in Derrida's oeuvre. Addressing it requires one to treat what Rodolphe Gasché calls the "problematic of consciousness in the context of an analysis of violence and writing" (2016, 70), and that one do so, moreover, in a way that avoids the twin pitfalls of religious belief and philosophical idealism. To be sure, such a treatment cannot give rise to a determinate standard of critique, but it can explain the quasi-ethical imperative to deconstruct. It can explain, in particular, what is "normative" about *exposing* the violence that produces the appearance of self-presence, a violence that results in turn in racism, sexism, xenophobia, chauvinism and so many other attacks against difference (Gasché 2016, 79).

Since what has been in question all along is the *desire* for reason, the most obvious resource for this treatment is psychoanalysis. Sigmund Freud was the first to fully demonstrate that individuals are impelled by unconscious motives, and that these motives are shaped by social and cultural forces. The revelation of heteronomous forces hidden from consciousness but at work within it unseats the traditional category of the subject immediately. It strikes a "wounding blow" to "human megalomania," as Freud says, because it proves the ego "is not even master in its own house" (Freud 1916–17, 284–5). In one of his late interviews, similarly, Derrida comments that, despite his reservations about "the grand conceptual framework" of psychoanalysis, Freudian thought bears a revolutionary force, most especially because "it always involves the affirmation of a reason 'without alibi'" (Derrida and Roudinesco 2004, 172). Now, Freudian theory is riddled with problems, to be sure; it manifests numerous instances of sexism, heterosexism, Eurocentrism and racism of its own, instances which are particularly apparent today. I address these issues of bias in detail below. Nonetheless, Freud did show why "the subject is not what says it is," and he thereby inaugurated a powerful discourse through which subjectivity can be historically contextualized and understood.

Of particular relevance is Freud's insight that there is something irrational about the way in which modern individuals answer to the principle of reason. He explicitly associated "Kant's categorical imperative" of morality with taboos, for example, insofar as the imperative "operates in a compulsive fashion and rejects any conscious motives" (Freud 1912–13, xiv). And by the time he published *The Ego and the Id* ten years later, Freud would assert that "the ego submits to the categorical imperative of its superego" just "as the child was once under a compulsion to obey its parents" (1923, 48–9). In this sense, "Kant's Categorical Imperative is the direct heir of the Oedipus Complex" (1924b, 167). Thus, behind the imperative of reason that characterizes philosophical responsibility, Freud diagnoses a deeper psychological complex. His intent was to explain not only why the categorical imperative imposes itself on modern subjects, but why any moral imperative might do so, at any given place or time. In fact, reason plays only an indirect role in Freud's own theory of morality; for him, Kantian morality is merely the contingent, contemporary manifestation of the dictates of the superego, not the necessary form those dictates will take. Freud's question, in short, is how "conscience" (the guilt one feels when one fails to repress unbridled libido or aggression) is possible at all. His answer centres on the emergence of a superegoic agency in the course of individual psychological development. Consequently, it is necessary to consider Freud's theory of conscience in relation to his theories concerning the genesis and development of the ego – in relation to *self*-consciousness, that is – more generally.

If one does so, however, one will see that Freud's explanation of moral responsibility in terms of the Oedipus complex is irreparably flawed. The theory is beset by a number of problems, in fact, but the most damaging among them is the veritable impossibility at the root of the subject itself. In particular, if one attends closely to the theory of ego development in which Freud's understanding of "conscience" is embedded, one discovers two opposing yet intricately entwined developmental trajectories. These are the "narcissism" and the "melancholic" trajectories of egoic development respectively. On the narcissism account, to which Freud repeatedly refers and which underlies the later "death drive" hypothesis, there is an originary cathexis of a unified *self* (*das Ich*), a primary narcissistic investment, which is eventually parcelled out to the others (from in here to out there). In the absence of primary narcissism, no attachment, and no sexual object, is possible at all. Yet narcissism, it emerges, is preceded and made possible by heteronomy. Drawing on Jean Laplanche's reconstruction of Freudian psychoanalysis, I show that self-generated subjectivity is impossible (both logically and psychologically). On the melancholic account, in contrast, which underlines Freud's oedipal theory of morality, what comes first is the internalization of the paternal other (from out there to in here) and, thus, the constitution of an ego (and a superego) from without, through a process of identification. And yet, contradictorily, heteronomy will be shown to have been preceded by narcissism too, as interventions by Laplanche and Judith Butler make clear. The two trajectories are not only mutually exclusive, therefore, but are also problematic independently. Read together, they indicate an impossible splitting at the origin of the ego, and thus an irreducibly aporetic subjective structure.

This reading of Freudian theory is the first of two necessary steps: it reveals the ego as aporetic, thus exposing an arguable truth about modern, Western subjectivity. For the point is not merely that Freud's failure to account for the emergence of the ego in a non-contradictory way undermines his gender-laden explanation of the oedipal basis of conscience. More importantly, I will argue, the paradox that emerges is the essential clue as to how reason imposes itself categorically. Specifically, in Chapter 12 I show in a second step why this aporia matters. I submit that the "life" of the ego requires the binding of heteronomous forces, that the principle of reason is instrumental with respect to how this binding occurs, and that the process as a whole is morally-imbued due to the vagaries of psychosexual development. The final chapter thus demonstrates how unconscious drives impel both the attachment to, and the ethical characterization of, the categorical imperative of reason – or, to put it succinctly, how the ethical *effects* of subjectivity and responsibility obtain. We can thereby see why deconstruction's radical faithfulness to the rational principles of completeness and non-contradiction appears in a normative light. To begin, however, let us follow Freud's "narcissism" and his "melancholic" explications of the genesis of the ego.

Narcissism

Freud's "narcissistic" account of subjectivity begins by modelling the infant as a self-enclosed, monadic entity endowed with a fundamental capacity for self-preservation. This capacity provokes the gradual development of an ego – which is to say, a representation of itself as an "I" (*das*

Ich) – as well as a sexual drive. The sexual drive is at first bound up with self-preservation and is no more than the attachment of libidinal energy to oneself. This is what Freud calls "primary narcissism." But the sexual drive eventually deviates from the (self-preservative) "ego-drive," redirects libidinal energy externally towards others, and ultimately comes into conflict with self-preservation. Since each of these claims is problematic in its own way, it will be useful to approach them separately.

The first dimension of Freud's narrative is that the ego develops strictly as a consequence of the innate, biological instinct for self-preservation. To begin with, infants are entirely self-contained, physiologically and psychologically. When a vital need first produces discomfort, the infant hallucinates its satisfaction in order to regain a state of pleasure as quickly as possible. However, this strategy leads quickly to "unpleasure," which is the unwelcome increase of tension rather than its abatement (1900, 598; 1911, 219), because it fails. This provokes the development of a secondary system, that of consciousness, which replaces the hallucination with a thought (1900, 566). The task of the secondary system is to bind the energy issuing from the primary system by connecting it with "verbal residues," thereby making "thinking" "perceptible to consciousness" (1911, 221), and it is on this basis that the ego evolves. Freud writes:

> a new functioning was thus introduced; what was presented in the mind was no longer what was agreeable but what was real, even if it happened to be disagreeable. This setting up of a *reality principle* proved to be a momentous step. (1911, 219; emphasis his)

This advance inaugurates the possibility of ego development, while simultaneously ensuring the preservation of the biological organism.

Now, as an explanation of infantile development, this narrative is entirely lacking in credibility. Even Freud does not believe it should be taken literally since, as he acknowledges, "an organization which was a slave to the pleasure principle and neglected the reality of the external world could not maintain itself alive for the shortest time, so that *it could not have come into existence at all*" (1911, 219, nt.4; emphasis added). However, Freud avers, the "fiction" that the infant is originally self-enclosed is justified on the grounds that the infant "does *almost* realize a psychical system of this kind" – provided, that is, that "one includes with it the care it receives from its mother" (ibid.; emphasis added). In other words, the argument that the ego develops autonomously from within an enclosed "psychical system" in order to ensure the organism's biological preservation can be taken to stand, as long as we remember that an enclosed psychical system is biologically unsustainable and counter-factual, and that no infant can survive without assistance and care from another person. The dimension of the narcissism thesis that concerns the autonomous development of the ego is thus belied by the irreducibility of the infant's heteronomy, a point to which I return below.

The substance of the second point – that a sexual drive also develops from the drive to self-preservation – is equally inconceivable. Freud suggests that the infant manufactures its own body (or parts thereof) as a sexual object for itself *from* the object-less state of instinctual satisfaction (from the "sensual sucking" associated with the self-preservative function of eating). A distinct sexual drive emerges endogenously, Freud argues, by "leaning" or "propping" itself on the vital, bodily register of self-preservation which "has as yet no sexual object" (Freud 1905, 182; qtd. in Laplanche 1976, 19). For, while the vital register may have "no sexual object" yet, on Freud's view, it is already imbued with libidinal energy. Freud calls this energy "ego-libido," and he associates it with "primary narcissism." As he explains, primary narcissism is merely "the libidinal complement to the egoism of the instinct for self-preservation, a measure of which may be found in every living creature" (1914, 73–4). Specifically, as it evolves the ego takes itself as its own object; it idealizes itself in the form of an "ideal ego" against which the 'self' (*Ich*) is later judged, and *thereby* becomes a coherent agency capable of relating to others in a healthy, non-pathological way (1914, 88, 89, 138). At work here is thus a distinction between "primary" narcissism, which is at work in every individual as the precondition for any object cathexis, and "secondary" narcissism, "which arises through the drawing in of object-cathexes" and is "superimposed" upon the primary (non-pathological) one "by a number of different influences" (1914, 75). Thus, Freud writes,

> we form the idea of there being *an original libidinal cathexis of the ego*, from which some is later given off to objects, but which fundamentally persists and is related to object-cathexis much as the body of an amoeba is related to the pseudopodia which it puts out. (1914, 75; emphasis added).

The gist of this argument is that the sexual drive is at first bound up with and dependent upon the narcissistic (sexualized) "ego-drive" of self-preservation (1905, 182; 1923, 40). Ego-libido and object-libido are thus initially indistinguishable, but they come into opposition later, after object-attachment has been enabled by virtue of a process that unfolds over time. In this sense, the ego is not inborn *as*, but *becomes*, the primary object of libidinal investment, and this development then paves the way for the later split between ego-libido ('hunger,' or self-preservation), and object-libido ('love,' or sexuality).

The primary issue with this second argument is that self-preservation and sexuality cannot both be characterized as "drives" (*Triebe*). To begin with, our rudimentary self-preservative "instinct" (*Instinkt*), such as it is, is not a "drive" (*Trieb*) in the psychoanalytic sense. Unlike an instinct, a drive is defined psychoanalytically as an internal source of excitation that is relatively indeterminate in terms of both its object and its aim

(Laplanche and Pontalis 1973, 214).[2] And second, as Laplanche notes, Freud himself observed that human beings do not have much in the way of survival "instincts" at all (Laplanche 2004, 457). "Innately, children seem to have very little true realistic anxiety," Freud writes; "It would have been a very good thing if they had inherited more of such life preserving instincts [here *Instinkt* in the original, Strachey notes]" (1916–17, 407, 408; compare 1926, 168). More plausibly, therefore, Laplanche postulates that all infants begin with is some basic "psycho-physiological wiring" (2004, 466), but the instinctual wiring is "so defective that in certain cases it can be almost virtual and cannot be made active other than at the moment when … [sexuality], as it is called, arouses it" (Laplanche 1984, 16).

If the difference between the vital order of self-preservation and the order of sexuality is crucially important, therefore (Laplanche 1995, 680), this is not because they are in conflict (ego *versus* object libido). It is because the self-preservative "instincts" are so inadequate that they are taken over by the sexual "drive" completely. As Laplanche puts it,

> The dominance of human needs, undeniable but truly minimal in the domain of biological life, is completely covered over by culture. The biological individual, the living human, is saturated head to foot by the invasion of the cultural, which is by definition intrusive, stimulating, and sexual. (1999a, 225)

The difference thus hinges on the fact that these two dimensions of human experience are not analogous. The sexual drive is "a *deviate version* of self-preservation," not its correlate (Laplanche 1984, 25; emphasis added).

This brings us to the third point, which is that sexuality is said to "be generated as it were *ex nihilo*, by a stroke of some magic wand" (Laplanche 1976, 18). Again, as Laplanche points out, this is to posit that "the human individual must thus 'open up' to his world – things as well as individuals – starting from what we are tempted to call a state of biological idealism" (Laplanche 1976, 18–19). Against this view, Laplanche insists that,

> It is inconceivable that sexuality should emerge biologically from self-preservation, even if it were to be by virtue of a displacement affecting both aim and object. This is the last word in Crusoesque enterprises, by which I mean the attempt to reconstruct the world of culture on the basis of the endogenous resources of the solitary baby Robinson. (1999a, 128–9 and 77nt. 53)

Thus, the process by which the self-preservative instincts become (sexual) ego-*drives* must be otherwise explained.

In this respect, Laplanche's notion of "primal seduction" is decisively important. Laplanche argues that Freud's notion of self-preservation must be reformulated to include care and attachment, specifically on the part of the adult or adults entrusted with the infant's well-being, as these are necessary for the infant's survival. For him, therefore, self-preservation is better qualified and "enlarged" as a "relation" (1976, 66–79; 2000, 39) rather than as a biological "instinct." He specifies,

> My formula, then, is this: the only truth of "leaning-on" is primal seduction. It is because the adult's gestures of self-preservation are the bearers of sexual messages that are unconscious for the adult and unmasterable by the child that, in the so-called erogenous zones, they produce the movement of splitting and drifting that may lead to auto-erotic activity. (1999a, 129)

This reformulation of self-preservation as "attachment" allows Laplanche to extend the range of the infant's needs beyond those of mere nourishment to a variety of relations, and it marks the replacement of Freud's "biological and ipsocentric model" of sexual development with an "intersubjective version of Freud's theory" (Van Haute and Geyskens 2004, 123). Laplanche thereby opens the door to an explanation of the exogenous source of infantile sexuality and, concomitantly, of the sexualization of self-preservation. As Philippe Van Haute summarizes the point, with the model of primary seduction,

> Sexuality no longer just "emerges" in the child, but it is rather introduced into the child from the outside. The "emergence" of sexuality can still be considered as a *Nebenprodukt* [by-product] of the satisfaction of the instincts of self-preservation, but the *Nebenprodukt* cannot occur without an active – albeit mostly unconscious – seduction by the other. (1995, 8)

I will return in the next chapter to Laplanche's notion of primal seduction, as it is crucial to an understanding of the formation of the ego and, relatedly, to the "must" of reason, with which I am concerned. At this point, however, it is important to underscore that Laplanche's reading of Freud illuminates both the way in which the sexual drive is "implanted" in the infant by the caretaking adult rather than self-generated, and how this implantation inaugurates a process whereby the infant's limited and insufficient self-preservative instincts are essentially taken over or largely absorbed from a very early stage by the (phantasmatic) ego, which unifies the sexual drives, and which "is itself the prototype of a unitary object" (Laplanche 2004, 461). Thus, the self-preservative ego function remains closely tied to sexuality, but on Laplanche's view this is because the so-called biological or "vital" register has been displaced by the narcissistic phantasm of the (sexualized) egoic object. It is this *phantasmatic object*, the *idea* of the organism as an autonomous ego, towards which the self-preservative "drives" will subsequently aim.[3]

Yet it is still unclear just what kind of object the ego is supposed to be, or how it is supposed to transition from a psychical border to an object worthy or capable of libidinal investment. For Freud, it should be recalled, the ego is both a "surface entity" (1923, 26) – a unity or "coherent organization of mental processes" (1923, 17) – *and* that which unifies, or exerts a "logical force" (1900, 55). While the ego is in one sense only a border between psychical and empirical "reality," in other words, it is *also* "itself the projection of a surface" (1923, 26); as a representation, it is also a possible object of cathexis. But, whence this representation? It would appear that, in order to idealize itself (its "self" as *such*), the organism must already have formed some kind of representation *of* itself, however rudimentary. As Laplanche proposes, "We are thus led to admit the existence of an identity that is both extremely early and probably also extremely sketchy in its initial phase, *an identification with a form conceived as a limit*, or a sack: a sack of skin" or, alternatively, as "a *network* of cathected neurons" – "a kind of *Gestalt*, or *form*" (1976, 81, 62; emphases added). Similarly, Karyn Ball proposes that Freud's argument in the "Narcissism" essay "anticipates an understanding of the ego *as the object of a fantasy of unity*" (2009, 169; emphasis added).

Jacques Lacan's notion of the mirror stage is illuminating in this regard, as Laplanche remarks, because Lacan undertakes an "elaborate attempt to fill the gap left by Freud's notion of the ego" (1976, 81). Lacan proposes that between 6 and 18 months the infant interiorizes an image of itself as a unified form, notwithstanding "the turbulent movements with which the subject feels he animates it." As Lacan elaborates,

> The jubilant assumption [*assomption*] of his specular image by the kind of being – still trapped in his motor impotence and nursling dependence – the little man is at the *infans* stage thus seems to me to manifest in an exemplary situation the symbolic matrix in which the *I* is precipitated in a primordial form, prior to being objectified in the dialectic of identification with the other, and before language restores to it, in the universal, its function as subject. (Lacan 2002, 76)

Significantly, this development does not depend on an actual visual experience or on the material presence of a mirror.[4] As Laplanche clarifies,

> The scenario of the child at the mirror is only the index of something that occurs, in any event, without that apparatus: the recognition of the *form of another human* and the concomitant precipitation within the individual of a first *outline of that form*. (1976, 81; emphases added)

Thus, the narcissistically-cathected ego is to begin with no more than a *form* of unity and, significantly, the assumption of this form is provoked from without.

It is hard to see, too, how the *ideal* ego can be a *pre*-linguistic form. In other words, the Freudian text makes it difficult to distinguish sharply between an imago that is prior to objectification in language, and the subsequent linguistic assumption of the "I" which Lacan sees as restoring the infant's subjectivity. For cathexis entails the binding of energy in the form of a representation in *words*. In *The Interpretation of Dreams*, for example, Freud explains that while the "primary process endeavors to bring about a discharge of excitation in order that … it may establish a 'perceptual identity' [with the experience of satisfaction]," the secondary process abandons "this intention and [takes] on another in its place – the establishment of a '*thought* identity' [with that experience]" (1900, 602; original emphasis). And thinking itself, Freud insists, only becomes conscious when it is bound to "verbal residues" (1911, 221; cf. 1900, 594, 602, 617). Indeed, Freud specifies elsewhere,

> by being linked with words, cathexes can be provided with quality even when they represent only *relations* between presentations of objects and are thus unable to derive any quality from perceptions. Such relations, which become comprehensible only through words, form a major part of our thought-processes. (1915b, 202)

Significantly, therefore, the process of binding through which the ego is constituted and consolidated as a potential libidinal *object* depends on the acquisition of language, because the secondary process only achieves its purpose by replacing a thing-representation with a word-representation, and word representations are essential for conscious thought (see Weber 1982, 37, 44; 1991, 87).

Once this is understood, it becomes clear that the rudimentary ego is essentially a purely formal concept; the "I" in which narcissistic libido is invested is the *idea* of unity – indeed, it is the ideal concept of the purely logical coherence of form. As an object of narcissistic love, in other words, the ego is idealized as a unity that coheres, and it persists by virtue of a libidinal, narcissistic drive to "preserve" itself. The idea of coherence, as such, constitutes the "ideal" against which the ego is judged, and upon which the individual expends its efforts of maintenance and preservation. For as we have seen, the ego-drive is fundamentally related to the self-preservative instincts – that is, the ego itself comes to be identified as the psychological representative of the individual's vital life. As Freud says, in order to be able to negotiate between the id and the external world without becoming a target of destructive psychic forces, the ego "has had itself to become filled with libido; it thus itself becomes the representative of Eros and thenceforth desires to live and be loved" (1923, 56; compare 58). This in turn, I contend, means corresponding with its unitary ideal.

The point comes across clearly when Freud transposes his analysis of the individual psyche onto that of the social group as a whole. In order to exist, Freud explains, the group must entail continuity of either a material or a systemic (structural) sort, and it must have a "definite idea … of [its] nature, composition, function and capacities"; it must also be able to interact with other similar but differing groups, and it must "possess traditions, customs and habits, and especially such as determine the relations of its members to one another" (1921, 86). Modifying these requirements somewhat, Freud goes on to argue that what holds a group together is the "illusion … of there being a head – in the Catholic Church Christ, in an army its Commander-in-Chief – who loves all the individuals in the group with an equal love" (1921, 94). Thus, Freud theorizes, "the essence of a group lies in the libidinal ties existing in it," and this is nowhere more obvious than in the case of panic, which arises, "if a group of that kind becomes disintegrated" (1921, 95–6). In other words, the survival of the entity *as* an entity is tied directly to its libidinal investment in a unifying figure through which it represents itself.

And, as for the group, so for the individual. Freud writes,

> In the undisguised antipathies and aversions which people feel towards strangers with whom they have to do we may recognize the expression of self-love – of narcissism. This self-love works for the preservation of the individual, and behaves as though the occurrence of any divergence from his own particular lines of development involved a criticism of them and a demand for their alteration. (1921, 102)

The individual ego, no less than that of the group, fears its own dissolution – indeed, it is panic-struck or made anxious by that threat – and goes to great lengths to maintain its own integrity, especially in the face of difference or outright contradiction. One can thus draw a direct correlation between the individual and the group's defensive response to alterity: the source of anxiety is in both cases arguably the same. As Laplanche remarks with respect to analyses of racism,

> what is lacking … is any consideration of the internal split inherent in the other himself: it is this *internal alterity* which is at the root of the anxiety provoked by external alterity; it is this that one needs to reduce at any price. (1999a, 230, nt. 21; emphasis his)

Now if the ideal ego is, before anything else, essentially a logically coherent form, its maintenance will require that it can offer an account of itself – in particular, that differences or divisions within the ego are rejected or expelled, that self-contradictions are disavowed or resolved, and that the questions of its origins and its impulses are determined. As I explain in the next chapter, the fundaments of the rational imperative are situated here.

Finally, given that the ego is initially an element of language through which "I" is represented as an organization, the *method* of its preservation becomes clearer as well. In effect, Freud's theory of narcissism would seem to lead to the conclusion that it is only through the discursive performance of the self, the repetition of the signifier "I," that a simulacrum of identity is achieved (cf. Weber 1991, 88–9). I borrow the term "simulacrum" from Samuel Weber. What is required to explain the link between language and subjectivity, he explains, is "a metaleptic sleight of hand." This linguistic operation, "is nothing other than the *recitation of a proper name* as the translation of an anonymous other, in which origin and end, individual and general converge in a 'simulacrum' of identity" (1992, 251; emphasis his). Derek Sayer makes the same point when he argues that one can only know oneself as a self that is primary or *first*, as an ego, insofar as one loses oneself in the simulacrum of the "I," which is to say, in an "act of objectification" or "primordial estrangement." Quoting Lacan, Sayer continues:

> "I identify in language, but only by losing myself in it like an object." Not that this I, *qua* subject, could ever have had any choice in the matter ... It is not that there was an already existent I who decided to enter language, an original self that was ever there to lose. The subject is only created in this act ... It is found(ed) ... in this original loss. (2004, 68)

In order to see more clearly how the "I" is simultaneously idealized and lost through a staged process of identification, it will be necessary to rework and develop the Lacanian interpretation of the formation of the ego in language. I return to this in Chapter 12. For now, however, it is important to underline that even at the most rudimentary stage of its development, the ego is already constituted at least minimally as a unit or form of bound psychic energy, and this form is given from without. It is in its character *as* a unitary form that the ego can serve on one hand to either repress or sublimate what Freud calls the "freely mobile" energy of the unconscious, and on the other hand, itself, to embody libidinal investment. And it is by virtue of such an investment that one is impelled, so to speak, to cohere. If the ego is constituted through identification with an ideal, it cannot be said to originate endogenously; thus, the very process of *becoming* an "I" is the same process through which the possibility of *being* a coherent unit, of accounting for myself by being my own source, is lost.

Once put in these terms, it becomes clear that the narcissistic account of ego formation is inseparable from the second developmental trajectory Freud describes, this one based originally on melancholic identification rather than on primary, narcissistic ego-cathexis. Yet not only does Freud neglect to probe the depths of their co-implication, he offers a parallel account of the constitution of the ego based on melancholia, notwithstanding its incompatibilities with the theory of primary narcissism.

Melancholia

Just as the narcissistic ego arguably depends on melancholic identification, so the melancholic account of the origin of conscience seems to stem from narcissism. This second trajectory of ego development begins from the supposition that the individual does not evolve an ego by itself, endogenously, but rather exogenously, through its conflictual relations with others. On this account, egoic consolidation occurs in conjunction with the emergence of a "superego," and it is explained as the outcome of the notorious Oedipus crisis. A conflict ostensibly arises when "the boy's sexual wishes in regard to his mother become more intense and his father is perceived as an obstacle to them" (1923, 32). The boy's intensifying hostility towards his father, together with his attachment to his mother, are dealt with through an identification with the father and an introjection or incorporation into his own ego of the boy's own ambivalence.

The subsequent resolution of the Oedipus complex (if all goes well) thus entails a modification of the subject's own ego; the (always) male subject internalizes both the figure of the father and the ambivalence he feels towards him, along with the threat that the father represents and more general social norms and values, as a newly incorporated part of his "self." Insofar as the lost or forbidden other (the ambivalently loved, same-sex parent) is internalized whole rather than being de-cathected (which is said to happen in normal mourning), the process is characterized as a "melancholic" one. The parental other then becomes a part of the ego itself, in the form of its 'nucleus,' namely, as the *ego ideal*. The ego is thus said to develop a new, specialized 'part,' the superego (*über-Ich*). It is this newly internalized ego *ideal* against which the ego is judged, or more precisely, against which the ego judges itself, in its capacity as "conscience" (1917, 247).

Setting aside for a moment this crucially important discussion of the emergence of a superego through primary melancholia, one notices that this version of ego formation contradicts the thesis of primary narcissism in a number of significant ways. First, the narcissistically-cathected ego was said to produce (or become) its *own* ideal (hence, "ideal *ego*"), whereas in this case the ideal to which conscience aspires and with which the ego identifies is based on an external object (the ego *ideal*). Moreover, beyond "the first of these identifications," which produces the superego, the ego itself is now said to be "formed to a great extent out of identifications which take the place of abandoned cathexes by the id" (1923, 48). As Laplanche and Pontalis remark, "In Freud's work the concept of identification comes little by little to have the central importance which makes it, not simply one psychical mechanism among others, but the operation itself whereby the human subject is constituted" (1973, 206). Thus, we find in the melancholic trajectory the description of an *exogenous* source of the ego in conjunction with the superego, namely, the original parental authorities, whereas the theory of narcissism posits endogeny.

A second contradiction is that in the melancholic account identification with an external figure *precedes* the cathexis of ego *and* object, whereas in the theory of primary narcissism the original cathexis of the ego was given as the condition *for* attachment to objects. To be sure, in the "Melancholia" essay Freud supports references he consistently makes elsewhere to the ego-based, amoeba-like structure of libidinal energy; he describes melancholic identification there as a "*regression* from object-cathexis to the still *narcissistic* oral phase of the libido" (1917, 250, emphases added). In fact, narcissistic object-choice is even postulated as an essential condition for melancholia. He writes,

> We have elsewhere shown that identification is a preliminary stage of object-choice, that it is the first way – and one that is expressed in an ambivalent fashion – in which the ego picks out an object. The ego wants to incorporate this object into itself, and, in accordance with the oral or cannibalistic phase of libidinal development in which it is, it wants to do so by devouring it. (1917, 249–50, 258)

If this is so, however, it is a very different form of narcissism than was given in the earlier (1914) account, whereby the ego as a whole was said to be the first and primary libidinal object. For in this case the ego is not yet (according to Freud) differentiated as a distinct entity; therefore, it cannot be seen as the original object of libidinal investment. On the contrary, at the oral or cannibalistic phase – from which issue what Freud calls "the oldest" of the instinctual impulses, those of "the infant at the breast" – there is not yet any distinction between 'the ego and the external world as the source of the sensations flowing in' (1925a, 237; see also 1930, 67), nor is there as yet any sharp distinction between the sexual (libidinal) and the self-preservative aims (1905, 198; 1923, 29). Rather, Freud postulates, it is only *through* the distinction between everything that is good and is to be "introjected" into oneself, and everything that is bad and that is to be "projected" from oneself, that the ego and the external world are separated at all (1925a, 237 and 1915a, 136). The separation between the self and the world is itself a consequence of the development of an ego which, among other things, allows the individual to distinguish its inside from its outside, and which only begins to take form, on this account, through the identification with an *other*. Given this argument, one can only assume that the narcissism Freud has in mind in "Mourning and Melancholia," unlike that of the "Narcissism" essay, entails the internalization of the identificatory relationship as a whole, and that the withdrawal of libido from an object onto the ego should here be understood as a "secondary" rather than as a primary event (1923, 46; compare Laplanche and Pontalis 1973, 255–6).

Indeed, if we follow Freud's thinking with regard to the melancholic trajectory, it emerges that the ego is initially an inadequate target for libidinal investment in the way Freud describes in the "Narcissism" essay, since it is not yet a distinct ideational object at all. On the contrary, when Freud develops the theory of identification in *The Ego and the Id*, he argues that

> When the ego assumes the features of the object, it is forcing itself, so to speak, upon the id as a love-object and is trying to make good the id's loss by saying: "Look, you can love me too – I am so like the object." (1923, 30)

This clearly indicates that the ego only becomes a libidinal object through the identificatory process. As Freud puts it elsewhere, it is at this "preliminary stage" of love (1915a, 139) – identification through incorporation, *prior* to object cathexes proper – that the ego itself is "altered" and can "*henceforth* be judged by a special agency, *as though it were an object, the forsaken object*" (1917, 249; emphases added).

The "full significance" of the process of identification is thus that it determines the ego's "form" and "character" (1923, 28), and that it is rooted in the ego's capacity to wrest object-libido *from the id* (which is here given as the "great reservoir of libido" and the original agent of object-cathexis), and to redirect that libido onto itself (1923, 30, nt.1, 29, 28).[5] From this point of view it is clear that melancholic identification should not be seen as pathological either; on the contrary, identification with an ego ideal is described as "a common and typical" process. But this brings a third contradiction into view.

As opposed to the process whereby attachment to objects is understood as dependent upon the primary, narcissistic attachment to the ego, Freud is now describing a process whereby a "preliminary stage of object-choice," identification via incorporation, not only determines the subsequent development of the ego, but also enables object-love of the later, more mature kind (1917, 249). As he clarifies in 1923,

> behind [the ego ideal] there lies hidden an individual's first and most important identification, his identification with the father in his own original prehistory. This is apparently not in the first instance the consequence or outcome of an object-cathexis; it is a direct and immediate identification and takes place *earlier than any object-cathexis.* (1923, 31, emphasis added; see also 1917, 249 and 1933, 63, 103)

Moreover, in *The Ego and the Id* Freud goes so far as to say that "it may be that this identification is the sole condition under which the id can give up its objects," and that this "makes it possible to suppose that the character of the ego is a precipitate of abandoned object-cathexes and that it contains the history of those object choices" (1923, 29). One only thereby becomes capable of cathecting (love, attachment) and de-cathecting (detaching, moving on) normally – which is to say, becomes capable of loving or mourning at all – *rather* than succumbing to melancholia in its secondary, pathological sense

These contradictions between narcissism and melancholia signal an impossibility at the root of subjectivity that is of particular salience for my argument here, since this impossibility, I will argue, drives the subject's attempts to cohere. To make that case, however, it is necessary to examine Freud's theory concerning the emergence of the superego. For, even if one ignores the contradictions between the two developmental trajectories, it remains that the melancholia account of the emergence of conscience is rife with its own problems. Specifically, the insistence that the original identification (the primary melancholia) that establishes the superego is driven by loss suggests that melancholic identification implicates narcissism in a way Freud has failed to theorize. Thus, the theory of primary melancholia no more stands alone as an account of the genesis of the ego than does the theory of primary narcissism; on the contrary, the ego is constitutively split between its 'inside' and its 'outside' on this account as well.

In particular, I propose that the renunciation of the desire for the mother and the quelling of the (purported) urge to kill the father presuppose the presence of at least a rudimentary (or infantile) ego, because an anxiety concerning self-preservation is already at stake prior to, and as a motive for, the formation of the super-ego. In other words, I contend that the identification through which the Oedipus crisis is resolved (or, in the case of girls, inaugurated, according to Freud) must have been propelled by a prior anxiety about loss and a desire for love, that is, by ego-based, self-preservative impulses that are endogenous rather than exogenous in nature. If this is so, it means that melancholia is inseparable from narcissism.

This suggestion is provoked by the logical circularity of Freud's argument. On one hand, both ego-cathexis and object attachment are said to be enabled by primary, melancholic identification – that is, by the *resolution* of the Oedipus complex. On the other hand, a melancholic form of identification is said to be undertaken when "the small boy's" *narcissistic* attachment to his penis (which he "values so highly," which he had hitherto assumed is a feature of every other creature like himself, and which he fears "will be taken away from him") comes into conflict with "the libidinal cathexis of his parental objects" (1924a, 176; 1905, 195). The thesis is thus that a prior set of ego and object investments *inaugurate* an (Oedipus) crisis (1912–13, 130), and that the resolution of this crisis makes these ego and object investments possible *as a result*.

The same circularity attends Freud's account of the Oedipus crisis in girls, notwithstanding other differences. Since in girls, Freud insists, "castration … has already been carried out," "has already had its effect" (1925b, 256), and is therefore already "an accomplished fact" (1924a, 178), and since in their case what is at stake is an anxiety concerning "a loss of love" (ibid.), a narcissistic and object-related motivation for identification is found there as well. In this case the motivation is said to be a "narcissistic wound" rather than a narcissistic benefit (1925b, 253), and is therefore even less plausible.[6] Regardless, it remains that, for both sexes, ego and object-cathexis are simultaneously given as both the cause and the effect of melancholic identification. The problem is that the ego cannot be, so to speak, in two places at once – both present in "infantile" form to the extent that one is already capable of deep object and narcissistic attachments, and also "formed to a great extent out of identifications" that make those object attachments and that narcissism possible (1923, 34, 48). *Something* must be at work behind the moment of a "primary" melancholia, something apparently impels a profound renunciation and apparently provokes (for the most part) a constitutive identification with the parent of the same sex. But the fear (or purported effect) of castration cannot be what it is.

We can find an important clue from the awkward way in which Freud's 1917 story of melancholic ego-formation is pressed into service to support his 1923 oedipal story of how the super-ego is instantiated. For while Freud's theory of conscience does follow from his earlier theory of melancholic identification, there is also a fundamental discrepancy. Melancholia, we recall, is a process through which the individual withdraws an erotic cathexis from an object and transfers it to the ego, in order not to lose "the love for the object," even though the object itself must be given up (1917, 250, 251). An "identification of the ego" is thus established "with the abandoned object" (1917, 249). Furthermore, in *The Ego and the Id* Freud specifies clearly that, in its simplified form, the process is one whereby, "along with the demolition of the Oedipus complex, the boy's object-cathexis of his mother must be given up" (1923, 32). If the abandoned object is the *mother*, however, then why does Freud insist that the first and most important identification that lies behind the ego ideal is the individual's "identification with the *father* in his own personal prehistory" (1923, 32; emphasis added)? According to the theory of melancholic introjection, one would anticipate that the (heterosexual) boy would identify with his mother, since she is the object he must 'forsake' when his father (as rival) is perceived as a threat.

If many (most?) boys do ultimately identify with their fathers nonetheless, Freud explains, this is because we are not being confronted with the Oedipus complex in its 'simplified or schematized' form. What is at issue, rather, is "the more complete Oedipus complex" (1923, 33). In its more complete form, children of both sexes are initially attached to both of their (sexually-differentiated) parents, because all children at the infantile stage are constitutionally bisexual (1923, 31) and "polymorphously perverse" (1905, 234). All children are also, therefore, simultaneously hostile to both parents – since each parent is at once both an object of desire *and* a rival for the attention of the other.[7] Thus the Oedipus complex is comprised of four trends which may ultimately be resolved in terms of "the normal positive Oedipus complex" (normative gender identity and sexual preference), the "inverted negative" Oedipus complex (transgender identity and/or homosexuality) or in terms of some intermediate position between the two (1923, 33–4). According to Freud, it is ultimately the "relative strength [or 'preponderance'] of the masculine and feminine sexual disposition" – an innate constitutional determinant – that regulates the final outcome of the sexual drive (ibid.). And this suggests that the gender identity and sexual aim that are supposed to have been consolidated by virtue of the *resolution* of the Oedipus complex both motivate the conflict to begin with and predetermine its outcome.

If gender identity and sexual aims are fundamentally dispositional on Freud's view, however, then one would have to discard his theory of the perversions entirely, since perversions entail the fixation on, rather than the overcoming of, infantile, component drives. For, as Freud specifies in the *Three Essays on Sexuality*, the erogenous zones are initially disjointed and have no determinate objects, and "the disposition to the perversions" (which is "innate in *everyone*," Freud adds few lines down), "is itself no great rarity but must form a part of what passes as the normal constitution" (1905, 171, 231–3). As a consequence of the oedipal crisis and its resolution, the ground is established for later (post-oedipal) development, whereby the sexual drives are unified in terms of a primary erogenous zone (or not), and through which they become focussed in an organized way on a particular libidinal object that is external to the child (1905, 197). Since the psychological process through which all this occurs is ostensibly so precarious, and since sexuality is supposedly so disjointed and incoherent at the infantile stage, the theoretical recourse to an innate, biological disposition that determines both an object and an aim *prior* to the latency stage of sexual development makes no sense. It suggests that we have been dealing with the "simplified and schematized" Oedipus complex all along, one which cannot account for same-sex (son–father) identification.

A central difficulty with Freud's oedipal theory of morality thus comes into view. It is that he fails to specify what actually impels the profound renunciation and the ego-constituting identification that characterize primary melancholia – and, through it, the instantiation of the super-ego, the assumption of a determinate gender identity, and the determination of any particular sexual object or aim. As we have seen, there are four distinct trends which the child must sort out: his (or her) attachment to an object of *both* sexes, and his (or her) hostility towards *both* of those same libidinal objects. Given Freud's theory that infantile sexuality is disjointed and undirected (polymorphously perverse), it is not obvious why normative gender or sexual identity would be the most common outcome. On the contrary, the theory of melancholia that he describes suggests that male children would be just as inclined to introject their mothers as their fathers in response to this crisis. What is obvious, though, is that if melancholic introjection is a strategic response to an unassimilable loss, and if the fear of castration cannot be both the cause and the effect of that strategy, then something *else* must be at stake to explain the normative outcome.

So, what does the infant fear is at risk and what does, therefore, impel the melancholic identifications that Freud describes? Judith Butler offers a compelling answer to this question. She speculates that the primacy of the phallus and the cultural valuation of this organ can only be internalized *after* a prior taboo on homosexuality has been addressed. Specifically, Butler posits that the desire for love – which is a condition for self-preservation (a narcissistic impulse) – impels the renunciation of an unavowed and unavowable homosexual desire (or its potential). This enables the assumption of the appropriate gender identity in the first place, and thereby confirms the social valuation of masculinity that Freud takes at face value (Butler 1997, 132–7; 1990). The father, not the mother, therefore must be the object of a boy's renunciation, just as the mother, not the father, must be given up by girls, in order for children to avoid contravening the taboos against homosexuality and gender nonconformity.

Butler's insight illuminates two points. The first is that there arguably *is* a form of narcissism underlying melancholic identification, but it is not the "narcissism" Freud originally described. What appears to be at stake is the small child's helplessness and its irreducible dependence on its parents or caretakers, not its auto-erotic self-enclosure as a coherent and autonomous organism. It is particularly interesting, therefore, that Freud himself specifies that we cannot properly "speak of conscience or a sense of guilt" prior to the formation of the superego through melancholic introjection, since the infant has no natural capacity to distinguish good from bad (1930, 125). He admits that there must be an "extraneous influence" that impels the child to submit to parental injunctions and prohibitions. This motive, he continues, is "easily discovered"

> in his [the infant or child's] helplessness and his dependence on other people, and it can best be designated as fear of loss of love. If he loses the love of another person upon whom he is dependent, he also ceases to be protected from a variety of dangers. Above all he is exposed to the danger that this stronger person will show his superiority in the form of punishment. At the beginning, therefore, what is bad is whatever causes one to be threatened with loss of love. (1930, 124)

Freud's explanation is clearly reductive. Children do not require love or fear its loss simply to avoid danger, but for their very physiological and psychological well-being. They also have no reason to assume, *prima facie*, that the withdrawal of love will automatically issue in the infliction of punishment. If anything, the withdrawal of love would more likely be experienced *as* an infliction of punishment, as Freud himself observes (1914, 102).

Nonetheless, the point is well taken: long before children have any vague intimation of how the binary categories of gender and the polymorphous varieties of sexual desire are supposed to map onto their anatomically specific bodies according to social norms, they need love and are, thus, profoundly susceptible to parental (or adult) injunctions. Indeed, according to Jacques André, Freud was led to his theory of *Hilflösigkeit* (helplessness) because the problematic of castration does not account for female anxiety. Furthermore, as André says, "anxiety due to loss of love … is first and foremost the anxiety of infants, regardless of gender" (2011, 217). Thus, it seems plausible that a narcissistic need for love (an intersubjective "narcissism" of self-preservation) provokes the renunciation of homosexual object choice and the assumption of gender identity in the first place, since without love (for itself) the infant cannot survive at all. As Laplanche writes, "While self-preservation [an *instinctual* behavioural pattern] does have a role to play, it must be quite categorically stated that it is not a protagonist in psychical conflict. We do not renounce sexuality for fear of losing our lives, but we do renounce it for other reasons; for example, fear of not being loved" (1989, 141).

The second point that Butler illuminates is that the self-preservative, narcissistic impulse cannot be linked in the *first* instance to the significance of the male genitalia. One does not assume the "right" gender because of the overvaluation of the penis – symbolized as this is by the boy's irrational fear of castration or the girl's equally inexplicable and implausible mourning of its occurrence – since the so-called primacy of the phallus is a consequence of heteronormativity that *has yet to be taken on*, not its foundation. Even if identificatory possibilities were to be extended to include "perverse" attachments and/or equally "perverse" (atypical) objects of renunciation, it would still remain that the assumption (*or* refusal) of normative (*or* transgressive) gender identity, based as it is on the prior prohibition of homosexuality, would have to *precede* rather than succeed the Oedipus complex and any of its various "resolutions." The child would *already* have to have adopted as its own a particular relation to the meaning of gender – that is, to the taboo against homosexual objects and aims – before the Oedipus complex could be resolved one way or another. Thus, the motivation to assume one's (appropriate) gender is more readily explained by a narcissistic anxiety provoked by a threat to the ego than it is by the force of phallocentrism; on the contrary, phallocentrism would be the effect of normative sexuality rather than its cause.

From this point of view, identification with a given (parental) figure must be understood as a consequence of narcissistic investment in oneself (as manifest in the self-preservative ego-*drive*), that is, as due to an *endogenous* anxiety about losing the love that is necessary for egoic survival, rather than as a response to (real or imagined) *exogenous* conditions or threats. And this means that the boy's (melancholic) identification (or lack thereof) with the masculine ego *ideal*, and the girl's (melancholic) identification (or lack thereof) with the feminine ego *ideal* can only take place *after* the formation of one's ideal *ego*, which is to say, after the initial formation of one's (however rudimentary) narcissistically-cathected *self*, since that is what is being protected from the start. In short, it is only insofar as narcissistic anxiety (a threat of dissolution, which is to say, the potential 'death' of the ego) is *already* in play that identification (so-called 'primary' melancholia) can get underway, for the "life" of the ego is already at stake in the way in which the Oedipus conflict is (or is not adequately) resolved.

The melancholic and the narcissism accounts of ego formation thus form a chiasmus. On one hand, I have argued, there is an *endogenous* narcissistic (libidinal) interest in parental love at the root of the melancholic incorporation of the exogenous object. This is the ego *drive*, which serves self-preservation. The drive that launches melancholic identification does implicate a *certain* theory of narcissism to be sure; however, it cannot be said to implicate "primary narcissism," if this is understood in terms of an absolute biological and psychological self-enclosure. For such a state is not only biologically untenable, as even Freud admits (1911, 219, nt.4; compare Laplanche 1989, 38). It is also theoretically untenable, inasmuch as the narcissistic investment *in* the ego requires the prior representation of the individual *as* an ego, which comes from without. Specifically, I have argued that the self-representation on which narcissism depends is first acquired *exogenously*, through the recognition of the form of another human being, and through identification with that form as conceptualized in language. On the other hand, therefore, the endogenous account of the genesis of the ego is equally incomplete, because the narcissistic objectification of the ego presupposes the *prior* identification with an *exogenous* object, which is subsequently represented by the ideational form of the word "I."

So not only do these two linear trajectories of ego development contradict one another insofar as their directions are opposed, but each account also requires the supplementation of its counterpart in order to be complete. Neither a "primary" narcissism *nor* a "primary" melancholia can logically obtain as the first moment (the true genesis) of the constitution of the ego. This aporia at the root of subjectivity does not itself explain why the force of the principle of reason obtains and why, therefore, deconstruction should be characterized as a quasi-ethical form of critique. But it does provide the essential first step. To see why this aporia gives rise to a quasi-normative attachment to reason, we shall have to turn to Laplanche.

Notes

1 The full quotation is as follows: "It is necessary to question this authority of the being-present, but the question itself neither offers the first nor the last word, as I have tried to show for example in *De L'esprit*, but also everywhere I have spoken of the 'Yes, yes,' of the 'Come' or of the affirmation that is not addressed first of all to a subject. This vigil or beyond of the question is anything but precritical. Beyond even the force of critique, it situates a responsibility as

irreducible to and rebellious toward the traditional category of 'subject.' Such a vigil leads us to recognize the processes of *différance*, trace, iterability, ex-appropriation, and so on" (Derrida 1991b, 109).

2 For further elaboration on the difference between "instincts" and "drives" see Laplanche (1976, 9–10; 2004 456–7). Tiina Koivikko (2017) provides an overview of recent debates about Freud's drive theory.

3 See Michael Naas for a fascinating discussion of the concept of the "phantasm" in Derrida's work (2008, 187–212, esp. 199).

4 According to Michael Billig, clinical evidence was already available that showed that pleasure or "jubilation" at mirror images, including the imitative gestures of the infant's movements made by parents or caretakers, can precede the capacity for self-recognition, and that such imitative "playfulness" is crucial for the development (which occurs gradually, rather than as an instantaneous *Gestalt*) of that capacity. What is needed, Billig therefore argues, is a different "mirror trope" – one that accentuates the importance of imitation for development (with or without an actual mirror), and the active role of *the parents* in that development (2006, esp. 14–18, 21).

5 Freud never ceased to equivocate about this (see "Appendix B" to *The Ego and the Id*, 1923, 63–6), and for good reason. For the purposes of supporting the theory that a process of primary identification resolves the Oedipus crisis, and for the related purpose of showing that this leads to the instantiation of the superego as the seat of moral conscience, Freud posits the *id* as the original "reservoir" of libido. This allows him to argue that in taking on the libido of the *id*, the ego *becomes* a compensatory object in lieu of the lost one and is altered as a result. For the purposes of defending "primary narcissism," conversely, Freud postulates that "the *ego* is the true and original reservoir of libido," and insists on the "libidinal character" of self-preservation. This drive, as part and parcel of the ego, is a "manifestation of the force of the sexual instinct" (1920, 51–2; emphasis added). The thesis of narcissism is shelved for a number of years, but it is resurrected to support the final theory of the instincts as represented by the conflict between the life drives and the "death" drive.

6 Freud associates the "narcissistic scar" attending a "permanent injury to self-regard" (due to loss of love, in particular) with the inferiority that "is so common in neurotics" (1920, 20–21). Notably, if women are 'narcissistically wounded' by definition, they are also *by definition* neurotic. One need not belabour the point of how problematic this theory is.

7 Freud presupposes a nuclear family comprised of two parents of opposite sexes. It is not clear from Freud's text itself how the scenario would change in the context of one parent, multiple parents or same-sex parent families. A good line of investigation, however, is opened by the question of the broader social forces through which the normative myths of heterosexuality and phallocentrism are communicated and imposed, regardless of the sex and gender composition of any individual familial unit. I treat this question in Chapter 12.

12 The Desire for Reason

> Following a well-known pronouncement of Kant's which couples the conscience within us with the starry heavens, a pious man might be tempted to honour these two things as the masterpieces of creation. The stars are indeed magnificent, but as regards conscience God has done an uneven and careless piece of work, for a large majority of men have brought along with them only a modest amount of it, or scarcely enough to be worth mentioning. We are far from overlooking the portion of psychological truth that is contained in the assertion that conscience is of divine origin; but the thesis needs interpretation. Even if conscience is something "within us," yet it is not so from the first.
>
> (Freud, 1933, 61).

In the preceding analysis of Freud's metapsychology, I argued that a coherent and autonomous ego can only take form through a heteronomous process, whereby the infant first identifies with another person. As I elaborate here, this Laplanchean-inflected Lacanian insight undermines Freud's understanding of "primary" narcissism, as it gives it an entirely different meaning. I have also argued, however, that a rudimentary, narcissistically-cathected ego must be in place *prior* to the oedipal crisis, because the individual's egoic "life" is endangered when attachments to the same-sex parent become too strong, and when the need to adopt a(ny) particular gender identity is experienced as a result. This thesis, which builds on Butler's analysis of the social force of heteronormativity to recast the oedipal problematic in critical terms, undermines the Freudian explanation of "primary" melancholia, because it implies the ineradicability of narcissistic attachment in the identificatory process. It also destabilizes Freud's own notion of conscience, because it suggests that what for Freud constitutes the very essence of morality – the restriction or renunciation of unbound (pregenital, infantile) sexuality and the assumption of the appropriate gender identity that the resolution of the Oedipus complex purportedly signifies – will have been underway already, prior to the onset of that crisis. This analysis highlights an irreducible aporia at the heart of Freud's theory of the subject.

Freud's theories are riddled with century-old biases and otherwise implausible claims, to be sure. But they are also extremely instructive because, by virtue of their very contradictions, they reveal a possible psychological truth. It is that the modern individual subject understands and invests in itself (as an ideal *ego*) prior to identifying with another person, *and* that identification with another person (with an ego *ideal*) is constitutive of the ego's form and its character. If the theoretical protocols of sufficient reason and non-contradiction are stymied by this hypothesis, I contend, this is because what is at issue is an originary splitting of the subject – a fold or "*pli*" exactly *there*, there where its origin should be. Indeed, I explain in what follows, Laplanche's theoretical reconstruction of Freudian psychoanalysis shows why this fold is arguably what underlies the constitution of the ego.[1]

Yet with respect to the nature of deconstructive normativity, this aporia is exactly what should interest us here. For the very heteronomy that constitutes the ego as present to itself, without which one cannot become a 'self' at all – namely, the identification with and the interiorization of the form of another person – also conditions the ego (*das Ich*) as the phantasmatic representation of a unified, autonomous whole. In other words, I argue below, what heteronomy enables is the emergence of the ego as a phantasmatic representation of autonomy (completeness) and coherence (non-contradiction). If this is so, it means that the ego-*drive* will be the fundamental drive to cohere. Insofar as the ego is libidinally cathected, in short, the ego (every ego) will be *driven* by the principle of reason, which is to say that every subject so constituted will be driven by "the enigmatic desire for vigilance, for the lucid vigil, for elucidation, for critique and truth" (Derrida 1983a, 22), despite the constitutive impossibility of ever fulfilling that demand. This constitutive impossibility, I submit, both opens the subject to the putative responsibility that deconstruction honours most faithfully, and is what so many theories of morality, including Freud's own, ignore.

Laplanchean psychoanalysis supports this argument because it encompasses both of Freud's theses (concerning the ego's impossible unity and the phantasmatic unity that prevails) without reducing either of them to the other. It explains, in particular, how the ego can be constitutively split and thus indebted to another, and yet still appear as an autonomous agency that can and must answer for itself. These contradictory claims can only be articulated together, however, if we mobilize the temporal logic of *Nachträglichkeit* – what Laplanche refers to in French as "*après-coup*" and in English as "afterwardsness" (2001, para. 12; 1999a, 263; Fletcher 2000, 100) – in the context of his general theory of "primal seduction." We will then be able to see why subjects are compelled to cohere, and why, accordingly, the desire for vigilance that attends deconstruction ties it to normative critique.

Primal seduction and the logic of "afterwardsness"

The German word *Nachträglichkeit* is a composite of "*tragen*," which is to bear, carry or "bring to fruition," and "*nach*," which means after or behind (Laplanche 1992, 42). In English it is generally rendered either as "deferred action" (Laplanche 2001, para. 11) – which suggests a "progressive causality" (Fletcher 1999, 15), such as when plans are laid down now and executed later – or as "belatedness," understood as the retrospective reinterpretation of what has already happened (Laplanche 2001, paras. 11–13; 1999a, 261). But in psychoanalysis the term connotes a more complicated form of temporality. Freud used it in 1895 to explain the bidirectional nature of a sexually traumatic event.

The case study of "Emma" illustrates this temporal logic, whereby trauma occurs *between* two scenes rather than at either the earlier or the later determinable moment. As Freud recounts, young Emma, aged 8, is assaulted (twice) by a store owner when she buys some candies. The store owner had apparently groped her through her clothing; however, she has no initial memory of the events. Later, at the age of 12, she enters a shop and sees two sales clerks laughing. She understands that they are laughing at her clothing, and she runs out of the store in terror. At this time, she develops a neurotic fear of entering stores alone, even though the phobic nature of her fear cannot be explained by the second event. The puzzle of why shopping by herself is so terrifying is only solved when, through analysis, Emma recalls the earlier sexual molestation. In both cases (at age 8 and age 12) she had been in the store alone, both times there was a sexual feeling (although it was not recognizable as such initially), both times there was laughter (or the grin of the earlier shopkeeper, with which she associates the laughing clerks) and both times clothing was involved. Thus, Emma connected the two events through a set of associations. The fright of the first event, which she perceived as dangerous and unpleasantly 'exciting' but which was not repressed, was attached to the second event, which was not only *not* frightening, but was actually banal (Laplanche 1976, 41).

This case is interesting, because neither the original incidents of molestation nor the later encounter with the laughing clerks explains the traumatic effect. In fact, Laplanche writes, "we never manage to fix the traumatic event historically" (1976, 41). The trauma is only produced retroactively, when the second event, which occurs after puberty, reactivates the *memory* of the first instance. The memory is reactivated through the lens of a sexual meaning that was not available to Emma when she was 8, but which became available to her during the interim. As Freud explains,

> Here we have the case of a memory arousing an affect which it did not arouse as an experience, because in the meantime the change [brought about] in puberty had made possible a different [or "new"] understanding of what was remembered.
>
> Now this case is typical of repression in hysteria. We invariably find that a memory is repressed which has only become a trauma by *deferred action* [i.e., *Nachträglichkeit*, or "after the event"]. (1950, 356; original emphasis)

Freud's point is that the trauma is neither purely deterministically progressive (*first* she was assaulted, and *then* she later experienced the trauma of that original experience), nor purely retrospective (*after* puberty she reinterpreted or created a story about an original event). It is not a matter of "simply opposing external and internal causality," as Laplanche says (2001, para. 6). Rather, "the first moment must be internalized, and then afterwards relived, revivified, in order to become an internal trauma." Thus, Laplanche continues, "it is not the first act which is traumatic, *it is the internal reviviscence of this memory that becomes traumatic*" (2001, para. 7; emphasis added). In this sense, "external events derive their effectiveness," as Laplanche and Pontalis explain, "from the phantasies they activate and from the influx of instinctual [i.e., libidinal] excitation they provoke" (1973, 468). As Laplanche puts it elsewhere, "This two-stage theory shows that it is only because it becomes *auto-traumatic* that a trauma has a pathogenic effect" (1989, 112; emphasis his).

As is well known, in 1897 Freud abandoned his "theory of seduction," in which he linked hysteria to sexual abuse, and posited an endogenous origin of sexuality instead. In so doing, however, he lost sight of the exogenous source of human sexuality and the logic of "afterwardsness" through which it emerges. These are the neglected dimensions of Freud's "special theory of seduction" that Laplanche incorporates into what he calls his "general theory of seduction" (1989, 114). For, quite apart from issues arising from specific incidents of sexual abuse, Laplanche suggests that all infants are born into a *structural* situation in which a kind of "primal" seduction takes place, and that this is the source of the sexual drives (*le sexual*).[2] The Freudian concept of *Nachträglichkeit* is essential to how he makes this case.

We saw in the previous chapter that infants are born into a "fundamental anthropological situation," according to Laplanche (2000, 36), whereby unconscious sexuality is literally embedded in their bodies, before the acquisition of language, by the caretaking ministrations of parents or caretakers. It is necessary to explain now, however, that bound, narcissistic ego-libido is opposed by what Laplanche calls "unbound (erotic) sexuality" (2004, 466),[3] which is the major constituent of the unconscious, and that the logic of afterwardsness destabilizes any possible priority regarding the inside and the outside, and the before and the after, with respect to them both. For there are, according to Laplanche, always two protagonists in the primal situation. One is the newborn infant, which is from the start a "bio-psychical" or communicative individual that is "aware of the world" and supplied with a set of "regulatory patterns," by which Laplanche means rudimentary self-preservative instincts. But it is "ill-equipped" to adapt to or to survive in its environment. This lack of adaptive capacity is bound up with its prematuration; infants need the care of adults to survive, because they are born in a state of *Hilflösigkeit*, a helpless or distressful state (Laplanche 1989, 92–7). When it experiences an intolerable level of disequilibrium, therefore, the child "cries and it kicks and it shouts, and its mother [or caretaker] very quickly learns to recognize this is a cry for help" (1989, 98).

The other protagonist is thus the caretaking adult, who provides for the physiological and psychological preservation of the infant by "feeding, cleaning [and] fondling" it, among other things (Fletcher 2000, 102). In so doing, the adult conveys "messages" that are "suffused with sexual meanings, unconscious meanings, which are unconscious for the transmitter of the message himself; messages perceived as enigmatic, that is as a 'to be translated'" (Laplanche 1992, 175). Laplanche clarifies,

> [I]n the enigmatic signifier, there is not only an explicit message, but also an implicit message, and the child cannot but understand there is something hidden in it. He doesn't understand it exactly, has no idea of what the fantasies of the mother are (about sexual pleasure in the breast and so on), but it is impossible in this relationship that something is not perceived of that "normal parapraxis"; what is perceived is that this gesture has something of another meaning, another meaning which is even unknown to the mother herself. (1992, 22)

Enigmatic signifiers, then, are not only or even primarily conveyed in words, but rather in "gestures, comportments, expressions and so on" (1992, 57). They are the "noise," or the "excess," of the "code of attachment" as well as of the social codes, which is to say, their content exceeds what is communicated through the adult's normal and essential caretaking of the infant's bodily needs and of the adult's association with the child (Laplanche 2011, 175–6, 109).

Because they are doubly enigmatic (both to the child and also to the adult), these messages are not signifiers *of* any determinate meaning, but merely signifiers *to* their initially passive, infant addressees (Laplanche 1989, 44–5). As John Fletcher elaborates,

> the enigmatic signifier is one that has been *de-signified*, whose signified is lost, without losing its power to signify to, to summon or address its recipient. It is enigmatic, not just because the adult world poses questions that are beyond the child's power to grasp or answer, but because of the role of the adult or parental unconscious. (2000, 101–2, emphasis his)

From the infant's point of view, it is only known *that*, not *what*, they signify (Laplanche 1989, 44–5). There is from the first (day), in other words, enigmatic, communicational 'noise' that is experienced as excess excitation, and that conveys unconscious fragments of the adult's own repressed, infantile sexuality, fragments that are reactivated in the adult when he or she cares for a child (2007, 215; 2011, 108).

This is why Laplanche refers to the fundamental anthropological situation as a scene of "primal seduction." What is at stake is the sexual fantasy of the adult (1995, 665), which is unconsciously but actively conveyed to the initially passive child (1992, 175; 1997, 660).[4] The situation is "seductive" because what is communicated is the adult's sexuality. These enigmas "break in," so to speak; they are traumatic (1999a, 211), and they seduce, "pervert" or lead the self-preservative instinct astray (1976, 23; 1995, 677). The situation is also "primal" because it is fundamental to the very constitution of the human being (1989, 157). As Laplanche elaborates, seduction "is grounded in a situation from which no human being is exempt … This fundamental anthropological situation is the adult-*infans* relation" (2011, 102). What confronts the child from the very first moments of its interaction with the adult world, then, is the enigmatic sexual noise associated with primal seduction. It plays a crucial role in the development of the child's ego and its unconscious.

The ego and "primary" repression

The ego and the id both emerge, on Laplanche's account, in response to the scene of primal seduction and, in keeping with the temporal logic of *Nachträglichkeit*, they are both effects after the fact. Specifically, according to Laplanche, individuals become subjects through the interaction of two moments, the second of which retroactively revivifies, reinterprets and simultaneously "represses" the first. The small "self-interpreting, self-theorizing, self-symbolizing" human being (Peter Dews, in Laplanche 1992, 68) begins as a "Copernican," Laplanche says, "circulating around the other's message," but he "has to internalize this." And so, "he Ptolemizes himself"; "he builds an inside in order to internalize" (2001, para. 30). The formation of an ego thus results from the infant's attempt to make sense of (to "bind") the largely incomprehensible, intolerable excitations it receives as messages. For the sexual messages that are initially implanted on its "skin-ego" (Fletcher 2000, 102) are not immediately apprehended. It is only at a second moment, when the infant responds and attempts to symbolize them, that the messages (the sexual excitations) are retroactively, and always only partially, interpreted. This moment, at which repression first occurs and an ego is correspondingly constituted, marks the second 'scene' of the seduction.

Because the messages are only partially "translated," then, this second scene has a dual character. It is simultaneously a process of translation and repression. Here "repression" is not a turning away, as Freud sometimes describes it, nor is it strictly speaking the inhibition of an originally-cathected representation. Initially there are no representations. Rather, Laplanche argues, repression must be understood in terms of an attempted "translation" and its "failure" (1989, 114; 1999b, 16–17). These first attempts fragment the libidinal energy that is enigmatically communicated into its codified (represented, or sublimated[5]) and its untranslatable (unrepresentable, repressed) parts. The term "translation" (2001, para. 108), therefore, should be understood as a *process* rather than an event. It produces over time a split that is at once both topographical (conscious/preconscious vs. unconscious) and temporal (an original implantation vs. a later interiorization). What Laplanche finds productive in Freud's concept of *Nachträglichkeit* is thus the structural quality of belatedness, whereby the interpretive moment always comes after the fact and reconfigures that fact (or, 'leads it astray,' seduces it [1995, 677]), afterwards, on the psychic level of fantasy.

Laplanche explains the emergence of an "ego" with this temporal process in mind. As he cryptically puts it, the ego appears "between these two phases" of "implantation" and "introjection" (1989, 113). For, initially, the infant's resources are few. There is merely what Laplanche identifies as "something in the order of consciousness, a presence in the world, or a sort of conscious-preconscious system" (1989, 95). But the "noise" of the adult's sexuality provokes in the newborn "an incorrigible yearning for synthesis" (Laplanche 1996, 12). It does so not because it is meaningful, but, on the contrary, because it is not, and it does so categorically, all before the infant has any linguistic, emotional or intellectual resources of its own. While it is still on the receiving end of initial communiques that are largely gestural, therefore, the infant will have to "[find] its own way" into "a pre-existing language" which it "inhabits" from the start (1989, 125) but which it does not yet speak. It does so by actively producing images or representations with which to symbolize the enigmatic sensations and communications it is passively receiving on the periphery of its body. An image of a breast, for example, may symbolize the sensation of milk in its mouth (attended as this is with the mother's own unconscious sexual energy), just as an image of its own form, based on the visual perception of another person, may represent the boundary being excited.

The first and most rudimentary form of the ego is thus merely the image of a corporeal envelope, "an identification with a form conceived as a limit" (1976, 82), as I have said. Laplanche calls this an "auto object" in the sense that it is "always an internal, 'reflected' object" (1989, 71); the "body-ego" is no more than the (internal) projection of the surface of the skin. More specifically, the imagined surface is the representation of an ontologically distinct form (a 'me') that is produced through "a play of interlocking images" (ibid.; compare Laplanche 1976, 54), images that reflect both the body of the child *and* that of its adult caretaker, "the human other" (Laplanche 1989, 49; 1976, 83), and that constitute the very earliest idea of the ego, namely, the organism's representation of itself as a unified whole.

This initial image, however, is overwritten quickly. For even if the initial body-ego is no more than a projected surface, the infant can only become conscious of itself *as* an individual self by virtue of some degree of access to language. As Laplanche says, it is "language that supplies the word-presentations which allow chains of thought to become conscious" (1989, 42). Becoming-conscious, in turn, implies the emergence of the ego-as-agency, because it implies self-reflexivity. On one hand, then, there is a body-ego, which is a metaphorical representation *of* the biological whole. On the other hand, there is the ego-as-agency which acts *on behalf of* the whole (individual), and which takes over the vital functions of self-preservation. Thus, although the ego may well be "initially a body-ego" (Laplanche 1999a, 129), and although verbal language must necessarily be *secondary*, as far as self-consciousness is concerned language must necessarily come first.[6]

Yet Laplanche's account of how the "I" is simultaneously idealized and lost in language during the process of identification differs from Lacan's significantly. For Laplanche draws on the logic of *Nachträglichkeit* to illuminate the complex process through which a body-ego (which is chronologically first) *will have been* "a projection of the organism" only *afterwards*. The body-ego will have become the "projection of a surface" (as Freud had put it) belatedly – thus psychologically in the second place – because it can be perceived as such (as 'me') only *after* the ego-as-agency – what Freud calls a "surface entity" (1923, 26) that functions as "*an apparatus of the organism* … the [differentiated] part charged with the organism's relations to the external world" – has already emerged (Laplanche 1999b, 176; emphasis his). Moreover, as *Ich* the body-ego is no longer implicated in the form of the other, from which it originally derived. Since what is found (the body-ego) is therefore not what was lost (the interplaying images of self and other), this is not a case of straightforward deferral. But neither is it purely a case of endogenous fantasy, because the source of that translation, the form of the other, has come from without. Understood in the temporal terms of *Nachträglichkeit* (rather than in the Lacanian terms of an instantaneous *Gestalt*), a certain rudimentary stage of identification (with the form of another person) *can* be seen to precede originary narcissism, but it also follows from it. In other words, the ego was not there first, but it appears (to self-consciousness) phantasmatically as what *will have been* the origin of the individual, because access to anything that precedes this (non-originary) 'origin' is unavailable to consciousness. Thus, although the ego does not begin as the agent of its own development, it appears (to itself) as the author and the centre of the narrative it constructs.

The burgeoning ego as a unified representation thus begins to take form. Essentially, a self-preservative relation loaded with (or contaminated by) sexuality is "translated" into a self-representation (a representation of the individual as an ego) loaded with bound libido. The ego is "a rudimentary or false image of a living thing" (2016, 57) that is charged with energy, and built out of certain privileged and enigmatic perceptions 'offered up' by the inter-human world of signification in which the child is "totally immersed from the outset" (1999a, 126). Its role is to maintain a constant level of energy that is "lower than that of its surroundings," and that is therefore "incommensurate with the energies outside it" (1989, 25), for the sake of its psychical equilibrium. As Laplanche explains,

> The ego thus turns out to be what introduces into the circulation of fantasy a certain ballast, a process of *binding*, which retains a certain energy and causes it to stagnate in the fantasmatic system, preventing it from circulating in an absolutely free and mad manner. Such is the appearance of the *secondary process*, a process which is but the result induced by the existence of an initial mass that is itself bound, the ego, which is literally *bound* by a limit, an envelope. (1976, 63–4, emphases his)

Here we see directly how the inadequate self-preservative *instinct* becomes an ego-*drive*: the infant draws on and mobilizes the sexual energy that enters from without in order to preserve itself. Specifically, Laplanche says, "what may be observed ... is a kind of reassumption of vital functions, in their feebleness and immaturity, by the ego and its libidinal support" (1976, 82). The ego-as-agency *takes over* the work of translation (1995, 678) and the activity of perception (1976, 83), as well as such other functions as censorship and thought processes (1981, 86; Freud 1923, 17), and it does so with the express purpose of maintaining its life. As a *representative* of the organism, however, the life that the ego-drive preserves is not biological but phantasmatic. For if the self-preservative instinct has become an ego-drive (a sexual drive), as Laplanche supposes, this means that the vital imperative is now operating on the level of fantasy.

This is why *the* "I" (ego-as-agency) is best understood as the fictional protagonist of its own story; the ego is the individual's theory or idea of itself, of which it is (self-reflectively) conscious. For Laplanche describes "translation" variously as theorization, temporalization, symbolization and narrativization, among others, and it is precisely through such narrativization that the child first establishes itself as an "I" with both a history and a future. In his fascinating recasting of the problematic of mourning, for example, Laplanche (1992, 172–3) makes the point that the ego, together with one's attachments to others, are always part of a narrative, an ongoing history and an anticipated future, which one fabricates or theorizes for oneself. "The translation of messages is in essence the production of a history, more or less coherent" (2011, 208).

The individual's (his)story is built up not only out of the "the relational codes" associated with self-preservation (attachment), but also out of "preformed narrative schemas" that are provided by the familial and the more general "cultural environment" (2011, 217). "One could speak here," Laplanche underlines, "of a veritable 'aid to translation' offered by the surrounding culture" (2011, 217). For of course, at what Laplanche calls the "very first moment of introjection," there is nothing yet as elaborate as a logical, non-contradictory account of oneself or one's world. And, while a "minimum of structure" is already implicit in attachment (1999b, 102), it is insufficient to decode the unconscious, adult 'noise' that has been communicated along with it (2011, 216–17). The infant therefore mobilizes as well as it can (1999a, 159) whatever material there is: its own tactile, auditory and visual perceptions (or some combination thereof), and the immediately available social codes.

Among these codes, castration and oedipal fantasies will have been transmitted by adults already. Laplanche specifies, "Even in the primal situation, a code like Oedipus is present. It is proposed by the adult world, not only by this or that adult, but by the adult world, also through language" (2000, 40). On one hand, then, these myths and codes, these "little stories" and "romances" (2004, 464–5) will be readily available to the child as "aids" for its translation. Indeed, what Freud identified as the "sexual theories of children" are primal translations, and they are made possible by the cultural narratives and schemas that permeate the infant's social world. On the other hand, one must also consider linguistic syntax in this regard. For, insofar as "man is a linguistic animal," the adult's pre- or para-linguistic messages are always already contaminated by "the complexity of verbal language," even if they are not communicated solely (or even at all) in words (2011, 18; 1989, 124). Moreover, as I argued much earlier, grammar and logic are co-extensive (de Man 1982, 14). It is therefore plausible that the syntactical logic embedded in language provides additional coding through which the infant's initial and subsequent translations will be structured.

Thus, the overwhelming affect (the indeterminate anxiety) produced by the implantation of enigmatic messages is 'translated' into ideational representatives with the help of the 'code of castration' and the logic of syntax. Among those communications, sexuality and gender – or gender assignment, more precisely – are chief among the social messages that are conveyed to the child, and gender is initially enigmatic for approximately the first 15 months (Laplanche 2011, 176). As I explained in the previous chapter, a child is designated as a boy or a girl from the moment of its birth (or sooner), but this message requires translation. First, there is no indication that infants actually perceive their biological sex during the first few months (2011, 172). And second, gender is not binary but plural, both "in the history of languages and in social evolution," as Laplanche specifies (2011, 159), and also in terms of the cultural practices, attitudes, dispositions and behaviours of the sexes through which children first encounter the distinctions (2011, 168; see also 309). This is why, behind the assignment of gender, there lingers "an enigmatic, masked difference immediately presented by the adult as a message to decipher" (1996, 9).

By virtue of the available codes, the enigma of gender can be reduced to the "binary, phallic logic" of the presence or absence of the male sex organ

(1996, 9; 1999b, 22). As a "way of organizing the world around the principle of contradiction" (1992, 81), in other words, phallic logic as code enables what Laplanche calls "an early genital phase" or "castration reaction," whereby the difference between the sexes is reduced to "a difference of sex," based on a popular, perceptual and "even purely illusory" anatomy (2011, 177). This is "actually a reaction by means of the castration complex," he clarifies (2011, 179), and it predates the narrative of negation, in which there is a real or imagined threat. It is only at a later, oedipal stage of development, during approximately the fourth or fifth year, that the phallic basis of binary sexuation will be further elaborated in terms of the narrative of castration as *negation*, that is, of the threat of the severance of a bodily part. As I elaborate below, this later identification, which constitutes *secondary* repression, is impelled by a narcissistic, self-preservative drive, because the child will already have taken on the meaning of gender and the sexual prohibitions it entails.

Before I return to the question of secondary repression, however, it is important to underline that the primary stage of "identification" is the moment at which, as Fletcher succinctly puts it, "the problematic of gender and the problematic of the ego – primary identification and primary narcissism – converge in an attempted organizing of the erogenous zones in an ideal, unified self-representation" (2000, 106). If this is plausible, it suggests a psychological truth underlying the contradictory trajectories of ego development we found in Freud: the ego's narcissistic self-representation as its own origin, and the identificatory incorporation that constitutes the individual as a gendered subject, are fundamentally connected and coterminous; *neither* is primary or first. The identificatory (phallic) dimension of infantile development, moreover – through which the narcissistic ego is constituted through its gender identification (presence or absence of the penis) – lays the ground for the later acquisition of oedipal morality. That is the moment when the binary logic of presence/absence will be overlaid with the (infantile) *theory* that in one of the sexes the sexual organ has already been cut off.

Prior to that later evolution, however, it must be recalled that the infant's translations are partial and incomplete. Thus, the second moment of primary seduction entails both translation proper – through which the phantasmatic ego (*das Ich*) emerges as an "agency" during the "period of primary narcissism" (Laplanche 1989, 134) – *and* primal repression, which produces de-signified, fragmented remains. The unconscious on Laplanche's account is thus comprised of the "waste products" of translation (1999a, 89). He calls these the "source-objects" of the drive, because what is at issue now is an internalized, foreign object, a de-signified representation or "thing-presentation" that acts as a force *on* the ego (from where it least expects it, from within). This is the force that will henceforth compel the ego to contain itself by continuing to undertake the theorization through which it is preserved (see Laplanche 1992, 71, 73).

Above all, the internalized remnants that constitute this force are fragmentary scenes, memories, fantasies, imaginings and "imagos" (2004, 465; 1997, 658; 1999a, 120). These representations, which are sexual in nature, make up "what is called the id" (1999a, 129). Their constitution marks the moment at which the trauma of the primal seduction has been internalized and has become auto-traumatizing. For what distinguishes mental from physical trauma, Laplanche says, is "the fact that psychical trauma comes from within," from a kind of "*internal-external* instance" that has been formed: a "spine in the flesh" (1976, 42; emphasis his). As he writes elsewhere, "The 'drive' is to the ego what pain is to the body," insofar as "the source-object of the drive is 'stuck' in the envelope of the ego like a splinter in the skin" (1999a, 209, 129; compare 1997, 662).

The moment of introjection thus constitutes *afterwards* both the primal (sexual) unconscious and the libidinally-cathected ('primarily' narcissistic, sexual) ego. Or, to put this differently, the 'primary' becomes primary "*from the moment when an unconscious comes to exist*" (1999a, 69, nt. 33), and its (the id's) existence is the product of the living being's immediate efforts to define itself against an "excess" of message. One must hold to a set of apparently contradictory claims, as Laplanche says: "the relation to the world comes first" and yet, nonetheless, the "internal world comes first." "The real object is lost and the sexual fantasy originates in this loss" and yet, nonetheless, the "fantasy-object" is "only some unrecognizably remote derivative of the primary object of attachment" (1981, 84; compare Laplanche 1976, 42–3). The contradiction is explicable once we understand that what was outside *will have been* metabolized, changed, translated and incorporated such that it is *no longer* what it was (the simultaneously and enigmatically exciting and nourishing breast, for example, or the interplay of bodily images). What is 'inside' now appears *as if* it were first (as *my* cathected object, *my* primal fantasy, or *my* ego), as if having been 'there' all along. In each case the second moment, the moment of introjection, retroactively revivifies, reinterprets and simultaneously represses the first.

"Afterwardsness" is thus implicated in primal repression in this specific sense: it is only 'afterwards', when at the second moment an attempt to translate has already been undertaken, that we can speak of "primary narcissism" *or* primal repression. As in Freud's theory of seduction, the trauma is temporally indeterminable; the ego and its (the *id*'s) repressed remains are temporally staggered in a discontinuous, retroactive staging. Just as the body-ego is temporally prior but psychologically subsequent to the ego-as-agency, so the exogenous sources of sexual fantasy are *temporally* prior to the formation of an unconscious system (and an ego) but, as source-objects, *psychologically* subsequent to their metabolization. The 'source-objects' of the drive are endogenous *after* the fact, because they will be – they are retroactively 'always already' – primary for the individual.

Once it has *become* primary, moreover, this unconscious force will continue to drive the ego to translate, and its work will be *imperative*. What characterizes a categorical imperative, Laplanche explains, is that it "contains no *if* clause. It states, 'You must do this, full stop'" (1989, 138). The obligation to translate is "categorical" in just this sense: "you must translate because it's untranslatable" (1992, 204). The point is particularly pertinent with respect to the superego, as we shall see, but it also applies more generally to the way in which the ego is compulsively driven to bind itself through the theoretical work of translation. The drive (*Trieb*) of the message itself "demands translation" (1995, 679), and it continues to do so after it has been metabolized and repressed. This is why there is always a tendency "to recompose a unity, to re-translate, to recast a synthetic vision of [oneself] and [one's] future" (1992, 171). The ego-*drive*, in short, is the drive to preserve oneself (one's self) through the repetitive, compulsive enactment of its own, ongoing and largely unconscious, defence (Laplanche and Pontalis 1973, 139; Laplanche 1999b, 137).

This imperative drive (to translate) gives rise to an intellectual construction (a theory), however rudimentary, of the ego as a total (autonomous and complete) object. In particular, the ego is conceived both as the agent *that* theorizes (*the* 'I'), and as the object *of* that theorization ('me,' or the whole individual). And, if there is a tendency to unify and to bind right from the start, then there also is instantiated right from the start a drive that can ultimately take form – at a much higher level of formality and abstraction, of course – as the principle of reason. The ego (will have been) constituted in its autonomy, in other words, insofar as it is a *complete* or total object (1981, 85) that is the agent of its own activities. And it (will have been) constituted as logically coherent (*non-contradictory*) insofar the elements and fragments of sexual fantasy that have been implanted on its body as excitations, but which cannot be systematically incorporated into the story of itself, will have been repressed.

As Laplanche says, "The internal aggressor is *not* the external, and afterwards the internalized, aggressor: it is aggressive and anxiety-producing *because* it is internal and because, as Freud puts it, it attacks the ego where the latter doesn't expect it" (1981, 84–5). For the contents of the id are the chaotic, unbound fragments of represented (symbolized) affect. This unbound energy threatens the ego by its very nature, since it can always overwhelm the ego's relatively fragile, synthetic work, by virtue of which it has become a phantasmatic representation of what the organism *is*. What is at issue for the ego, therefore, is nothing less than its life. One does not confront the objective danger of death, Laplanche says, but rather the subjective danger of annihilation, of being "fragmented by the attack of the drive" (1999b, 208). For the ego, dissolution *means* its death. What is at issue is precisely life and death, in short, but at a *meta-psychological*, not a biological level. The ego is bound, and compulsively so, by the laws of its narrativization, and it must (imperatively) defend itself against the unbound lawlessness of its fragmentary remains. However, this primal imperative to cohere in a complete and non-contradictory way only takes on *moral* colour in conjunction with the secondary repressions.

"Secondary" repression, *afterwards*

Let us examine more closely, therefore, the relationship between so-called "primal repression" and the subsequent (nominally "secondary") repressions, which Laplanche calls "repression in the true sense" (1989, 133). Most importantly, "afterwardsness" (*après-coup*) "intervenes in primal repression itself." Specifically, "secondary repression is needed" to 'seal' primary repression "if it is to be maintained" (1989, 136). This somewhat cryptic claim becomes a bit clearer once we recognize that the process of primal repression is no more than an elementary "attempt to bind something that isn't bound" (1992, 74). In order to be consolidated, therefore, "there needs to be a counter-investment (Strachey's 'counter-cathexis') – that is, something which keeps in place that which ceaselessly seeks to rise up again" (1999b, 71). It is only with what Freud called "after pressure," in other words, that primal repression can be sustained, and it is only such "after pressure" that constitutes "repression in the true sense."

Specifically, the source-objects of the drive – which are, essentially, forces of unbound sexual energy – produce anxiety (that is, they *affect* the body and the ego); consequently, the (now) *auto*-traumatic reminiscence will provoke further translations and repressions. As Dominique Scarfone helpfully explains:

> Intransitive primal repression, rightly so called, will be the founding act, displacing the line of defence against excitation, from the frontier with the external world (in relation to the enigmatic signifier) towards the internal frontier, which is thereby established as such. Secondary repression will be charged with reinforcing that line of defence against the *other thing*, henceforth installed in the interior: that external-internal *other*, that Laplanche calls the source-object of the drive. (1994, 71)

Indeed, it is only by virtue of the symptoms of counter-investments and defences that primal repression can be ascertained (1999b, 63) – as a "trace" *afterwards* – since it is not directly accessible to consciousness. This is why "secondary" repression, too, will have come "first."

The concept of "after-pressure" is particularly salient here. Laplanche identifies "obsessional 'character' formations" as among its "best illustrations" (1999b, 63), and this is important, because what is at issue is the way in which the ego itself can become a symptom, precisely as a counter-investment, as it were, of the id's repressed and unmasterable contents. First of all, we know that the mark of the unconscious is the "compulsive character" of the behaviour (Laplanche and Pontalis 1973, 79) and that, as Freud has emphasized, repression is necessary for compulsive force (Laplanche 1995, 677; compare Freud 1939, 101). Second, the ego's defensive strategies against the onslaught of the drive indicated to Freud that there is "something in the ego itself which is also unconscious," not merely in the sense that the subject is unaware of them, but in that "they present a compulsive, repetitive and unrealistic aspect" (Laplanche and Pontalis 1973, 138–9). Thus, the resistance of the ego is not only a sign that repression has taken place; these defences are themselves "comparable to the very repressed against which they are struggling" (Laplanche and Pontalis 1973, 139). Indeed, Freud argued that, in repression, the ego itself "begins to function in the mode of 'all or nothing,' according to the model of total discharge, which is precisely that of unconscious fantasy or the primary process" (Laplanche 1999b, 137). These largely *unconscious* ego defences are, thus, the means of the 'secondary' repressions, and they suggest that the ego itself has become a symptom of repression.

What is most interesting about secondary processes of repression, in other words, is that they re-translate the ego in a particular (and in a particularly "originary") way. For in order to bind the anxiety that is now coming from within – the experience of an indeterminate, subjective danger that cannot be represented – the individual will attempt to attach it to an objective representation that can be "isolated and mastered" (1999a, 105–6). Thus, anxiety will often be 'fixed' to (or fixated on) an "anxiety occasioned by the real," as Laplanche puts it (1989, 167, nt. 17) – here using the term ("real") in its everyday, not its Lacanian, sense. For example, the infant may well bind its subjective anxiety to the objective fear of a loss of love, as I explained earlier, because the loss of love represents to the infantile ego a threat to its (phantasmatic) "life." In other words, an *objective* threat of the loss of parental love may represent the infant's *subjective* danger (the danger that the ego will be annihilated by the attack of the drive). If so, however, then we can see why the self-preservative ego-drive that impels the melancholic identification Freud described – the process he associates with the acquisition of morality at an oedipal stage – is actually imperative. The process of melancholic (gender) identification (that instantiates the superego) does bear directly on the issue of conscience, in other words, but Laplanchean theory allows us to explain it more plausibly.

For Laplanche, moral imperatives are a consequence of what he calls "intromission," which is a violent form of implantation. In particular, Laplanche understands moral imperatives as unworked, unmetabolized "chunks" of messages that remain "enclaved" in the psyche. He writes, "the superego will be immediately connected to verbal traces, the traces of the parental 'word'" (1999a, 247; compare 1992, 12). These are messages that not only have not been translated yet, but that cannot be translated at all, because they have been imposed violently, in a such a way that translation is blocked or prohibited (1999a, 136). This is what Laplanche understands as a categorical imperative: it "is untranslatable into anything other than itself, being impossible to metabolize: 'you must because you must'" (2011, 211).

The parallel Freud draws in *Totem and Taboo* between morality and taboo is telling in this regard. For Freud describes the taboo as, in Laplanche's words, "a closed space" – something "that looks a little like a collective psychotic enclave" (1992, 36). Such enclaves can result in particular, Laplanche says, "from an intergenerational transmission" (2011, 211). This occurs most regularly, one imagines, with respect to cultural taboos, norms and prohibitions regarding homosexuality and gender nonconformity, given that these are so pervasive cross-culturally and transhistorically. If such messages are conveyed violently (as is often the case), and if they are therefore walled off from any interrogative or translational work, then "verbal traces" of these parental words would remain "trapped between the two stages [i.e., implantation and translation] of primal repression" (1989, 139). They would be "untranslatable into anything other than [themselves]" (2011, 211).

In short, the indeterminable excitations that infants experience, which are variously translatable and untranslatable, will in the first place be "soldered" to a particular representation (1999b, 19) such as the fear of loss of love, just as the enigmatic message of gender may be soldered to the phallic logic of absence/presence. For there is no question that taboos surrounding sexuality and gender impose enormous pressure on children to take on their identities in a socially appropriate way. This imposition may well impel the child to adopt, in the second place and for its own preservation, the great cultural narratives concerning kinship and family structure that are immediately available and particularly privileged. The child will do so by incorporating these schemas into its own narrative of itself, thereby mastering the *subjective* anxiety it is experiencing and, at the same time, safeguarding itself from the perceived *objective* threat of parental disapprobation or harm. The child's renunciation of same-sex attachments as per the taboo of homosexuality, and its melancholic identification with an appropriate gender role, serve both of these (ultimately narcissistic) purposes at once.

Something like an Oedipus complex is therefore likely to play a central role in the development of a moral conscience for many individuals at a given historical time and within a given cultural context. The "pseudo-unconscious of the mythic-symbolic" (1999a, 164, nt. 23) is one way, as Laplanche says, for the individual to synthesize "*his* existence *for himself*: approximately but also compulsively" for the purpose of warding off anxiety (1999a, 161; emphasis his). But this particular narrative is neither a necessary nor a deciding factor in the development of moral conscience. On the contrary, the so-called "law of the father" is merely as a "privileged system of self-theorization" (1999a, 164, nt. 23), not an intrinsic (or endogenous) feature of the unconscious; it is just one way that morality can take shape.[7] Consequently, one ought to separate the "form" of the ego from its substance, that is, from its particular and contingent "character."

With respect to its form, we have seen, the ego initially develops by virtue of an originary process of translation–repression. This development is the consequence of an imperative (a self-preservative imperative) *to* cohere that was impelled by exciting, enigmatic messages that have been implanted by (concrete) others, adults, who care for the child. The response to these messages is the staged process of "Ptolemization" or centring of itself, whereby the ego gradually takes shape as a coherent and agential whole that represents the individual as a subject. The "character" of the ego, on the other hand, continues to evolve later, during what Freud called the oedipal period, but what might be better characterized as the period during which social norms concerning sexuality and gender (whichever they may be) are taken on. This is when the child internalizes and makes his or her own the specific protocols *of* its egoic coherence.

For, by the time children are approximately 4 or 5 years old, when they are already beset by the attacks (the anxiety-producing effects) of internalized "source-objects," the impact of social prohibitions and norms will also have begun to make themselves felt (see Laplanche 1976, 45). This is likely why, as Freud theorized, a crisis manifests itself at this point. It is the moment at which children understand (inchoately), for example, that they must sacrifice an erotic cathexis of an adult caretaker of the same sex (since this is taboo in any cultural milieu in which heterosexuality is strictly enforced) as well as their feelings of hostility towards adults perceived as sexual rivals. These potential conflicts must ultimately be overcome if the child is to avoid the danger that its parents (or caretakers) will withdraw their love in response to its unacceptable sexuality or gender identification.[8]

This later stage inaugurates the *secondary* processes of repression, because it is only by virtue of the formation of anti-cathexes that the developing ego can be consolidated and enforced as an adequate defence. Moral codes, social taboos, gender and sexuality regulations and, notably, the protocols of communicative reason (to borrow Habermas's phrase) of one's culture provide the means for that consolidation. The process results in a fully-formed, Ptolemic self-representation, the character of which is (now) socially recognizable. It is only at the secondary stage of later repressions, therefore, that there will have emerged an ego that is compelled to cohere in a *particular way* that corresponds with social norms and values.

For Freud, of course, this moment represents the resolution of the Oedipus conflict, the instantiation of the superego, and thus the inauguration of "conscience." We can leave aside the claim (with which I dealt in the previous chapter) that the "preponderance" of specific sexual "dispositions" determines the final nature of the sexual drive in male and female children alike. Instead, let us just underline this:

> The broad general outcome of the sexual phase dominated by the Oedipus complex may, therefore, be taken to be the forming of a precipitate in the ego, consisting of these two identifications [paternal and maternal] in some way united with each other. This modification of the ego retains its special position; it confronts the other contents of the ego as an ego ideal or super-ego. (1923, 34, emphasis omitted)

In other words, the result of the identification with an ego ideal is nothing less than an alteration of the ego itself. Importantly, then, this is a process whereby the ego – driven as it is by a categorical imperative to translate that is (constantly) impelled by the source-objects of the id – will draw on the character of the sacrificed (parental) object to theorize *for* itself a new 'translation' *of* itself. The individual thereby gains a self-regulating, critical faculty (a "conscience") that was not there before, and that in a certain way stands *against* his or her self-representation. A new representation or phantasmatic-object, the ego *ideal*, is now juxtaposed against the 'original' representation (the ideal *ego*), and the phantasmatic ego is transformed as a result.

This is why, as I said earlier, secondary repressions are associated with reaction-formations. For Freud, specifically, "the erection of the superego" is the same thing as "the formation of a conscience" (1930, 128), and conscience is manifest in a number of new character traits. There emerges on the one hand, conscientiousness (for example), which is a reaction-formation in the ego, and on the other hand, a "fear of conscience" (1923, 57), which is the anxiety provoked by the superego in its capacity as judge. The implication here is thus that "conscience" *is* a reaction-formation; it is the way the ego defends against anxiety stemming from the id, and it is maintained with the unconscious force of compulsion.

The processes of "secondary" repression thus serve a series of interrelated purposes. In the first place, they consolidate the primary translation–repression. Second, they rewrite the individual's narrative of itself and thereby re-translate the story of the ego into its later, *conscientious* form. And third, they transform the categorical imperative *to* translate (which produced the ego as a phantasmatic, formal entity) into a *moral* imperative (that is, into an imperative that shapes the ego's "character"). Significantly, this means that secondary repression results in the imperative *to translate in a particular way*, one that is indisputably culturally and historically specific. For the "momentous objects" that the superego has "introduced into the ego" (1923, 48) cannot be anything other than the protocols of reason and the norms governing sexuality and gender through which the individual can make him or herself recognizable (or 'readable') as a subject, that is, as coherent (non-contradictory) and unified (complete) self. These protocols will now be imbued with morality.

What ensues from the resolution of the crisis, in short, is the transformation of the self-preservative drive to cohere *into* a moral injunction to cohere 'as such.' Subsequent to the resolution of the crisis, one is compelled to cohere by way of a specific set of protocols that concern both the logical form (the principle of reason, the Law of the Father, the imperative of 'castration' with its "phallic logic" as an interpretive schema, and so on), *and* the behavioural characteristics (gender norms, social prohibitions, and so on) of the ego.

We can see quite clearly, therefore, the way in which the principle of reason takes psychological root in the human mind. For although the drive to unify and to bind is instantiated right from the start of human consciousness, according to Laplanche, this tendency will not have given rise to a fully logical, non-contradictory account of oneself while the child is still an infant. What distinguishes the secondary repressions, however, is that they are provoked when categorical choices (in both senses) must be made. With the aid of the formal resources of logic, language and communicational norms, as well as the "great narrative schemas" provided by the cultural milieu, these infantile ego-representations will subsequently be refined or even radically rewritten in accordance with the social structures that underlie individuals' subjective possibilities. In particular, the dictates of Aristotelian logic, which have governed communicational norms in the Western world (at least) for over 2000 years, will at this stage begin to be internalized, and to be brought to bear on the self-preservative impulse itself.

How each individual takes on (or in) each of these protocols is, of course, open to infinite variation. For instance, as Freud specifies, identification may involve the imitation of a person who is loved or a person who is not loved, and one may take on only a particular trait or the entirety of the other person's character (1921, 107). The possibilities and permutations of (gendered) character development are far too numerous and too varied to itemize, and in any case such an elaboration would require additional anthropological and sociological support. The point is merely that there is a relationship between an originary "drive to translate" (oneself) and a secondary imperative to translate (oneself) according to pre-given protocols and norms. For, regardless of one's anatomical sex, it is nonetheless imperative that one coheres as a subject (as a logical entity, an "I") more or less "completely," and in a more or less "non-contradictory," autonomous way. This imperative is indeed "categorical" for every modern subject (at the very least), regardless of the particular social and ethical norms that are in place. And, to the extent that the psychical demands of rational coherence are met, it is indeed possible to say that responsibility in its customary sense – namely, as a 'response-ability' to the law of reason – obtains.

Precisely because the secondary repressions will overwrite the primary binding of the ego, however, the imperative to bind and the norms though which it is undertaken will (have) be(come) inseparable. In other words, after the secondary repressions, the phantasms that were produced in conjunction with primal repression (namely, those concerning the ego and its ideal) will no longer be distinguishable from the social norms *through which* they will have been (*après-coup*) re-elaborated. As Laplanche was to clarify years later,

> What Freud designates on occasion as "primal repression" is nothing other than the result of what can legitimately be called the proto-historization of the human being: his manner of auto-theorizing from the start, of responding to what I designate as "enigmatic signifiers" with a world view, and thereby entering into time by means of translation, which is at once a taking oneself forward and a leaving behind. Soon the new translations will cover up this archaic to-be-translated. The succession of developmental stages, infinitely more complex than the tenets of the manuals of psychoanalysis would have it, is finally only this movement of detranslation-retranslation of an "originary" (an adult originary, then the originary of the individual unconscious), according to the available idioms: the "languages" of orality, anality, genitality, etc. (1992, 176)

This retroactive effect (*après-coup*), I submit, results in the experience of the ego as an *origin*, a "me" that was "there" all along. Not only will the subject have become an origin *afterwards*, but the imperative to render reason will impose itself categorically, and in a commanding way, as if it were of "divine origin" (1933, 61). Moreover, it will be mixed with the original ideal of a complete form that was introjected at a much earlier stage. And this transformed entity, I submit, will now be (for modern, Western subjects) the "I" that not only accounts for itself, but that does so imperatively, relentlessly rendering reason, and ceaselessly seeking its ground.

*

A notable virtue of Laplanche's theory is that it illuminates the historically and politically contingent forces that shape gender and sexuality. In my view, Laplanche's description of a fundamental anthropological (adult–infant) situation and his related "general theory of seduction" account for the origin of infantile sexuality in a highly plausible way. The theory as a whole is therefore a decided advance over Freud's, which is grounded on phylogenetically-transmitted primal fantasies and the "fact" of female castration, among other controversial assumptions. More importantly for my argument here, however, Laplanche also illuminates the paradoxical truth behind Freud's contradictory accounts of ego development. In so doing, he allows us to see what might be subjectively compelling and apparently normative about the critical need to deconstruct.

Specifically, I have shown how the retroactive logic of *Nachträglichkeit* applies to the two Freudian theses, namely, that narcissistic self-enclosure (autonomy) and melancholic introjection (heteronomy) *both* mark the "origin" of the ego. These statements, which signal an aporetic subject when taken together, are arguably both correct. For, although heteronymous identification – identification with the form of another person as expressed by the linguistic concept "I" – does enable the semblance of egoic coherence first *chronologically*, the narcissistic phantasm of self-enclosed autonomy will always be "first" *psychologically*. This is because whatever came before the instantiation of a rudimentary ego *will have been* (afterwards) repressed. We have also seen that, at the "primary" stage of translation–repression, the rudimentary egoic form (a form of bound, sexual energy) serves as a kind of ballast against the enigmatic, traumatic, adult "noise" that breaks in on the infant's skin. The ego is said in this sense to 'take over' the instinct of self-preservation, and thus to be associated with a drive (*Trieb*) to preserve oneself.

Insofar as *I* am driven *as* a subject to preserve myself, what is at stake is the ego's unity and form, since the "life" at issue is phantasmatic. So, there is already in play a drive that appears as a demand for completeness and non-contradiction. This basic compulsion to cohere logically will be imbued with and overwritten by a moral quality, however, at a subsequent stage of "secondary" repressions. This is when the child confronts the new and more profound danger of parental condemnation associated with the risk of failing to conform to socially-imperative norms, and when it resolves that conflict through the production of the reaction-formation that appears as moral "conscience." On one hand, the subject will always *already* have depended on another person (an other), and so the need to account for itself and thereby to complete itself in a non-contradictory way can never be satisfied. On the other hand, the subject so constituted will be continually driven to try. This is the subject, in a nutshell, for whom the principle of reason *matters* and for whom, consequently, responsibility demands critique.

There is, of course, no ultimate basis on which to insist that subjectivity must be constituted in the way that Laplanche, following Freud, describes (that is, beyond the basic adult–infant relationship that grounds the anthropological thesis) or that egos, so understood, always have been or perpetually will be reproduced in this way. Thus, the Laplanchian version of how subjects are constituted does not provide a universal explanation of the desire for reason either. Nonetheless, Laplanche's reformulation of Freudian psychoanalysis does illuminate the drive manifest in Western philosophy to answer to reason's imperatives. This subjective exigency cannot be generalized or ultimately justified, because subjective formation is necessarily culturally contingent; as we have seen, the protocols of subjective coherence are historically and socially variable. For this reason, the imperatives that drive subjectivity today are only seemingly stable and only relatively sedimented or fixed. But what I have characterized as a 'desire for reason' is clearly manifest in theoretical work today. It is therefore evident that this subject does obtain now, at least insofar as we (theorists) do experience ourselves as unified "selves," that is, as subjectively constituted through a subjection to the demands of unity and logical coherence. To this extent, not more but not less, the responsibility to deconstruct is imperative. Critical analysis is interminable, as Derrida says, but this is also why the chance of thinking remains.

Notes

1 Derrida has questioned the continuing relevance of the "ego," the "id" and the other major Freudian categories (Derrida and Roudinesco 2004, 172). Once loosened from the Freudian edifice in which they are lodged, however, these terms are invaluable indices. The term "ego" provides an indispensable way of talking about the basic image all individuals seem to have of themselves as more or less self-directing, closed, agential entities. It is the fact of this phenomenon, rather than the term that announces it, that matters here. "Id," similarly, is an index of the non-rational or irrational forces that seem so often to inform individuals' motivations and actions. Insofar as these forces are never fully amenable to one's *own* (to *egoic*), conscious reconstruction, they are 'it-like' within one. The "superego" can likewise be seen as an index of the way in which moral responsibility (however conceived) is experienced as subjectively compelling and, conversely, of why the failure to honour the prevalent norms is generally discomfiting. The deconstruction to which I have subjected Freudian metapsychology does not obviate the usefulness of his terms or validate their rejection, therefore, any more than to deconstruct the subject means to deny its existence.

2 Laplanche calls this "*le sexual*," using the German word instead of the French one (*le sexuel*) to specify that he means unconscious, infantile sexuality, not human sexual behaviour or sexual preference in general (see Sauvayre 2017, esp. 130–31).

3 Laplanche thus reformulates the Freudian distinction between the "life drive" and the "death drive" in terms of a difference between a (vital) "principle of binding" (the secondary process), which constitutes the "sexual life drive" and a "principle of unbinding" (the primary process), which he refers to as "the sexual death drive." The conflict at issue is thus not between the metaphysical forces of "life" and "death," but rather between the binding undertaken by the narcissistically-cathected ego, through which the self-preservative interests are represented and supported, on the one hand, and the forces of "unbound sexuality" that constitute the unconscious, on the other (2004, 465, 466).

4 As Dominique Scarfone underscores, the child's "passivity pertains strictly to the sexual domain; in every other aspect, the child is seen as active by Laplanche" (personal correspondence, February 11, 2015).

5 In Laplanche's view, "sublimation" is not a separate process, but simply "the normal process of acculturation by which the ego attempts to drain the Zuyderzee of the id, partly transposing death drives into life drives" (2015, 269–70). He continues, "this progression of Eros, principally by way of symbolization, is hard to distinguish from sublimation. It is sublimation itself: the integration of anarchic sexual aims into a 'socially valued' perspective" (2015, 270). These passages suggest that for Laplanche "sublimation" is essentially the process of "translating" the anarchic sexual "messages" that have been implanted from without. John Fletcher provides a similar view (2007, 1257).

6 Laplanche explains that language is secondary historically (it succeeds the preverbal stage in every individual and perhaps also in human civilization), topographically (it succeeds a state without the unconscious [1999b, 64], that is, the pre-egoic, pre-split stage of infantile development), and economically (it succeeds the circulation without end that would render meaning impossible [1989, 42]).

7 Laplanche refers to the intriguing case of the Na of China, for example, which has no concept of paternity or of a "paternal function" (in the Lacanian sense) at all, even though the mechanism of reproduction is understood. (2011, 152; see also Blake 2003).

8 The opposite-sex identifications entailed in some (but not all) cases of homosexual desire and in cases of transsexual identity 'resolve' these psychical conflicts as well, but they are presumably more complicated, given the more nuanced ways in which non-conforming individuals have to negotiate between immediate familial messages, broader social and cultural expectations, and their own psychical needs.

Conclusion

The Risk of a Certain Critique

> Thanks to the impulse of the initial Freudian send-off [*coup d'envoi*], one can, for example, renew the question of responsibility; in place of a subject conscious of himself, answering for himself in a sovereign manner before the law, one can introduce the idea of a divided, differentiated "subject" who cannot be reduced to a conscious, egological intentionality. And the idea of a "subject" installing, progressively, laboriously, always imperfectly, the *stabilized* – that is, non-natural, essentially and always *unstable* – conditions of his or her autonomy: against the inexhaustible and invincible background of heteronomy.
>
> (Derrida and Roudinesco 2004, 176)

Laplanche's reconstruction of Freudian thought allows us to discern why, for Western modern individuals (at least), reason always already *matters*. The theory thus illuminates the way in which the hyperbolic fidelity to reason that characterizes deconstruction (the radically *critical* move of turning reason back upon itself) will qualify as quasi-ethical, that is, as "normative" in a certain sense. Specifically, one can extrapolate from Laplanche's theory, first, an understanding of how the concrete individual, situated historically in the context of Western modernity, is *driven* (unconsciously, and only more or less) to preserve itself as a complete and non-contradictory egoic whole. One can also extrapolate, second, how this need for logical coherence, the imperative to assert the primacy of the "I" by denying constitutive heteronomous forces, comes to be associated with moral responsibility. Laplanche's account of how the effects of subjectivity obtain thereby clarifies what I am calling the "quasi-responsibility" that underlies deconstructive vigilance. This psychoanalytic account allows us to see, in other words, why deconstruction is peculiarly "normative," even if it does not entail a prescription for political action, and even if it cannot be rationally (or otherwise) alibied.

The argument I have presented is essentially that, in response to an unconscious drive to cohere, the infant draws on (among others) the principles of completeness and non-contradiction that are conveyed by adults through linguistic and para-linguistic messages. The principle of reason is present in rudimentary form to begin with, in other words, because it serves the self-preservative function of an "aid to translation." The fundaments of reason are subsequently imbued with moral value, however, when the small child has to deal with conflicts between its own (narcissistic) needs and desires, and external prohibitions and norms. Insofar as these conflicts are resolved through processes of identification with external social roles and values, the child's sense of itself as a "self" or an ego is fundamentally changed. This is when the convergence of the ego (an ideal *ego*) and the identification with gender (with an ego *ideal*) is entrenched and revivified as a moral imperative. As one's self-representation, the ego becomes, as it were, a reaction-formation insofar as one develops a "conscience"; this is, afterwards, a symptom of (secondary) repressions, to which compulsive impulses are attached. These ever-present impulses, which compel one to assert oneself as an autonomous "self" against the threat of fragmentation, continue to serve self-preservation, I contend, because what is at stake is the maintenance of the ego *as* a coherent form. But the compulsion to cohere appears as a moral injunction, because it *will have been* (*après-coup*) caught up with, and overwritten by, the existing moral codes and socially-regulatory norms through which subjects are recognized.

This account of "the problematic of [self-] consciousness" (Gasché 2016, 70, cited above) fills a lacuna in Derrida's oeuvre. It allows one to see – without recourse to religion or metaphysics – not only what compels the radical critique of reason that characterizes deconstruction, but also why that impulse might seem to bear transcendental, a priori, or messianic force. Specifically, a fidelity to the protocols and principles of critique – or, as Derrida puts it, an acknowledgement of "the spirit of Enlightenment that must not be renounced" (1994, 88, cited above) – appears to manifest responsibility, because in order to establish one's standing as a freely acting subject, one has to be able to account for oneself. To be a "responsible" subject, in other words, is to "render reason" (for oneself) by completing or systematizing one's narrative of oneself, and this also means dealing, in some way, with any differences or inconsistencies that can potentially undermine it. And yet, because the *cause* of this imperative is logically indeterminable and unavailable to consciousness (it comes from "one knows not where"), the demand for reason becomes (again, *après-coup*) that for which no reason can or need be given. This is why, I aver, when one moves from the level of individual psychology to the level of formal philosophy, whereby one seeks to establish logical conditions of possibility as grounds, the nature of so-called "critical responsibility" seems to be self-evident. Indeed, we have seen, the search for epistemological grounds, *notwithstanding* their impossibility, is what philosophical responsibility has meant all along.

As I have argued, a rigorous deconstructive analysis exemplifies this understanding of responsibility. It does so by showing that the epistemological grounds of ethical–political claims cannot be logically established without an unwarranted appeal to a transcendental essence and, thus, not without obfuscating the specific political interests they entail. This is the *political* point that was missed during the original "modernism–postmodernism" debate, and it is why it was necessary to revisit it. What is political about deconstruction, I have argued, is that it discloses the irreducible violence that inheres in every moral claim, edict or law. This is why one can find evidence throughout Derrida's oeuvre, as Michael Naas asserts, of an "overwhelming orientation … toward the deconstruction of all kinds of religious and metaphysical dogmatisms, chauvinisms, racisms, and so on" (2009, 64). It is not because deconstruction advocates a moral principle of *différance* or because it provides a philosophical justification for some sort of ethical hospitality to those who are radically other. It is because deconstruction radicalizes the critical philosophical imperative to provide grounds, or the ethical–legal imperative to seek justice, by submitting those very spheres to their own normative presuppositions. Contrary to critical and political theorists who continue to rail against what they mistakenly characterize as a "literary" or relativist approach to politics, therefore, there is nothing nihilistic, irresponsible or destructive about deconstruction at all. Deconstruction simply enacts the most vigilant response that is possible to the demand, whether ethical, political or critical, that already *has* been or *is* being affirmed.

After demonstrating how deconstructive reading radicalizes the protocols of critique, therefore, and after investigating the consequences of this for emancipatory political thought, I have interrogated the nature and source of the affirmation that underlies it. In particular, I have attempted to "renew the question of responsibility," as Derrida puts it in the epigraph above, by investigating what might give rise in an aporetic subject to its enigmatic desire for vigilance, given that this is a "'subject' who cannot be reduced to a conscious, egological intentionality." What emerges from my investigation is a psychoanalytic explanation of an unconscious drive (*Trieb*) to honour the principle of reason. This leads by extension to an understanding of deconstruction as normative in a *certain* way (as quasi-responsible). Specifically, deconstruction emerges as quasi-responsible solely insofar as it entails a *hyperbolically*-responsible interrogation of responsibility, not because it produces any prescriptions. As I have shown, deconstruction cannot establish what we ought (legitimately) to do and, indeed, any political theory that tries to do so will, by virtue of that fact, have already repudiated the critical impulse behind it for the sake of its political end. A rigorous deconstructive analysis, therefore, cannot satisfy the political need for a standard of judgement by virtue of which the "ought" can be determined. It can only enact the unconditional injunction – that is, what appears to be and is accepted as an unconditional – to practise the lucid vigilance of critique.

This separation between normativity and prescription has implications for the field of Derrida Studies directly, as well as for emancipatory theories of education and politics more broadly. With respect to the field of Derrida Studies, for example, the separation between normativity and prescription suggests that current discussions about the so-called "ethics" of deconstruction somewhat miss the point. On one hand, for example, the consequence of my analysis is that it is correct to say, as Martin Hägglund does, that "no *prescriptions* can be derived from the logic of deconstruction" (2008, 203; emphasis added). On the other hand, however, it does not follow from this that no "intrinsic *normativity*" can be associated with deconstruction at all (2008, 232 nt.4; emphasis added).

To be sure, it is widely assumed that if a critical theory is to go beyond mere description, its fundamental task will be to establish norms with which contemporary conditions can be judged. Hägglund's "radically atheistic" intervention into debates about Derrida's thought is therefore important, because it contests both positive and negative theological readings of Derrida as well as secular interpretations of deconstructive normativity. Against Matthias Fritsch for example – who has developed an intergenerational, environmentally-conscious conception of justice based on deconstruction (2002, 2015, 2018) – Hägglund argues that deconstruction cannot provide a normative justification for political action. Hägglund's argument concerning the strictly logical character of deconstruction is compelling, but it also overstates the case; he mistakenly assumes that the critical interrogation of grounds and the political determination of norms *are the same thing*. This was the error in Simon Critchley's approach to the ethics of deconstruction originally (1992), and it appears to have set the stage for reiterations of the same error today. As I have tried to show, what is not adequately appreciated, yet, is that it is one thing to analyze the undecidability at the root of political decisions and norms, and it is quite another to try to establish them. This is why "explicit prescriptions" are indeed difficult to find in Derrida's oeuvre (Naas 2009, 64), but why a quasi-normative impulse, a *desire*, to deconstruct, can be found nonetheless.

Indeed, Naas implies, something like this, something more than mere logic, must be driving Hägglund's own analysis as well. Hägglund claims that his "project of radical atheism" is "not to convert anyone," but merely "to describe the exigencies that are at work whatever we do and however we live" (Hägglund 2009, 250). In this, as Naas says, Hägglund's strategy is similar to the "strategy of metaphysics itself," insofar as Hägglund is trying "to get behind the appearance of … absolutes or to the bottom of … claims to identity either to reveal their true nature or to clarify the conditions of their appearance" (Naas 2009, 50). The question that Naas poses, however, is why Hägglund would undertake to *make* the case for "radical atheism" if it is *already* the case is that "nothing … can ever be exempt from the movement of time" (Naas 2009, 48), and therefore that all we can really want is "radically atheist" to begin with. In other words, why deconstruct the metaphysics of theism and the phantasm of immortality it promises at all? Would not this project, too, evidence a hyperbolic responsibility? Would it not, too, manifest the same normative imperative to honour the principle of reason – the same (old) principle of reason rather than a "new" conception of it (Hägglund 2008, 24) – precisely because it entails questioning the condition of possibility *of* those normative claims, and this for the sake of exposing the phantasms that still populate our thought?

Normative the inquiry may be, therefore, but still it is not prescriptive. Of course, the injunction to be vigilant – which is to say, the injunction to engage in the "perpetual critique of absolutes" (Naas 2009, 63) – may be all that Naas has in mind when he identifies, consequently, a "minimal" deconstructive prescription (2009, 65). Nass's point, that Hägglund's work is a performative response to that very injunction, is exactly on the mark (2009, 65–6). To be clear, however, if this is a political imperative, it is fundamentally indeterminate, as Naas is certainly aware. It is not a criterion for decision, since it states no more than that one must respond to one's responsibilities, which means in this case only that one must affirm (as Hägglund obviously does) the *normative* necessity of critique. However, as soon as one seeks to establish a particular ethical or political value, one will have confused the critical *interrogation* of norms with their determination.

This is why one should approach with caution the suggestion that one should "attempt to cultivate cosmopolitanism's international spirit" (Naas 2008, 70), for example, or the endorsement of a particular way of inheriting democracy (Haddad 2013, esp. 67), the appeal to "a 'promise' of unconditional welcoming of the unknowable 'to come'" (Anderson 2012, 110), or the argument that animal vulnerability calls for "unconditional hospitality" and friendship (Lawlor 2007, 3, 8). For, no matter how minimally determined, qualified, ambiguous or uncertainly named those norms are, it remains that no determination can ever be made outside of a system of differences, as we have seen. This will apply to any foundational value, whether it is named "life" or "faith," whether it is positivist (as in speculative realism) or ethical (as in Levinasian thinking) (Colebrook 2011, 62), and whether it claims post-secular reason or precarious life (Butler 2004, 30) as the basis for a new intervention. Deconstruction is not purely logical, we have seen, but it is not *substantively* normative either. Thus, its peculiar quality of criticality will have to be formulated differently.

Specifically, I have argued that a qualified kind of normativity accompanies the deconstruction of the political categories that structure our lives. Deconstruction is not simply neutral, as Derrida once provocatively said, but intervenes (1981b, 93). It follows from this that deconstruction does constitute a certain form of ethical–political critique, and that it therefore has implications for emancipatory political thought in general. Most significantly, the critical–theoretical consequence of my analysis is that, rather than attempting to produce an alternative norm in, for example, post-metaphysical, post-secular or new materialist terms, the critical theorist can only undertake an unrelenting, vigilant interrogation of ethical–political norms that are already espoused. In other words, the point and the value of critical theory, on this view, is to reveal the politics of emancipatory thought itself, that is, to expose its hidden or unacknowledged stakes. This is what makes deconstruction "critical" in the radical sense I have described, and this, I submit, is what many recent scholars appear to overlook.

Also overlooked is the way in which deconstruction (so understood) can be situated in sympathetic relation to the critical theory tradition that was inaugurated by Frankfurt School thinkers, rather than as in contention with it. More specifically, we can see deconstruction as a continuation and advancement of Theodor Adorno's original and radical version of critical theory, before his insights were obscured by the second generation's Kantian and Hegelian (re)turns, such as those undertaken by Jürgen Habermas and Axel Honneth, among others (see Allen 2016). One might now explore, for example, the way in which Derrida and Adorno both radicalize critique in a similar way, and how in both cases the meaning of critique is informed by a psychoanalytic understanding of the relation between reason and the constitution of subjectivity in the context of late modernity. Most importantly, Derrida like Adorno turns the laser-like inquiry into conditions of possibility – that is, the traditional philosophical demand *for* grounds – *onto* the epistemological and ontological grounds of political norms themselves, thereby revealing, as I have said, their ethical and political stakes. In contrast to Adornian critical theory, however, the "negative" understanding of deconstruction as critique that I have developed here is based on a significantly revised and updated, Laplanchean understanding of Freudian psychoanalysis. This new understanding of the relationship between subjectivity and Enlightenment reason thus opens up a fascinating line of inquiry concerning affinities between Derrida and Adorno, which so far have gone unremarked.

If Enlightenment reason is subjected to the critical interrogation that deconstruction entails, of course, this will have important implications for an emancipatory project of education as well. Emancipatory educational theories, we have seen, stem from the Enlightenment ideal of critical consciousness, and this is based in turn on the determination of a standard of judgement by virtue of which the difference between justice and ideology can be known. In the absence of this standard, there is no criterion of judgement, and therefore the promised inculcation of criticality (so understood) cannot obtain. Conversely, however, any such standard will be subject to the "postmodern" challenge to modern legitimacy that I have described. This is why the logical grounds of a critical or radical theory of education cannot be discarded, but they cannot be justified by a theory of critical consciousness either.

Moreover, we have seen, the vulnerability to deconstruction does not pertain only to critical educational theories that explicitly rely on Kant. Rather, the significance of deconstruction in this context is that it undermines the ideological purity of *any* standard of critique, regardless of whether the criterion at issue is purportedly transcendental or not. This outcome is revealed when one examines how various alternatives to the Kantian value of "freedom" within the field of radical educational and pedagogical theory depend on the original Kantian link between ethics and epistemology that establishes moral legitimacy. In each case, I have argued, the alternative value can only be established through an ideological restriction of the subject to its ostensible essence (again, whether this restriction is explicitly acknowledged or not). In every instance, in short, the criterion of political judgement must be rationally determinable and normatively justified, or else it cannot be taught. And this is why, I have claimed, one must rethink the ends of education as well.

Specifically, just as a critical approach to society that takes the deconstructive radicalization of the principle of reason seriously will undertake to *expose* the politics of emancipatory thought, rather than to establish them, so by extension will a critical theory of education aim to instil a spirit of radical critique. In other words, on the view presented here a progressive or emancipatory approach to education is one which is committed to instilling resources for critical inquiry, not one which purports to teach the substance of what is morally right. For, no matter how "progressive" it seems, any determinate form of "critical consciousness" will have already closed the critical question, the question *of* grounds, because it will already have the political answer. And political answers, we have seen, are always intrinsically violent. A quasi-responsible approach to education as emancipation, therefore, will take the radical meaning of Enlightenment to heart: it will be based on the idea of reason as *self*-critique, rather than as the vehicle of moral or political truth.

To enact responsibility in this way, by undertaking the kind of critique that arises from an uncompromising interrogatory spirit, *would* be to intervene politically in the kinds of intractable problems that face us today. But it would be to do so in a way that is significantly different from how critical–theoretical interventions have been understood before. The point is not that political interventions are not urgently needed, but merely that they are always already political rather than critical in character. An emancipatory *critical* theory, in contrast, is one that will have to challenge what is claimed in the name of justice, notwithstanding the risk this always entails. It will have to do so without apology, without guarantee and without respite. This is what it means to deconstruct, and it is what it means to undertake a radical, ethical–political critique.

References

Adorno, Theodor. 1973. *Negative Dialectics.* Translated by E.B. Ashton. New York: The Continuum Publishing Company.

Allen, Amy. 2016. *The End of Progress: Decolonizing the Normative Foundations of Critical Theory.* New York: Columbia University Press.

Anderson, Nicole. 2012. *Derrida: Ethics Under Erasure.* London and New York: Continuum.

André, Jacques. 2011. "From Femininity to the Primitive Forms of Psychic Life." Translated by Alyson Bernard. *European Psychoanalytical Federation Bulletin* 65 (March 2012): 215–222.

Arcilla, René Vincente. 1995. "For the Stranger in My Home: Self-Knowledge, Cultural Recognition, and Philosophy of Education." In *Critical Conversations in Philosophy of Education*, edited Wendy Kohli, 159–172. New York and London: Routledge.

Arendt, Hannah. 1982. *Lectures on Kant's Political Philosophy.* Edited, with an interpretive essay by Ronald Beiner. Chicago: University of Chicago Press.

Aronowitz, Stanley. 1997. "A Different Perspective on Educational Inequality." In *Education and Cultural Studies: Toward a Performative Practice*, edited by Henry Giroux and Patrick Shannon, 179–196. New York and London: Routledge.

Aronowitz, Stanley and Giroux, Henry. 1991. *Postmodern Education: Politics, Culture, and Social Criticism.* Minneapolis: University of Minnesota Press.

Ball, Karyn. 2009. *Disciplining the Holocaust: Traumatic History as an Object of Inquiry and Desire.* Albany: State University of New York Press.

Beardsworth, Richard. 1996. *Derrida and the Political.* London and New York: Routledge.

Benhabib, Seyla. 1986. *Critique, Norm, and Utopia: A Study of the Foundations of Critical Theory.* New York: Columbia University Press.

Benhabib, Seyla. 1987. "The Generalized and the Concrete Other: The Kohlberg-Gilligan Controversy and Feminist Theory." In *Feminism as Critique: On the Politics of Gender*, edited by Seyla Benhabib and Drucilla Cornell, 77–95. Minneapolis: University of Minnesota Press.

Benhabib, Seyla. 1990. "Afterward: Communicative Ethics and Current Controversies in Practical Philosophy." In *The Communicative Ethics Controversy*, edited by Seyla Benhabib and Fred Dallmayr, 330–369. Cambridge, MA: The MIT Press.

Benhabib, Seyla. 1997. "On Reconciliation and Respect, Justice and the Good Life." *Philosophy & Social Criticism* 23, no. 5: 97–114.

Bennington, Geoffrey. 2016. "Embarrassing Ourselves." Review of the 40th Anniversary edition of *Of Grammatology*. *Los Angeles Review of Books*, March 20, 2016. https://lareviewofbooks.org/article/embarrassing-ourselves/

Bernard, Gaëlle. 2011. "On the 'Postmodern' Crisis of Legitimation and the Confusion of Reasons." Translated by Cadenza Academic Translations. https://www.cairn-int.info/article-E_CITE_045_0087–on-the-postmodern-crisis-of-legitimation.htm. First published as "Sur la crise 'postmoderne' de la légitimation et la confusion des raisons." *Cités* 1, no. 45(2011): 87–101.

Bernasconi, Robert. 1992. "No More Stories, Good or Bad: de Man's Criticisms of Derrida on Rousseau." In *Derrida: A Critical Reader*, edited by David Wood, 137–166. Oxford and Cambridge: Blackwell.

Bernasconi, Robert and Critchley, Simon, eds. 1991. *Re-Reading Levinas*. Bloomington and Indianapolis: Indiana University Press.

Berns, E.E. 1996. "Decision, Hegemony and Law: Derrida and Laclau." *Philosophy & Social Criticism* 22, no. 4: 71–80.

Billig, Michael. 2006. "Lacan's Misuse of Psychology: Evidence, Rhetoric and the Mirror Stage." *Theory, Culture & Society* 23, no. 4: 1–26,

Blake, Fred. 2003. "A Society Without Fathers or Husbands: The Na of China, by Hua Cha, Book Review." *China Review International* 10, no. 1: 103–106.

Blake, Nigel. 1996. "The Democracy We Need: Situation, Post-Foundationalism and Enlightenment." *Journal of Philosophy of Education* 30, no. 2: 215–238.

Blanchot, Maurice. 1988. *The Unavowable Community*. Translated by Pierre Joris. Barrytown, NY: Station Hill Press.

Borradori, Giovanna. 2003. *Philosophy in a Time of Terror: Dialogues with Jürgen Habermas and Jacques Derrida*. Chicago and London: University of Chicago Press.

Britzman, Deborah. 1998. *Lost Subjects, Contested Objects: Toward a Psychoanalytic Inquiry of Learning*. Albany: State University of New York Press.

Burbules, Nicholas. 1996. "Postmodern Doubt and Philosophy of Education." In *Philosophy of Education 1995*, edited by Alven Neiman, 3–48. Urbana, Illinois: Philosophy of Education Society.

Burbules, Nicholas and Rice, Suzanne. 1991. "Dialogue across Differences: Continuing the Conversation." *Harvard Educational Review* 61, no. 4: 393–416.

Burwood, Les. 1996. "How Should Schools Respond to the Plurality of Values in a Multi-cultural Society?" *Journal of Philosophy of Education* 30, no. 3: 415–427.

Butler, Judith. 1990. *Gender Trouble: Feminism and the Subversion of Identity*. New York and London: Routledge.

Butler, Judith. 1992. "Contingent Foundations: Feminism and the Question of 'Postmodernism'." In *Feminists Theorize the Political*, edited by Judith Butler and Joan Scott, 3–21. New York and London: Routledge.

Butler, Judith. 1997. *The Psychic Life of Power: Theories in Subjection*. Stanford CA: Stanford University Press.

Butler, Judith. 2004. *Precarious Life: The Powers of Mourning and Violence*. London and New York: Verso.

Butler, Judith. 2016. "Introduction." In *Of Grammatology*, 40th Anniversary edition, by Jacques Derrida, vii–xxiv. Translated by Gayatri Chakravorty Spivak. Baltimore: Johns Hopkins University Press.

Cachopo, João Pedro. 2013. "Disagreeing Before Acting: The Paradoxes of Critique and Politics from Adorno to Rancière." *Theoria and Praxis* 1, no. 1: 64–77.

Callinicos, Alex. 1996. "Messianic ruminations: Derrida, Stirner and Marx." *Radical Philosophy* 75 (Jan/Feb): 37–41.

Carr, Wilfred. 1995. "Education and Democracy: Confronting the Postmodernist Challenge." *Journal of Philosophy of Education* 29, no. 1: 75–91.

Carr, Wilfred. 1997. "Professing Education in a Postmodern Age." *Journal of Philosophy of Education* 31, no. 2: 309–327.

Chalier, Catherine. 1991. "Ethics and the Feminine." In *Re-Reading Levinas*, edited by Robert Bernasconi and Simon Critchley, 119–129. Bloomington and Indianapolis: Indiana University Press.

Cherryholmes, Cleo H. 1988. *Power and Criticism: Poststructural Investigations in Education*. New York and London: Teachers College Press.

Ciaramelli, Fabio. 1991. "Levinas's Ethical Discourse: Between Individuation and Universality." In *Re-Reading Levinas*, edited by Robert Bernasconi and Simon Critchley, 83–105. Bloomington and Indianapolis: Indiana University Press.

Colebrook, Claire. 1997. "Feminist Philosophy and the Philosophy of Feminism." *Hypatia* 12, no. 1: 79–98.

Colebrook, Claire. 2011. "Extinct Theory." In *Theory After 'Theory'*, edited by Jane Elliott and Derek Attridge, 62–71. London and New York: Routledge.

Coles, Romand. 1995. "Identity and Difference in the Ethical Positions of Adorno and Habermas." In *The Cambridge Companion to Habermas*, edited by Stephen K. White, 19–45. New York: Cambridge University Press.

Cornell, Drucilla. 1992a. *The Philosophy of the Limit*. New York and London: Routledge.

Cornell, Drucilla. 1992b. "The Philosophy of the Limit: Systems Theory and Feminist Legal Reform." In *Deconstruction and the Possibility of Justice*, edited by Drucilla Cornell, Michel Rosenfeld and David Gray Carlson, 68–91. New York: Routledge.

Critchley, Simon. 1992. *The Ethics of Deconstruction: Derrida and Levinas*. Oxford and Cambridge, MA: Blackwell Publishers.

Critchley, Simon. 1995. "On Derrida's *Specters of Marx*." *Philosophy & Social Criticism* 21, no. 3: 1–30.

Dallmayr, Fred. 1992. "Hermeneutics and the Rule of Law." In *Deconstruction and the Possibility of Justice*, edited by Drucilla Cornell, Michel Rosenfeld and David Gray Carlson, 283–304. New York: Routledge.

de Castell, Suzanne. 1995. "Textuality and the Designs of Theory." In *Critical Conversations in Philosophy of Education*, edited by Wendy Kohli, 241–257. New York and London: Routledge.

de Man, Paul. 1982. "The Resistance to Theory." *Yale French Studies* 63: 3–20.

Derrida, Jacques. 1976. *Of Grammatology*. Translated by Gayatri Chakravorty Spivak. Baltimore and London: The John Hopkins University Press. First published in French in 1967.

Derrida, Jacques. 1978. *Writing and Difference*. Translated, with an introduction and additional notes by Alan Bass. Chicago: University of Chicago Press.

Derrida, Jacques. 1981a. *Dissemination*. Translated, with an introduction and additional notes by Barbara Johnson. Chicago: University of Chicago Press.

Derrida, Jacques. 1981b. *Positions*. Translated and annotated by Alan Bass. Chicago: University of Chicago Press.

Derrida, Jacques. 1982. *Margins of Philosophy*. Translated, with additional notes by Alan Bass. Chicago: University of Chicago Press. First published in French 1972.

Derrida, Jacques. 1983a. "Of an Apocalyptic Tone Recently Adopted in Philosophy." Translated by JohnLeavey, Jr. *The Oxford Literary Review* 6, no. 2: 3–37.

Derrida, Jacques 1983b. "The Principle of Reason: The University in the Eyes of its Pupils." Translated by Catherine Porter and Edwards P. Morris. *diacritics* 13, no. 3: 3–21.

Derrida, Jacques. 1987. *The Post Card: From Socrates to Freud and Beyond*. Translated by Alan Bass. Chicago: University of Chicago Press.

Derrida, Jacques. 1988a. "Letter to a Japanese Friend." In *Derrida and Différance*, edited by David Wood and Robert Bernasconi, 1–5. Evanston, Il.: Northwestern University Press.

Derrida, Jacques. 1988b. *Limited Inc*. Translated by Samuel Weber. Evanston, Il.: Northwestern University Press. First published in French 1972. First published in English in 1977.

Derrida, Jacques. 1988c. "The Politics of Friendship." Translated by Gabriel Motzkin. *The Journal of Philosophy* 85, no. 11: 632–644.

Derrida, Jacques. 1991a. "At This Very Moment in This Work Here I Am." Translated by Ruben Berezdivin. In *Re-Reading Levinas*, edited by Robert Bernasconi and Simon Critchley, 11–48. Bloomington and Indianapolis: Indiana University Press.

Derrida, Jacques. 1991b. "'Eating Well,' or the Calculation of the Subject: An Interview with Jacques Derrida." In *Who Comes After the Subject?*, edited by Eduardo Cadava, Peter Connor and Jean-Luc Nancy, 96–119. New York and London: Routledge.

Derrida, Jacques. 1992a. "Force of Law: The 'Mystical Foundation of Authority'." In *Deconstruction and the Possibility of Justice*, edited by Drucilla Cornell, Michel Rosenfeld and David Gray Carlson, 3–67. New York and London: Routledge.

Derrida, Jacques. 1992b. "Passions: 'An Oblique Offering'." Translated by David Wood. In *Derrida: A Critical Reader*, edited by David Wood, 5–35. Cambridge: Blackwell.

Derrida, Jacques. 1994. *Specters of Marx: The State of the Debt, the Work of Mourning, and the New International*. Translated by Peggy Kamuf. Introduction by Bernd Magnus and Stephen Cullenberg. New York and London: Routledge.

Derrida, Jacques. 1995a. "A Certain 'Madness' Must Watch Over Thinking." Interview with François Ewald. *Educational Theory* 45, no. 3 (Summer): 273–291.

Derrida, Jacques. 1995b. *The Gift of Death*. Translated by David Wills. Chicago and London: University of Chicago Press.

Derrida, Jacques. 1996. "Remarks on Deconstruction and Pragmatism." Translated by Simon Critchley. In *Deconstruction and Pragmatism*, edited by Chantal Mouffe, 77–88. London and New York: Routledge.

Derrida, Jacques. 1998. *Resistances of Psychoanalysis*. Translated by Peggy Kamuf, Pascale-Anne Brault and Michael Naas. Stanford: Stanford University Press.

Derrida, Jacques. 2002a. "Psychoanalysis Searches the States of Its Soul: The Impossible Beyond of a Sovereign Cruelty." In *Without Alibi*, edited, translated and with an introduction by Peggy Kamuf, 238–280. Stanford: Stanford University Press.

Derrida, Jacques. 2002b. "The University Without Condition." In *Without Alibi*, edited, translated and with an introduction by Peggy Kamuf, 202–237. Stanford: Stanford University Press.

Derrida, Jacques. 2002c. *Without Alibi*. Edited, translated and with an introduction by Peggy Kamuf. Stanford: Stanford University Press.

Derrida, Jacques. 2005a. "As If It Were Possible, 'Within Such Limits'." In *Paper Machine*, 73–99. Translated by Rachel Bowlby. Stanford: Stanford University Press.

Derrida, Jacques. 2005b. "Fichus: Frankfurt Address." Translated by Rachel Bowlby. In *Paper Machine*, 164–181. Stanford: Stanford University Press.

Derrida, Jacques. 2005c. *Paper Machine*. Translated by Rachel Bowlby. Stanford: Stanford University Press.

Derrida, Jacques. 2005d. *Rogues: Two Essays on Reason*. Translated by Pascale-Anne Brault and Michael Naas. Stanford: Stanford University Press.

Derrida, Jacques, Gadamer, Hans-Georg and Lacoue-Labarthe, Philippe. 2016. *Heidegger, Philosophy, and Politics: The Heidelberg Conference*. Edited by Mireille Calle-Gruber, translated by Jeff Fort, foreword by Jean-Luc Nancy. New York, Fordham University Press.

Derrida, Jacques and Roudinesco, Elisabeth. 2004. *For What Tomorrow … A Dialogue*. Translated by Jeff Fort. Stanford: Stanford University Press.

Dews, Peter. 1987. *Logics of Distintegration: Poststructuralist Thought and the Claims of Critical Theory*. London: Verso.

Dews, Peter. 1995. *The Limits of Disenchantment: Essays on Contemporary European Philosophy*. London and New York: Verso.

Dews, Peter. 2004. "Resituating the Postmodern?" Review of Peter Bürger, *Ursprung des postmodernen Denkens. New Left Review* 25 (Jan–Feb): 136–144.

Ellsworth, Elizabeth. 1992. "Why Doesn't this Feel Empowering? Working Through the Repressive Myths of Critical Pedagogy." In *Feminisms and Critical Pedagogy*, edited by Carmen Luke and Jennifer Gore, 90–119. New York and London: Routledge.

Felman, Shoshana. 1982. "Psychoanalysis and Education: Teaching Terminable and Interminable." *Yale French Studies* 63: 21–44.

Flax, Jane. 1992. "The End of Innocence." In *Feminists Theorize the Political*, edited by Judith Butler and Joan Scott, 445–463. New York and London: Routledge.

Fletcher, John. 1999. "Introduction: Psychoanalysis and the Question of the Other." In *Essays on Otherness*, by Jean Laplanche, 1–51. Edited by John Fletcher. London and New York: Routledge.

Fletcher, John. 2000. "Gender, Sexuality and the Theory of Seduction." *Women: A Cultural Review* 11, no. 1/2: 95–108.

Fletcher, John. 2007. "Seduction and the Vicissitudes of Translation: The Work of Jean Laplanche." *Psychoanalytic Quarterly* LXXVI, no. 4: 1241–1291.

Forst, Rainer. 1997. "Situations of the Self: Reflections on Seyla Benhabib's version of critical theory." *Philosophy & Social Criticism* 23, no. 5: 79–96.

Foucault, Michel. 1980. *Power/Knowledge: Selected Interviews and Other Writings, 1972–1977*, edited by Colin Gordon. Translated by Colin Gordon, Leo Marshall, John Mepham, Kate Soper. New York: Pantheon Books.

Freire, Paulo. 1970. *Pedagogy of the Oppressed*. Translated by Myra Bergman Ramos. New York: Continuum.

Freire, Paulo. 1973. *Education for Critical Consciousness.* New York: The Seabury Press.
Freud, Sigmund. 1900. *The Interpretation of Dreams*, volumes 4–5 of *The Standard Edition of the Complete Psychological Works of Sigmund.* Translated and edited by James Strachey. 24 vols. London: Vintage Books, 2001. (Reprint of the original Standard Edition, London: Hogarth Press, 1953–1966).
Freud, Sigmund. 1905. *Three Essays on the Theory of Sexuality*, in *The Standard Edition* vol. 7.
Freud, Sigmund. 1911. "Formulations on the Two Principles of Mental Functioning." In *The Standard Edition* vol. 12, 215–226.
Freud, Sigmund. 1912–13. *Totem and Taboo*, in *The Standard Edition* vol. 13.
Freud, Sigmund. 1914. "On Narcissism: An Introduction." In *The Standard Edition* vol. 14, 67–102.
Freud, Sigmund. 1915a. "Instincts and Their Vicissitudes." In *The Standard Edition* vol. 14, 109–140.
Freud, Sigmund. 1915b. "The Unconscious." In *The Standard Edition* vol. 14, 159–215.
Freud, Sigmund. 1916–17. *Introductory Lectures on Psycho-Analysis*, in *The Standard Edition* vols. 15–16.
Freud, Sigmund. 1917. "Mourning and Melancholia." In *The Standard Edition* vol. 14, 237–258.
Freud, Sigmund. 1920. *Beyond the Pleasure Principle*, in *The Standard Edition* vol. 18.
Freud, Sigmund. 1921. *Group Psychology and the Analysis of the Ego*, in *The Standard Edition* vol. 18.
Freud, Sigmund. 1923. *The Ego and the Id*, in *The Standard Edition* vol. 19.
Freud, Sigmund. 1924a. "The Dissolution of the Oedipus Complex." In *The Standard Edition* vol. 19, 173–179.
Freud, Sigmund. 1924b. "The Economic Problem of Masochism." In *The Standard Edition* vol. 19, 157–170.
Freud, Sigmund. 1925a. "Negation." In *The Standard Edition* vol. 19, 235–239.
Freud, Sigmund. 1925b. "Some Psychical Consequences of the Anatomical Distinction Between the Sexes." In *The Standard Edition* vol. 19, 243–258.
Freud, Sigmund. 1926. *Inhibitions, Symptoms and Anxiety*, in *The Standard Edition* vol. 20.
Freud, Sigmund. 1930. *Civilization and Its Discontents*, in *The Standard Edition* vol. 21.
Freud, Sigmund. 1933. *New Introductory Lectures*, in *The Standard Edition* vol. 22.
Freud, Sigmund. 1939. *Moses and Monotheism: Three Essays*, in *The Standard Edition* vol. 23.
Freud, Sigmund. 1950 [1895]. "Project for a Scientific Psychology." In *The Standard Edition* vol. 1, 283–297.
Fritsch, Matthias. 2002. "Derrida's Democracy to Come." *Constellations* 9, no. 4: 574–597.
Fritsch, Matthias. 2015. "Democracy, Climate Change, and Environmental Justice." *Mosaic: A Journal for the Interdisciplinary Study of Literature* 48, no. 3: 27–45.
Fritsch, Matthias. 2018. *Taking Turns with the Earth: Phenomenology, Deconstruction, and Intergenerational Justice.* Stanford: Stanford University Press.
Gaon, Stella. 1998. "Pluralizing Universal 'Man': The Legacy of Transcendentalism and Teleology in Habermas's Discourse Ethics." *The Review of Politics* 60, no. 4: 685–718.

Gaon, Stella. 2018. "*Il la faut (la logique)*, Yes, yes: Deconstruction's critical force." *Derrida Today* 11, no. 2: 196–210.

Gasché, Rodolphe. 1986. *The Tain of the Mirror: Derrida and the Philosophy of Reflection*. Cambridge, MA and London: Harvard University Press.

Gasché, Rodolphe. 1987. "Infrastructures and Systematicity." In *Deconstruction and Philosophy: The Texts of Jacques Derrida*, edited by John Sallis, 3–20. Chicago and London: University of Chicago Press.

Gasché, Rodolphe. 1994. *Inventions of Difference: On Jacques Derrida*. Cambridge, MA: Harvard University Press.

Gasché, Rodolphe. 1995. "Possibilizations, in the Singular." In *Deconstruction is/in America: A New Sense of the Political*, edited by Anselm Haverkamp, 115–124. New York and London: New York University Press.

Gasché, Rodolphe. 2016. *Deconstruction, Its Force, Its Violence*. New York: State University of New York Press.

Giroux, Henry A. 1983. *Theory and Resistance in Education*. South Hadley, Mass.: Bergin and Garvey.

Giroux, Henry A. 1988a. "Border Pedagogy in the Age of Postmodernism." *Journal of Education* 170, no. 3: 162–181.

Giroux, Henry A. 1988b. "Literacy and the Pedagogy of Voice and Political Empowerment." *Educational Theory* 38, no. 1: 61–75.

Giroux, Henry A. 1991. "Introduction. Modernism, Postmodernism, and Feminism: Rethinking the Boundaries of Educational Discourse." In *Postmodernism, Feminism, and Cultural Politics: Redrawing Educational Boundaries*, edited by Henry A. Giroux, 1–59. Albany, New York: State University of New York Press.

Giroux, Henry A. 1993. "Literacy and the Politics of Difference." In *Critical Literacy: Politics, Praxis, and the Postmodern*, edited by Colin Lankshear and Peter McLaren, 367–377. Albany: State University of New York Press.

Gore, Jennifer. 1993. *The Struggle for Pedagogies: Critical and Feminist Discourses as Regimes of Truth*. New York and London: Routledge.

Gutmann, Amy, ed. 1994. *Multiculturalism: Examining the Politics of Recognition*. Princeton, NJ: Princeton University Press.

Habermas, Jürgen. 1982. "A Reply to my Critics." In *Habermas: Critical Debates*, edited by John Thompson and David Held, 219–283. Cambridge, MA: The MIT Press.

Habermas, Jürgen. 1987. *The Philosophical Discourse of Modernity: Twelve Lectures*. Translated by Frederick G. Lawrence. Cambridge, MA: The MIT Press (1985).

Habermas, Jürgen. 1990. *Moral Consciousness and Communicative Action*. Translated by Christian Lenhardt and Shierry Weber Nicholsen. Cambridge, MA: The MIT Press.

Habermas, Jürgen. 1993. *Justification and Application: Remarks on Discourse Ethics*. Translated by Ciaran P. Cronin. Cambridge, MA: The MIT Press.

Habermas, Jürgen. 2007. "How to Answer the Ethical Question." Translated by Bettina Bergo and Michael B. Smith. In *Judeities: Questions for Jacques Derrida*, edited by Bettina Bergo, Joseph Cohen and Raphael Zagury-Orly (eds.), 142–154. New York: Fordham University Press.

Haddad, Samir. 2013. *Derrida and the Inheritance of Democracy*. Bloomington and Indianapolis: Indiana University Press.

Hägglund, Martin. 2008. *Radical Atheism; Derrida and the Time of Life*. Stanford: Stanford University Press.

Hägglund, Martin. 2009. "The Challenge of Radical Atheism: A Response." *The New Centennial Review* 9, no. 1: 227–252.

Hare, William and Portelli, John P. eds. 1988. *Philosophy of Education: Introductory Readings.* Calgary: Detselig Enterprises Ltd.

Heath, Joseph. 1995. "The Problem of Foundationalism in Habermas's discourse ethics." *Philosophy & Social Criticism* 21, no. 1: 77–100.

Honneth, Axel. 1992. "Pluralization and Recognition: On the Self-Misunderstanding of Postmodern Social Theorists." In *Between Totalitarianism and Postmodernity*, edited by Peter Beilharz, Gillian Robinson and John Rundell, 163–172. Cambridge, Mass: The MIT Press.

Horkheimer, Max. 2002. "Traditional and Critical Theory." In *Critical Theory: Selected Essays.* Translated by Matthew J. O'Connell et al. New York: Continuum.

Horowitz, Asher. 2006. "Beyond Rational Peace: On the Possibility/Necessity of a Levinasian Hyperpolitics." In *Difficult Justice: Commentaries on Levinas and Politics*, edited by Asher Horowitz and Gad Horowitz, 27–47. Toronto: University of Toronto Press.

Houpt, Simon. 2003, June 27. "U.S. Supreme Court lifts ban on sodomy." *The Globe and Mail*, pp. A1, A11.

Inwood, Michael. 1992. *A Hegel Dictionary.* Cambridge, MA: Blackwell Publishers.

Irigaray, Luce. 1991. "Questions to Emmanuel Levinas: On the Divinity of Love." In *Re-Reading Levinas*, edited by Robert Bernasconi and Simon Critchley, 109–118. Bloomington and Indianapolis: Indiana University Press.

Kamuf, Peggy. 1995. "Going Public: The University in Deconstruction." In *Deconstruction is/in America: A New Sense of the Political*, edited by Anselm Haverkamp, 95–111. New York and London: New York University Press.

Kamuf, Peggy. 2002. "Introduction: Event of Resistance." In *Without Alibi* by Jacques Derrida, 1–27. Edited, translated and with an Introduction by Peggy Kamuf. Stanford: Stanford University Press.

Kant, Immanuel. 1929. *Critique of Pure Reason.* Translated by Norman Kemp Smith. London: MacMillan.

Kant, Immanuel. 1959. *Foundations of the Metaphysics of Morals and What Is Enlightenment.* Translated, with an introduction by Lewis White Beck. Indianapolis: Bobbs-Merrill Educational Publishing.

Kant, Immanuel. 1987. *Critique of Judgment.* Translated, with an introduction by Werner S. Pluhar. Indianapolis/Cambridge: Hackett Publishing Company.

Kant, Immanuel. 1993a. *Critique of Practical Reason.* 3rd Edition. Edited and translated, with notes and introductions by Lewis White Beck. New York: MacMillan Publishing Company.

Kant, Immanuel. 1993b. *Grounding for the Metaphysics of Morals, with On a Supposed Right to Lie Because of Philanthropic Concerns.* 3rd Edition. Translated by James W. Ellington. Indianapolis and Cambridge: Hackett Publishing Company.

Kant, Immanuel. 1998. *Critique of Pure Reason.* Translated and edited by Paul Guyer and Allen Wood. Cambridge UK: Cambridge University Press.

Kearney, Richard, ed. 1984. *Dialogues with Contemporary Continental Thinkers: The Phenomenological Heritage.* Manchester: Manchester University Press.

Keenan, Thomas. 1995. "Deconstruction and the Possibility of Justice." In *Critical Encounters: Reference and Responsibility in Deconstructive Writing*, edited by

Cathy Caruth and Deborah Esch, 262–274. New Brunswick and New Jersey: Rutgers University Press.

Keenan, Thomas. 1997. *Fables of Responsibility: Aberrations and Predicaments in Ethics and Politics*. Stanford: Stanford University Press.

Kohli, Wendy. 1995. "Educating for Emancipatory Rationality." In *Critical Conversations in Philosophy of Education*, edited by Wendy Kohli, 103–115. New York and London: Routledge.

Koivikko, Tiina. 2017. "Drives and objects – notes on the change of drive theory." *The Scandinavian Psychoanalytic Review* 40, no. 1: 19–28, DOI: doi:10.1080/01062301.2017.1377976.

Lacan, Jacques. 2002. "The Mirror Stage as Formative of the *I* Function as Revealed in Psychoanalytic Experience." In *Écrits: The First Complete Edition in English*. Translated by Bruce Fink, in collaboration with Héloïse Fink and Russell Grigg, 75–81. New York and London: W.W. Norton & Company.

Laclau, Ernesto. 1995. "The Time is Out of Joint." *diacritics* 25, no. 2: 86–96.

Lankshear, Colin and McLaren, Peter. 1993. "Introduction." In *Critical Literacy: Politics, Praxis, and the Postmodern*, edited by Colin Lankshear and Peter McLaren, 1–56. Albany: State University of New York Press.

Laplanche, Jean. 1976. *Life and Death in Psychoanalysis*. Translated, with an introduction by Jeffrey Mehlman. Baltimore and London: John Hopkins UP.

Laplanche, Jean. 1981. "A Metapsychology put to the Test of Anxiety." Translated by Philip Slotkin. *International Journal of Psychoanalysis* 62, no. 1: 81–89.

Laplanche, Jean. 1984. "To Situate Sublimation." Translated by Richard Miller. *October* 28 (Spring): 7–26.

Laplanche, Jean. 1989. *New Foundations for Psychoanalysis*. Translated by David Macey. Cambridge: Basil Blackwell.

Laplanche, Jean. 1992. *Jean Laplanche: Seduction, Translation and the Drives: A Dossier*. Edited by John Fletcher and Martin Stanton. Translations by Martin Stanton. London: Institute of Contemporary Arts.

Laplanche, Jean. 1995. "Seduction, Persecution, Revelation." Translated by Philip Slotkin. *The International Journal of Psychoanalysis* 76, no. 4: 663–682.

Laplanche, Jean. 1996. "Psychoanalysis as Anti-Hermeneutics." Translated by Luke Thurston. *Radical Philosophy* 79 (Sept/Oct): 7–12.

Laplanche, Jean. 1997. "The Theory of Seduction and the Problem of the Other." Translated by Luke Thurston. *International Journal of Psychoanalysis* 78, no. 4: 653–666.

Laplanche, Jean. 1999a. *Essays on Otherness*. Edited by John Fletcher. London and New York: Routledge.

Laplanche, Jean. 1999b. *The Unconscious and the Id*. Translated by Luke Thurston with Lindsey Watson. London: Rebus Press. First published in French in 1981.

Laplanche, Jean. 2000. "The Other Within: Rethinking Psychoanalysis." Interview with Jean Laplanche. By John Fletcher and Peter Osborne. *Radical Philosophy* 102 (July/Aug): 31–41.

Laplanche, Jean. 2001. "An Interview with Jean Laplanche." Interview with Cathy Caruth. *Postmodern Culture* 11, no. 2. http://pmc.iath.virginia.edu/text-only/issue.101/11.2caruth.txt

Laplanche, Jean. 2004. "The So-Called 'Death Drive': A Sexual Drive." *British Journal of Psychotherapy* 20, no. 4: 455–471.

Laplanche, Jean. 2007. "Gender, Sex, and the Sexual." Translated by Susan Fairfield. *Studies in Gender and Sexuality* 8, no. 2: 201–219.

Laplanche, Jean. 2011. *Freud and the Sexual: Essays 2000–2006*. Translated by John Fletcher, Jonathan House and Nicholas Ray. New York: International Psychoanalytic Books.

Laplanche, Jean. 2015. "Sublimation and/or Inspiration." In *Between Seduction and Inspiration: Man*. Translated and with an introduction by Jeffrey Mehlman. New York: The Unconscious in Translation.

Laplanche, Jean. 2016. *New Foundations for Psychoanalysis*. Translated by Jonathan House. New York: The Unconscious in Translation.

Laplanche, Jean and Pontalis, Jean-Bertrand. 1973. *The Language of Psychoanalysis*. Translated by Donald Nicholson-Smith. New York and London: W.W. Norton and Company.

Lather, Patti. 1991. *Getting Smart: Feminist Research and Pedagogy with/in the Postmodern*. New York and London: Routledge.

Lather, Patti. 1992. "Post-Critical Pedagogies: A Feminist Reading." In *Feminisms and Critical Pedagogy*, edited by Carmen Luke and Jennifer Gore, 120–137. New York and London: Routledge.

Lawlor, Leonard. 2007. *This is Not Sufficient: An Essay on Animality and Human Nature in Derrida*. New York: Columbia University Press.

Levinas, Emmanuel. 1981. *Otherwise than Being or Beyond Essence*. Translated by Alphonso Lingis. The Hague: Martinus Nijhoff.

Levinas, Emmanuel. 1989. *The Levinas Reader*. Edited by Sean Hand. Oxford and Cambridge, MA: Blackwell Publishers.

Levinas, Emmanuel. 1991. "Wholly Otherwise." Translated by Simon Critchley. In *Re-Reading Levinas*, edited by Robert Bernasconi and Simon Critchley, 3–10. Bloomington and Indianapolis: Indiana University Press.

Lüdemann, Susanne. 2014. *Politics of Deconstruction: A New Introduction to Jacques Derrida*. Translated by Erik Butler. Stanford: Stanford University Press.

Lyotard, Jean-François. 1984. *The Postmodern Condition: A Report on Knowledge*. Translated by Geoff Bennington and Brian Massumi, foreword by Fredric Jameson. Minneapolis: University of Minnesota Press.

Lyotard, Jean-François. 1991. *The Inhuman: Reflections on Time*. Translated by Geoffrey Bennington and Rachel Bowlby. Stanford: Stanford University Press.

McCarthy, Cameron. 1993. "After the Canon: Knowledge and Ideological Representation in the Multicultural Discourse on Curriculum Reform." In *Race, Identity, and Representation in Education*, edited by Cameron McCarthy and Warren Critchlow, 289–305. New York and London: Routledge.

McCarthy, Thomas. 1988. "On the Margins of Politics." *The Journal of Philosophy* 85, no. 11: 645–648.

McGee, Patrick. 1993. "Decolonization and the Curriculum of English." In *Race, Identity, and Representation in Education*, edited by Cameron McCarthy and Warren Critchlow, 280–288. New York and London: Routledge.

McLaren, Peter. 1988. "Schooling the Postmodern Body: Critical Pedagogy and the Politics of Enfleshment." *Journal of Education* 170, no. 3: 53–83.

McLaren, Peter. 1989a. *Life in Schools: An Introduction to Critical Pedagogy in the Foundations of Education*. New York and London: Longman Inc.

McLaren, Peter. 1989b. "On Ideology and Education: Critical Pedagogy and the Cultural Politics of Resistance." In *Critical Pedagogy, the State, and Cultural*

Struggle, edited by Henry Giroux and Peter McLaren, 174–202. Albany: State University of New York Press.

McLaren, Peter. 1995. "Collisions with Otherness: 'Traveling' Theory, Postcolonial Criticism, and the Politics of Ethnographic Practice – The Mission of the Wounded Ethnographer." In *Critical Theory and Educational Research*, edited by Peter McLaren and James Giarelli, 271–300. Albany: State University of New York Press.

McLaren, Peter and Giarelli, James. 1995. "Introduction: Critical Theory and Educational Research." In *Critical Theory and Educational Research*, edited by Peter McLaren and James Giarelli, 1–22. Albany: State University of New York Press.

McLaren, Peter and Lankshear, Colin. 1993. "Critical Literacy and the post-modern turn." In *Critical Literacy: Politics, Praxis, and the Postmodern*, edited by Colin Lankshear and Peter McLaren, 379–419. Albany: State University of New York Press.

Misgeld, Dieter. 1985. "Education and Cultural Invasion: Critical Social Theory, Education as Instruction, and the 'Pedagogy of the Oppressed.'" In *Critical Theory and Public Life*, edited by John Forester, 77–118. Cambridge, MA: The MIT Press.

Misgeld, Dieter. 1992. "Pedagogy and Politics: Some Critical Reflections on the Post-modern Turn in Critical Pedagogy." *Phenomenology and Pedagogy* 10: 125–142.

Mohanty, S.P. 1986. "Radical Teaching, Radical Theory: The Ambiguous Politics of Meaning." In *Theory in the Classroom*, edited by Cary Nelson, 149–176. Urbana and Chicago: University of Illinois Press.

Naas, Michael. 2008. *Derrida From Now On*. New York: Fordham University Press.

Naas, Michael. 2009. "An Atheism that (*Dieu merci*!) Still Leaves Something to be Desired." *The New Centennial Review* 9, no. 1: 45–68.

Nagl-Docekal, Herta. 1997. "Seyla Benhabib and the radical future of the Enlightenment." *Philosophy & Social Criticism* 23, no. 5: 63–78.

Norris, Christopher. 1992. "Deconstruction, Postmodernism and Philosophy: Habermas on Derrida." In *Derrida: A Critical Reader*, edited by David Wood, 167–192. Oxford and Cambridge: Blackwell.

Norris, Christopher. 1993. *The Truth About Postmodernism*. Oxford and Cambridge: Blackwell.

Norris, Christopher. 2004. "Postmodernism, Politics, and the Assault on Truth." *Journal of Critical Realism* 3, no. 2, 353–369.

Orner, Mimi. 1992. "Interrupting the Calls for Student Voice in 'Liberatory' Education: A Feminist Poststructuralist Perspective." In *Feminisms and Critical Pedagogy*, edited by Carmen Luke and Jennifer Gore, 74–89. New York and London: Routledge.

Payrow Shabani, Omid. 2003. *Democracy, Power, and Legitimacy: The Critical Theory of Jürgen Habermas*. Toronto, Buffalo and London: University of Toronto Press.

Perpich, Diane. 2008. *The Ethics of Emmanuel Levinas*. Stanford: Stanford University Press.

Peters, R.S. 1967. "What is an Educational Process?" In *The Concept of Education*, edited by R.S. Peters, 1–23. London: Routledge and Kegan Paul.

Peukert, Helmut. 1993. "Basic Problems of a Critical Theory of Education." Translated by Peter P. Kenny. *Journal of Philosophy of Education* 27, no. 2: 159–170.

Purcell, Sebastian. 2015. "Review of *Ricoeur and the Post-Structuralists: Bourdieu, Derrida, Deleuze, Foucault, Castoriadis*" by Johann Michel. *Notre Dame Philosophical Reviews*, 2015-03-37. Retrieved from http://ndpr.nd.edu/news/56620-ricoeur-and-the-post-structuralists-bourdieu-derrida-deleuze-foucault-castoriadis/

Readings, Bill. 1996. *The University in Ruins*. Cambridge, MA and London. England: Harvard University Press.

Rehg, William. 1994. *Insight and Solidarity: The Discourse Ethics of Jürgen Habermas*. Berkeley: University of California Press.

Robbins, Jill. 1991. "Visage, Figure: Reading Levinas's Totality and Infinity." *Yale French Studies* 79: 135–149.

Roberts, Peter. 1996. "Rethinking Conscientisation." *Journal of Philosophy of Education* 30, no. 2: 179–196.

Rockefeller, Steven. 1992. "John Dewey, Spiritual Democracy, and the Human Future." In *Revisioning Philosophy*, edited by James Oglivy, 165–190. Albany: State University of New York Press.

Rorty, Richard. 1989. *Contingency, Irony, and Solidarity*. New York: Cambridge University Press.

Rose, Gillian. 1984. *Dialectic of Nihilism: Poststructuralism and Law*. Oxford: Basil Blackwell.

Rose, Gillian. 2008. "Interview with Gillian Rose." Edited and introduced by Vincent Lloyd. *Theory, Culture & Society* 25, nos. 7–8: 201–218.

Rötzer, Florian, ed. 1995. *Conversations with French Philosophers*. Foreword by Rainer Rochlitz. Translated by Gary Aylesworth. New Jersey: Humanities Press.

Sauvayre, Pascal. 2017. "The Unconscious in Translation: Jean Laplanche." Review essay. *Contemporary Psychoanalysis* 53, no. 1: 112–139.

Sayer, Derek. 2004. "Incognito Ergo Sum: Language, Memory and the Subject." *Theory, Culture & Society* 21, no. 6: 67–89.

Scarfone, Dominique. 1994. "'It Was Not My Mother': From Seduction to Negation." *New Formations* 48, ed. by John Fletcher (2002–2003): 69–76.

Schrag, Calvin O. 1995. "Speculative Philosophy." In *The Cambridge Dictionary of Philosophy*, edited by Robert Audi, 758. Cambridge, England and New York: Cambridge University Press.

Shor, Ira. 1992. *Empowering Education: Critical Teaching for Social Change*. Chicago and London: University of Chicago Press.

Siegel, Harvey. 1988. *Educating Reason: Rationality, Critical Thinking, and Education*. New York and London: Routledge.

Siegel, Harvey. 1997. *Rationality Redeemed? Further Dialogues on an Educational Ideal*. New York and London: Routledge.

Smeyers, Paul. 1995a. "Education and the Educational Project I: The Atmosphere of Post-Modernism." *Journal of Philosophy of Education* 29, no. 1: 109–119.

Smeyers, Paul. 1995b. "Education and the Educational Project II: Do We Still Care About It?" *Journal of Philosophy of Education* 29, no. 3: 401–413.

Smith, Paul. 1988. *Discerning the Subject*. Foreword by John Mowitt. Minneapolis: University of Minnesota Press.

Soper, Kate. 1996. "Specters of Derrida: The Limits of Hauntology." *Radical Philosophy* 75 (Jan/Feb): 26–31.

Spivak, Gayatri Chakravorty. 1993. *Outside in the Teaching Machine*. New York and London: Routledge.

Strike, Kenneth. 1995. "Discourse Ethics and Restructuring." In *Philosophy of Education 1994*, edited by Michael S. Katz, 1–14. Urbana, Illinois: Philosophy of Education Society.

Taylor, Charles. 1989. *Sources of the Self: The Making of the Modern Identity.* Cambridge, MA: Harvard University Press.

Usher, Robin and Edwards, Richard. 1994. *Postmodernism and Education.* London and New York: Routledge.

Van Haute, Philippe. 1995. "Fatal Attraction: Jean Laplanche on Sexuality, Subjectivity and Singularity in the Work of Sigmund Freud." *Radical Philosophy* 73 (Jan/Feb): 5–12.

Van Haute, Philippe and Geyskens, Tomas. 2004. *Confusion of Tongues: The Primacy of Sexuality in Freud, Ferenczi, and Laplanche.* New York: Other Press.

Visker, Rudi. 1995. *Michel Foucault: Genealogy as Critique.* Translated by Chris Turner. London: Verso.

Wardekker, Willem and Miedema, Siebren. 1997. "Critical Pedagogy: An Evaluation and a Direction for Reformulation." *Curriculum Inquiry* 27, no. 1: 45–61.

Weber, Samuel. 1982. *The Legend of Freud.* Minneapolis: University of Minnesota Press.

Weber, Samuel. 1991. *Return to Freud: Jacques Lacan's Dislocation of Psychoanalysis.* Cambridge: University of Cambridge Press.

Weber, Samuel. 1992. "In the Name of the Law." In *Deconstruction and the Possibility of Justice*, edited by Drucilla Cornell, Michel Rosenfeld and David Gray Carlson, 232–257. New York: Routledge.

Wellmer, Albrecht. 1991. *The Persistence of Modernity: Essays on Aesthetics, Ethics, and Postmodernism.* Translated by David Midgley. Cambridge, MA: The MIT Press.

Wills, David. 2006. "Affirmation." In *A Dictionary of Continental Philosophy*, edited by John Protevi, 14–15. New Haven and London: Yale University Press.

Wortham, Simon. 1999. *Rethinking the University: Leverage and Deconstruction.* Manchester and New York: Manchester University Press.

Index

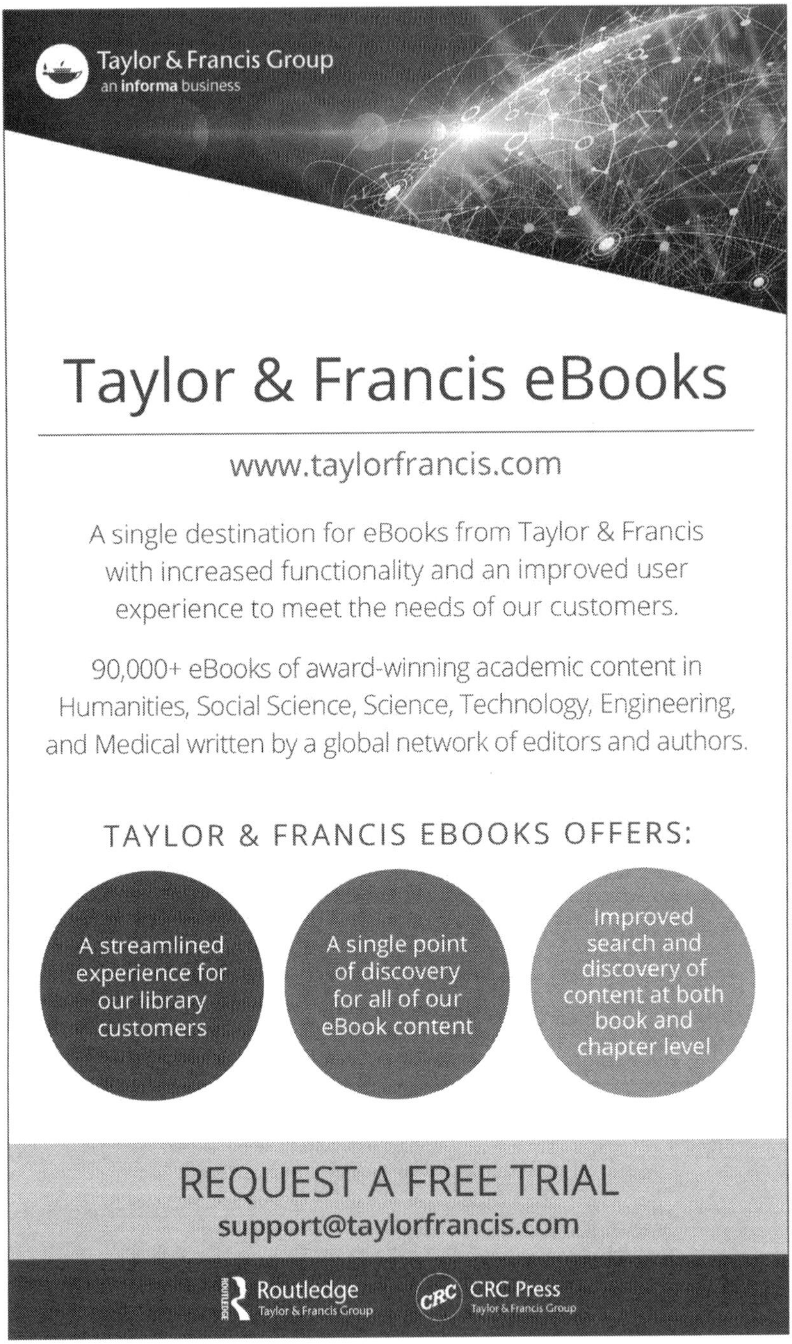
Taylor & Francis Group
an informa business
Taylor & Francis eBooks
www.taylorfrancis.com
A single destination for eBooks from Taylor & Francis with increased functionality and an improved user experience to meet the needs of our customers.
90,000+ eBooks of award-winning academic content in Humanities, Social Science, Science, Technology, Engineering, and Medical written by a global network of editors and authors.
TAYLOR & FRANCIS EBOOKS OFFERS:
A streamlined experience for our library customers
A single point of discovery for all of our eBook content
Improved search and discovery of content at both book and chapter level
REQUEST A FREE TRIAL
support@taylorfrancis.com
Routledge Taylor & Francis Group
CRC Press Taylor & Francis Group